LSHTM

REPRODUCTIVE TRACT INFECTIONS

GLOBAL IMPACT AND PRIORITIES FOR WOMEN'S REPRODUCTIVE HEALTH

REPRODUCTIVE BIOLOGY

Series Editor: Sheldon J. Segal

The Population Council
New York, New York

Current Volumes in this Series

AIDS AND WOMEN'S REPRODUCTIVE HEALTH
Edited by Lincoln C. Chen, Jaime Sepulveda Amor, and Sheldon J. Segal

AUTOCRINE AND PARACRINE MECHANISMS IN REPRODUCTIVE ENDOCRINOLOGY
Edited by Lewis C. Krey, Bela J. Gulyas, and John A. McCracken

CONTRACEPTIVE STEROIDS: Pharmacology and Safety
Edited by A. T. Gregoire and Richard P. Blye

DEMOGRAPHIC AND PROGRAMMATIC CONSEQUENCES OF CONTRACEPTIVE INNOVATIONS
Edited by Sheldon J. Segal, Amy O. Tsui, and Susan M. Rogers

ENDOCRINE AND BIOCHEMICAL DEVELOPMENT OF THE FETUS AND NEONATE
Edited by José M. Cuezva, Ana M. Pascual-Leone, and Mulchand S. Patel

GENETIC MARKERS OF SEX DIFFERENTIATION
Edited by Florence P. Haseltine, Michael E. McClure, and Ellen H. Goldberg

IMMUNOLOGICAL APPROACHES TO CONTRACEPTION AND PROMOTION OF FERTILITY
Edited by G. P. Talwar

REPRODUCTIVE TRACT INFECTIONS: Global Impact and Priorities for Women's Reproductive Health
Edited by Adrienne Germain, King K. Holmes, Peter Piot, and Judith N. Wasserheit

UTERINE AND EMBRYONIC FACTORS IN EARLY PREGNANCY
Edited by Jerome F. Strauss III and C. Richard Lyttle

A Continuation Order Plan is available for this series. A continuation order will bring delivery of each new volume immediately upon publication. Volumes are billed only upon actual shipment. For further information please contact the publisher.

REPRODUCTIVE TRACT INFECTIONS

GLOBAL IMPACT AND PRIORITIES FOR WOMEN'S REPRODUCTIVE HEALTH

Edited by

Adrienne Germain
International Women's Health Coalition
New York, New York

King K. Holmes
University of Washington
Seattle, Washington

Peter Piot
Institut de Medicina Tropicale
Antwerp, Belgium

Judith N. Wasserheit
National Institutes of Health
Bethesda, Maryland

Plenum Press · New York and London

Library of Congress Cataloging-in-Publication Data

Reproductive tract infections : global impact and priorities for
  women's reproductive health / edited by Adrienne Germain ... [et
  al.].
        p.   cm. -- (Reproductive biology)
     Papers from a conference held for Apr. 29-May 3, 1991, at the
  Bellagio Study and Conference Center, in Bellagio, Italy and co
  -sponsored by the International Women's Health Coalition and the
  Rockefeller Foundation.
     Includes bibliographical references and index.
     ISBN 0-306-44241-8
     1. Generative organs, Female--Infections--Developing countries-
  -Congresses. 2. Medical policy--Developing countries--Congresses.
  I. Germain, Adrienne. II. International Women's Health Coalition.
  III. Rockefeller Foundation. IV. Series.
     [DNLM: 1. Genital Diseases, Female--congresses. 2. Health Policy-
  -congresses. 3. Urinary Tract Infections--congresses. 4. Women's
  Health--congresses. 5. World Health--congresses.   WP 140 R425
  1991]
  RG218.R47   1992
  362.1'98142'0091724--dc20
  DNLM/DLC
  for Library of Congress   92-19797
                                                                  CIP

The International Women's Health Coalition is a private, non-profit organization
dedicated to improving women's reproductive health in the Third World. By supporting innovative health care projects, policy-oriented field research, and public
education, IWHC serves as an advocate and catalyst for change in national and
international policies and programs.

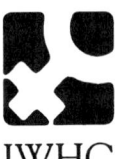

IWHC
International Women's Health Coalition

Fourteen papers commissioned for a conference entitled, "Reproductive Tract
Infections in Women in the Third World: National and International Policy
Implications," held April 29–May 3, 1991, at the Bellagio Study and Conference
Center, Bellagio, Italy, co-sponsored by the International Women's Health Coalition
and The Rockefeller Foundation

ISBN 0-306-44241-8

© 1992 Plenum Press, New York
A Division of Plenum Publishing Corporation
233 Spring Street, New York, N.Y. 10013

Printed in the United States of America

PREFACE

Reproductive tract infections (RTIs) have become a silent epidemic that is devastating women's lives. Each year, thousands of women die needlessly from the consequences of these infections, including cervical cancer, ectopic pregnancy, acute and chronic infections of the uterus and the fallopian tubes, and puerperal infections. For many women, this happens because they receive medical attention too late, if at all. The terrible irony of this tragedy is that early diagnosis of and treatment for many RTIs do not require high-technology health care.

For the hundreds of millions of women with chronic RTIs acquired from their sexual partners, life can become a living hell. Infection is a major cause of infertility, and it leads to scorn and rejection in many countries. These women may experience constant pain, have festering lesions of the genital tract, be at enhanced risk of secondary diseases, and endure social ostracism. The problems associated with RTIs have grown even greater in the past decade with the emergence of human immunodeficiency virus (HIV) and AIDS. Preexisting sexually transmitted disease, particularly when associated with genital tract ulcers, raises women's vulnerability to the transmission of HIV 3–5 fold.

The International Women's Health Coalition and The Rockefeller Foundation, concerned with this epidemic among women in Africa, Asia, and Latin America and the Caribbean, organized a multidisciplinary meeting on this subject. The meeting took place at the Foundation's Study and Conference Center in Bellagio, Italy, from April 29 to May 3, 1991. This book compiles the papers, conclusions, and recommendations of the meeting.

To our knowledge, this is the first comprehensive publication that focuses on the risks of RTIs among women in the general population and examines the interactions between RTIs and international health goals, such as family planning, safe motherhood and child survival. The book is intended as a reference for educators, the scientific community, health policy analysts, and women's health activists. It is directed especially to those involved in establishing priorities in international and national health programs and to health care providers who are charged with implementing programs.

RTIs take lives, and equally tragic, they destroy lives. The intent of this volume is to give voice to a silent epidemic and to call on health professionals, community leaders, and the international donor community to assign higher policy priority to prevention and control of RTIs.

Joan B. Dunlop
President
International Women's Health Coalition

Sheldon Segal
Former Director, Population Sciences
The Rockefeller Foundation

ACKNOWLEDGMENTS

We thank the many people and institutions whose talents and contributions have made this book possible.

The Rockefeller Foundation not only provided access to the Bellagio Study and Conference Center, but also gave grant support to the International Women's Health Coalition (IWHC). IWHC's nine general support donors, and The Commonwealth Fund, provided additional financial support.

Special thanks are due to Dr. Sheldon Segal, formerly Director of Population Sciences, The Rockefeller Foundation, for his sustained commitment, and for inviting us to publish these papers in the Plenum Press series, *Reproductive Biology*, which he edits. We appreciate, as well, the contributions of Dr. Katherine LaGuardia, Research Scientist for Population Sciences, The Rockefeller Foundation, to the conference agenda.

Staff of IWHC worked exceptionally hard to bring this book into being:

- **Kenneth Berg** helped develop the book's design and applied his talents in desktop publishing, through many drafts of the manuscript, to create the final camera-ready copy.
- **Anahita Sia Nowrojee** undertook the herculean task of coordinating the manuscript through every stage of production; reading and editing manuscripts for substantive issues; fielding queries; communicating with authors, consultants, and editors; and maintaining production schedules.
- **Jane Ordway** served as liaison to Plenum Press, negotiated the agreement with Plenum, developed production schedules, identified and hired necessary consultants, and provided project oversight.

We appreciate the work of Dore Hollander, consultant to IWHC, who applied her finely honed talents as an editor to standardizing text style and line-editing the manuscript, creating consistency and cohesion throughout the book.

Many thanks to our assistants Carmen Díaz-Olivo, Mary Fielder, and Helen Martin for patience and skill through the conference and production of the book.

Finally, we thank Patricia Vann, Editor at Plenum Press, for her advice and guidance, and Thomas Flood, Production Manager, for his technical assistance.

Adrienne Germain
King K. Holmes
Peter Piot
Judith N. Wasserheit

CONTENTS

PART III
ACTIONS FOR CONSIDERATION

PART IV
COUNTRY CASES

INTRODUCTION

Across the world, millions of girls and women needlessly suffer the severe consequences of reproductive tract infections (RTIs). For example, estimates from hospital data presented in this volume suggest that sexually transmitted diseases (STDs) may have directly affected 10 percent of the 1.2 million women who had live births in Kenya in 1987:

- Some 80,000 women developed postpartum pelvic infection.
- Of these women, 8,000–16,000 became infertile as a result of infection.
- Approximately 22,000 infants died or suffered permanent disabling sequelae; 4,000 stillbirths occurred; 10,000 infants acquired perinatal HIV.
- About 90,000 infants developed eye infections, and 10,000 of these were at risk of blindness; 10,000 infants acquired chlamydial pneumonia.

In the same year, thousands of additional women in Kenya, as in many other countries, died or became infertile from sepsis due to botched abortions or poor delivery services; still others died from ectopic pregnancy caused by the tubal scarring that results from infections of the upper reproductive tract; and uncounted thousands suffered acute and chronic illness due to these infections. By 1990, as Maggwa and Ngugi document in their paper, an estimated 100,000 Kenyan women were HIV-positive, and these women face certain death. Such suffering and death occur in virtually every country, especially where health services are inadequate, where women are restricted from using available services, and where sexual attitudes and behaviors leave women unable to protect themselves from unsafe and unwanted sex.

The International Women's Health Coalition (IWHC), our colleagues, and the women we serve have paid increasing attention to this problem, not only among "high-risk" women such as commercial sex workers, but among women in the general population. In 1987, IWHC began program work on RTIs, focussing on iatrogenic infections (those acquired during medical procedures such as abortion or delivery), endogenous infections (those caused by overgrowth of organisms normally present in the genital tract), and STDs, including AIDS.

By 1990, concern among our colleagues and their constituencies was sufficient to warrant a meeting with major donor agencies about the significance of RTIs among women in the general population and the feasibility of prevention and control programs. The papers in this volume were commissioned as background documents for the meeting, which was co-sponsored by IWHC and The Rockefeller Foundation in Bellagio, Italy, in April and May 1991.

This collection of papers breaks new ground by providing a comprehensive review of the implications of RTIs for established international health goals and programs, including family planning, maternal and child health (or MCH, which encompasses "child survival" and "safe motherhood"), and HIV prevention. In addition to reviewing the medical and public health dimensions of RTIs, the papers examine their multiple impacts on women's lives. Finally, they systematically assess the efficiency and cost-effectiveness of a range of possible actions to prevent and control RTIs, especially among women in the general population.

Overviews by Wasserheit and Holmes, and by Brunham and Embree, summarize currently available data on the magnitude of the problem. They also examine methodological, program, and policy issues, particularly the low priority given to RTI surveillance and control. The papers make clear that although RTIs seriously undermine the success of other health initiatives, they have been ignored because of widespread and erroneous beliefs that they are not serious, do not kill, or are too complicated and expensive to control. RTIs have also been neglected because deeply held attitudes and values make them socially taboo subjects among women and men at all levels of society. This "culture of silence" prevents changes in long-standing behaviors related to sexuality and gender, and has inhibited the development of effective information and services.

Many girls and women in resource-poor settings are at risk of serious infection because they lack access to necessary maternal health and family planning services, or they receive poor-quality services from providers who are untrained, poorly supervised, or ill equipped. Conventional STD control programs, directed primarily to men and to "high-risk" groups, are typically inaccessible to women in the general population. Women are constrained from using these services by the likelihood of social censure, and by financial and personal costs. At the same time, conventional STD programs, which serve mostly men, often fail to inform and serve the partners, especially the stable partners, of their clients. One of the better mechanisms for identifying and serving women at very high risk of infection is thus lost.

The papers by Meheus, Cates and Stone, Laga, and Schulz et al. assess these issues and describe numerous programmatic actions that should be taken. The authors emphasize that serving women in the general population, through existing health and family planning systems, is essential for RTI prevention and control. The case for integrated services—explored in depth in these four papers—is based on six points:

- Women using MCH and family planning programs are important in their own right and are increasingly at risk of RTIs.

- Because over half of women with RTIs are asymptomatic, integrated services are the most effective and efficient means of reaching infected women.

- STD information and services prevent and cure primary disease. As important, these services prevent upper tract infection and other serious consequences of untreated STDs.

- Although definitive cost data are not available, current analyses suggest that RTI prevention, education, and services are less costly than treatment of the consequences of RTIs.

- RTI information and services can provide a strategic link between related, but often separate, health delivery systems and, in so doing, can increase their efficiency and efficacy.

- Integrated RTI services are a primary means to collect necessary data on the scope and significance of infection among women in the general population, as well to develop effective and appropriate services.

The papers by Aral, Ronald and Aral, and Piot and Rowley examine some of the behavioral and sociocultural factors that make girls and women so vulnerable to RTIs, as well as the economic impact of these diseases. They review specific actions, including measures that can be taken immediately, provided political will is generated and resources are allocated. The authors describe research and actions required in the medium term, especially investment in the development and testing of medical and other technologies. In addition, they outline longer-term efforts to reduce underlying sociocultural, economic, political, and gender conditions that foster the spread of infections.

Finally, country-specific papers from Brazil, Kenya, Nigeria, India, and Mozambique indicate that commonalities as well as significant diversities exist in the underlying causes of infection, patterns of infection, and proposals for action across countries. These papers clearly indicate the severe data gaps and need for more systematic data collection. They present the dilemmas policymakers confront in allocating scarce human and financial resources. At the same time, they illustrate the urgent need to address RTIs more directly and extensively.

Discussions among the authors of these papers and staff of donor agencies at the Bellagio conference generated comprehensive recommendations, reproduced in full as Appendix 1. On the basis of their assessment of the scientific evidence and review of programmatic experience to date, conference participants identified six basic needs:

- Prioritize prevention and control of RTIs on national and international public health agendas.
- Integrate information, screening, and services for STDs and endogenous infection into ongoing health and family planning programs already serving women in the general population.
- Increase investments in training, supervision, and basic supplies to minimize procedure-related infections in these health and family planning programs.
- Increase attention to partner notification and services in STD programs.
- Undertake carefully selected research to develop products for the prevention, detection, and treatment of disease; to enhance understanding of the behavioral factors that promote infection; and to delineate cost-effective programmatic actions.
- Modify public policies on education, employment, and legal rights to foster women's ability to protect their sexual health, and to enable women and men to be caring, responsible, and respectful in sexual relationships, thus reducing the risk of infection.

Many of the detailed conference recommendations listed in the Appendix have been under consideration for some time. Their immediate implementation would begin to fill serious gaps that exist in services and knowledge. Other recommendations can be implemented only when questions such as the following have been addressed:

- How can infected women who do not have symptoms be identified at manageable cost?
- How can we reach women who are too poor to use health services, who are too distant from services, or who are prevented from using them by a number of factors, including the objections of their families and social stigmatization?

- How can sexually active women who have completed childbearing and no longer use family planning, child survival, or MCH services be reached?
- How can parents and policymakers be persuaded to allow adolescents and children access to information and services on safer, caring sex?
- Can substances or technologies that protect against RTIs be developed for women who want to conceive?
- How can we take effective demonstration projects to scale?
- What are effective means to change male sexual behavior and to adjust the balance of power between women and men in sexual relationships?
- How can we keep women's health in its own right at the center of the international health agenda?

Prevention and control of RTIs require profound changes in scientific approaches, sexual behavior, gender power relations, men's self-concepts, and women's status and self-esteem. Substantial political will and community leadership are needed to effect such changes. Women need support to organize so they can inform each other and become an effective constituency for women's health nationally and internationally. Scientific and medical policymakers need to include women's health advocates in their decision making, and to recognize socioeconomic and political factors in their models and their strategic thinking. They need also to achieve balance between public health priorities and the requirements of individual human beings.

These challenges are substantial, but the papers in this volume demonstrate that the likely rewards are more than worth the cost.

Adrienne Germain
Vice President
International Women's Health Coalition

PART I
OVERVIEW OF REPRODUCTIVE TRACT INFECTIONS

REPRODUCTIVE TRACT INFECTIONS: CHALLENGES FOR INTERNATIONAL HEALTH POLICY, PROGRAMS, AND RESEARCH

Dr. Judith N. Wasserheit
Chief, Sexually Transmitted Diseases Branch
National Institute of Allergy and Infectious Diseases
National Institutes of Health
Bethesda, Maryland 20892

Dr. King K. Holmes
Center for AIDS and STDs
University of Washington
Seattle, Washington 98122

INTRODUCTION

In resource-poor settings around the world, reproductive tract infections (RTIs) are extremely common, and the consequences for the health and social well-being of women and their children are frequent and potentially devastating.[1,2] RTIs include three types of infection: sexually transmitted diseases (STDs), such as chlamydial infection, gonorrhea, trichomoniasis, syphilis, chancroid, genital herpes, genital warts, and human immunodeficiency virus (HIV) infection; endogenous infections, which are caused by overgrowth of organisms that can be present in the genital tract of healthy women, such as bacterial vaginosis and vulvovaginal candidiasis; and iatrogenic infections, which are associated with medical procedures. All these infections are preventable or treatable causes of infertility, ectopic pregnancy, cervical cancer, fetal wastage, low birth weight, infant blindness, neonatal pneumonia, and mental retardation.[3,4] In addition, they facilitate transmission of HIV.[5,6] Because of sociocultural factors and structural barriers to care, both the incidence and the impact of RTI sequelae are likely to be particularly great in the Third World.

RTIs and their sequelae are also inextricably intertwined with key health-related development programs, such as those concerned with family planning, child survival, women's health, safe motherhood, and HIV prevention. RTI syndromes have profound implications for the success of each of these initiatives.[3-7] Conversely, each of these initiatives provides a critical opportunity for the prevention and control of RTIs.[2,7,8] From program and policy perspectives, therefore, RTIs offer a strategically important common element among reproductive health and development programs (Figure 1).

Reproductive Tract Infections, Edited by A. Germain *et al.*
Plenum Press, New York, 1992

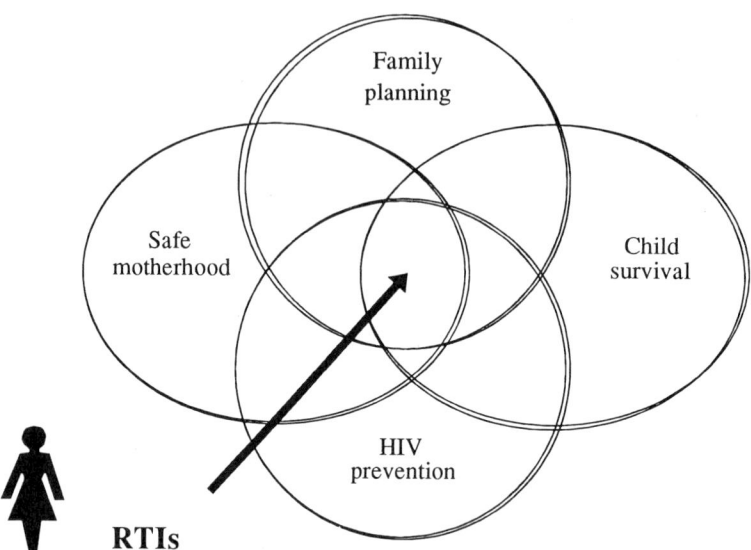

**Figure 1. RTIs: A Strategic Common Element in
Reproductive Health and Development Programs**

In view of their impact on all of these programs concerned with reproductive health, the degree to which RTIs have been neglected by the international health community is striking. In allocating scarce human and financial health resources for developing countries, most policymakers, program planners, and donor agencies consistently give low priority to control of these infections.[9] This paradox springs from the widely held perception that the financial costs and technical difficulty of interventions greatly outweigh the biomedical, social, and programmatic costs of these diseases. It is compounded by deep-rooted societal attitudes about sexuality and gender. Key barriers to addressing RTIs include:

1. The widespread misperception that RTIs rarely result in severe morbidity or in mortality
2. The belief that RTIs occur primarily among limited numbers of sexually promiscuous adults, such as commercial sex workers (CSWs), and are rarely a problem for the general population
3. The assumption that diagnosis and treatment of RTIs are too expensive and too technically sophisticated for developing countries
4. The position taken by many donor agencies against providing curative care, coupled with a failure to appreciate that STD treatment prevents secondary infections in partners of treated individuals and, therefore, ultimately results in declining disease prevalence and diminishing recurrent costs

5. The difficulty that many individuals and societies have in confronting issues related to sexuality and sexual behavior, and the resulting belief that addressing RTIs will stigmatize individuals, societies, and programs
6. The gender separation of existing health care services, in which AIDS prevention programs and STD clinics (where they exist) often fail to configure services to attract women, while family planning and maternal-child health (MCH) clinics generally do not serve men
7. The low status of women in many countries, which limits women's ability to control the conditions under which sexual intercourse occurs; gives low priority to diseases such as RTIs that disproportionately affect women; and nevertheless assigns women primary responsibility for safeguarding the couple from infection and unwanted pregnancy
8. In many settings, socially sanctioned male promiscuity

It is now time to reevaluate our long-standing assumptions about the impact and feasibility of systematic prevention and control efforts, and to examine critically the national and international policy implications of RTIs in the Third World. In the spirit of stimulating such a reassessment, this chapter examines the demographic, societal, biomedical, and technological developments that set the stage for addressing RTIs; summarizes the human and socioeconomic costs of RTIs in the developing world; and discusses program and policy implications.

RTIs: Why Now?

Several factors bring fresh urgency and motivation to addressing RTIs. During the past 40 years, these infections have become a bigger, more visible problem in many developing countries, while simultaneously, research advances in industrialized nations have provided new insights and options for solutions.

Demographic changes in the developing world have placed an ever greater proportion of these populations at risk for RTIs and their sequelae. Persistently high birthrates in the face of rapidly declining death rates—especially with improving child survival—have led to dramatic growth in the number of adolescent and young adult Third World women and men in the most sexually active years. Furthermore, the "momentum" of population growth created by the large numbers of individuals who are currently infants means that this trend will continue for several decades, even if fertility drops to replacement levels tomorrow.[10] In Sub-Saharan Africa, 15–44-year-old women constituted 73 percent of the adult female population in 1950 and 75 percent in 1980; the figure will probably be at least 76 percent by the year 2000. In absolute numbers, this represents roughly a doubling in each interval, from 36.9 million in 1950 to 77 million in 1980, to a projected 143.3 million at the turn of the millennium.[11] In terms of STD risk, the problem is compounded by rapid urbanization, often associated both with loosening of traditional restraints on sexual activity and with high male-to-female sex ratios. In the developing world exclusive of China, it is estimated that the proportion of the population in cities grew by 60 percent between 1950 and 1980, and will further increase by almost 25 percent by 2000. Comparable figures for industrialized countries are 25 percent and 9 percent, respectively.[10]

Societal changes in some parts of the developing world are beginning to alter women's expectations about their own health and productivity. As larger numbers of women become literate and are able to obtain jobs outside of the home, social as well as financial self-sufficiency is possible. In this context, acute and chronic infectious morbidity related to sex or reproduction, lack of access to health care, and commercial sex as a means of survival are less likely to be passively accepted by women both for themselves and for each other. Furthermore, as the status of women improves, RTI-related morbidity and premature mortality result in increased costs to society in terms of lost productivity. A recent analysis[12] showing that country-specific HIV seroprevalence in Africa is inversely correlated with the female-to-male secondary school enrollment ratio is consistent with these arguments. The interrelatedness of RTIs and other reproductive health and development issues is reinforced by the fact that these findings echo those on the relationship between fertility and measures of women's status such as female education.[13,14] Societal changes precipitated by the HIV epidemic are also responsible for the increasing willingness of some communities to acknowledge the prevalence of sexual behaviors that place people at risk for RTIs. Clearly, such openness markedly increases the feasibility of behavioral interventions.

Biomedical developments have provided critical insights into the impact of RTIs, have altered perceptions about the importance of RTI control, and are likely, in the near future, to result in increasing options for RTI diagnosis and treatment that are technologically and financially appropriate for the developing world. During the past 25 years, investigators have defined much of the clinical and epidemiological spectrum of syndromes associated with four of the major STD pathogens—Chlamydia trachomatis, herpes simplex virus, human papilloma virus (HPV), and HIV. They have greatly expanded our understanding of the role of RTIs in infertility, ectopic pregnancy, and HIV transmission; begun to elucidate the role of these infections in cervical cancer and adverse outcomes of pregnancy; and clarified many of the relationships between RTIs and contraceptive technologies.[3-7,15] These advances have highlighted the potential relationships between RTIs and existing reproductive health initiatives. Simultaneously, the HIV epidemic has lent new urgency to RTI prevention and control, and stimulated the development of models of interdisciplinary and intersectoral coordination in both clinical and research programs.[16,17] Additionally, the success of other international health initiatives, such as smallpox eradication, the Expanded Program on Immunizations (EPI), and diarrheal disease control, has led to more widespread expectation of healthy adulthood through the reproductive years.

All these changes are complemented by biotechnological and pharmaceutical innovations that suggest that within the next five years, simple, inexpensive, rapid tests and shorter-course therapies may be available for several RTIs. For example, approaches that detect unique chlamydial constituents or metabolites appear promising; syphilis immuno diagnostics that can be performed using finger-prick blood and require no ancillary equipment are being explored; and single-dose therapy for uncomplicated chlamydial infection is now available in the form of a new macrolide antibiotic, azithromycin.[18,19,20]

Finally, the technological revolution has greatly facilitated communication and travel. Increased opportunities for international intercourse have not been limited to the cultural, economic, and political spheres. RTIs, along with several other infectious diseases, have truly become international health problems and must be attacked as such.

DIMENSIONS OF THE PROBLEM

Prevalence of RTIs

As a result of problems in study design, reporting, specimen collection, and laboratory

methods, data on the prevalence of RTIs in the developing world are often difficult to
interpret in terms of both internal validity and generalizability. Nevertheless, five
observations appear consistently. First, RTIs are common in almost all of the developing
countries in which they have been investigated, even among asymptomatic populations and
low-risk individuals, such as family planning or antenatal clinic attendees and adults
sampled in population-based studies. Second, in most countries, STD rates are highest

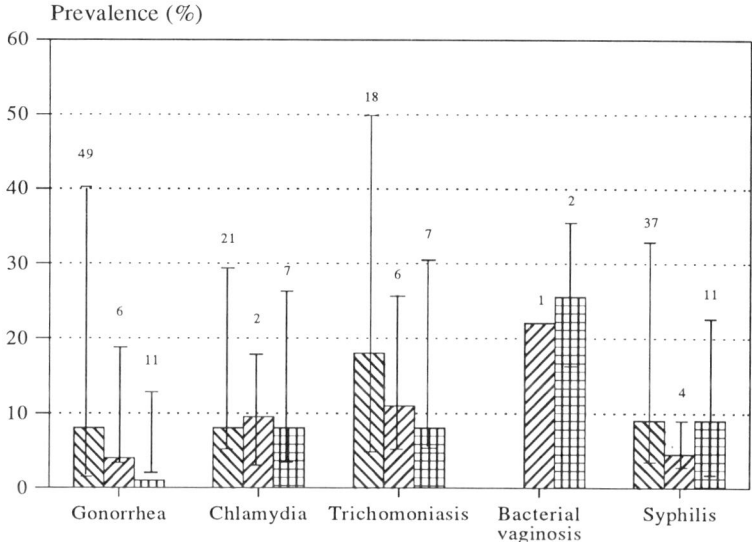

Figure 2. Median RTI Prevalence among
Low-risk Third World Women,* by Continent

among high-risk populations, such as commercial sex workers (among whom rates are
inversely related to socioeconomic status), STD clinic patients, and men in occupations
involving extended or recurrent separations from family (e.g., truck drivers and military
personnel). Third, although data are more limited for Asia and Latin America than for
Africa, and may therefore be misleading, the prevalence of some STDs appears to be greater
in Africa than in other parts of the developing world (Figure 2). For example, gonorrhea

---

*Antenatal, abortion, and family planning clients; peripartum women; participants in community surveys.
Note: Bars indicate median values; vertical lines indicate ranges; figures over lines indicate number of samples.
Source: references 1, 2, 4, 53–60.

rates among asymptomatic women are 2–3 times higher in Africa than in the other regions. Fourth, because serosurveys measure the cumulative burden of previous infection rather than current disease, they document higher prevalence rates than culture-based studies. Finally, chlamydial infections and bacterial vaginosis, despite their potential roles in upper tract infection, infertility, and adverse outcomes of pregnancy, remain largely ignored as causes of morbidity among Third World women.[1,2]

The prevalence of specific RTIs in high- and low-risk populations is summarized in Table 1. Interestingly, although the median RTI prevalences are generally higher for the former than for the latter, the ranges are roughly similar and are broad for both populations, suggesting an overlapping spectrum of risk factors in the two groups. It is noteworthy that the median prevalences for chlamydia and trichomoniasis in the high- and low-risk

Table 1. Median Prevalence of RTIs in the Third World

Disease	High-risk population		Low-risk population	
	Median (%)	Range (%)	Median (%)	Range (%)
Chlamydia	14	2–25	8	1–29
Gonorrhea	24	7–66	6	0.3–40
Trichomoniasis	17	4–20	12	3–50
Syphilis	15	4–32	8	0.01–33
Chancroid	9	3–16	NA	NA

Note: NA = not available.
Source: references 1–4 and 53–60.

categories are less disparate than those for gonorrhea and syphilis. This may be related to the relatively long duration of infectiousness in the former group, which makes it possible for these infections to persist in the absence of a core group of high-frequency transmitters.[1]

To put these prevalences into perspective and to emphasize the potential impact of successful control programs, it is useful to compare data for antenatal clinic attendees in developing and industrialized countries. Among pregnant women in the Third World, gonorrhea rates are 10–15 times higher, chlamydia rates 2–3 times higher, and syphilis rates 10–100 times higher than rates among comparable women in industrialized nations.[1,2,4,21] The lower differential for chlamydia than for the other STDs reflects the fact that many industrialized countries (including the United States) have not yet launched aggressive chlamydia control activities, while almost all have well-established gonorrhea and syphilis control programs.

A number of factors probably contribute to the high prevalence of RTIs found in many developing countries. As discussed above, population pyramids that are heavily weighted with young individuals, explosive urbanization, and low status of women are important. In addition, low levels of education and health information vacuums foster misconceptions about RTIs and discourage preventive practices. Certain customs or traditions—such as polygamy; proscriptions against intercourse during menses and for extended periods postpartum; high bride prices, which force men to postpone marriage until they can afford a wife; and socially sanctioned male promiscuity—result in patterns of sexual behavior characterized by multiple partners, often for a substantial proportion of men and a much smaller proportion of women.[1,2] Finally, limited access to care for STDs increases the prevalence of infection in the community and, therefore, the probability that any given sexual encounter will lead to exposure to an STD.

Biomedical Costs of RTIs

RTIs, and particularly STDs, disproportionately compromise the health of women. Women are less able to prevent exposure to an STD than men, because of the lack of available female-controlled barrier methods and because the power dynamic in sexual relationships frequently limits their ability to negotiate the conditions under which intercourse occurs. For anatomic reasons, transmission of HIV or discharge syndromes (e.g., gonorrhea, chlamydia, trichomoniasis) following exposure appears to be more efficient from male to female than from female to male.[22] When transmission occurs, women are far more likely than men to be asymptomatically infected and, as a result, not seek care. If a woman is "lucky" enough to develop symptoms, it is frequently socially unacceptable for her to seek care for a genital problem, particularly in an STD clinic. And even when the stigma associated with genital examination and STDs does not represent an insurmountable barrier to seeking care, diagnosis of a number of STDs is more difficult in women than in men. Furthermore, the potential for spread of infection to the upper genital tract (e.g., the uterus and fallopian tubes or the testicles) is greater in women than in men. Clearly, because of these factors, the probability of delayed treatment and the severity of complications of RTIs are far greater in women.

Infertility. One of the most common and potentially devastating complications of RTIs in women is infertility. It results from scarring of the fallopian tubes, following ascent of gonorrhea, chlamydia, or possibly bacterial vaginosis organisms into the upper genital tract which cause pelvic inflammatory disease (PID). Data from industrialized countries indicate that 10–40 percent of women with untreated chlamydial or gonococcal infection develop symptomatic PID[23,24,25] and that up to one quarter of those with PID will become infertile.[23] By contrast, post-PID infertility rates were 60–70 percent in the preantibiotic era,[26] a situation that may be analogous to that in many developing countries, where treatment is frequently delayed or is completely unavailable. Indeed, in parts of Sub-Saharan Africa, 30–50 percent of couples are unable to conceive.[27-30] In contrast, the generally accepted baseline infertility rate due to genetic, anatomic, or endocrine factors is 3–7 percent.[28,31] On the basis of fallopian tube abnormalities that highly suggest prior infection, it appears that much of the excess infertility is due to RTIs, and that the proportion of infertility that is RTI-related is markedly higher in Africa than in other Third World regions or in industrialized countries (Table 2).

Ectopic (Tubal) Pregnancy. This potentially fatal complication of RTIs is also associated with prior PID. In contrast to infertility, however, it probably follows incomplete occlusion of the tubal lumen. In industrialized countries, women who have had PID are 6–10 times as likely to develop an ectopic pregnancy as are those who have never had upper genital tract infection,[26,32,33] and case-fatality ratios are approximately 3–5 per 10,000 ectopics.[34] Where RTIs are common and access to health services is limited, it is likely that both the incidence of extrauterine pregnancies and the case-fatality ratio are much higher than these figures. In fact, in such settings, the vast majority of women with ectopic pregnancies probably die without ever coming to medical attention. In most developing countries, the true magnitude of the problem is unknown. However, ectopic pregnancy was the most common surgical emergency in one Kenyan hospital, and the ratio of ectopic to intrauterine pregnancy in countries such as Benin, Gabon, South Africa, and Uganda ranges from 1:91 to 1:62, substantially higher than the ratio of 1:133 in Sweden.[2,3]

Table 2. Proportion of Infertility Due to RTIs, by Region

Region	Proportion
Africa	50–80%
Asia	15–40%
Latin America	~ 35%
Industrialized countries	10–35%

Source: references 2, 3, 27–31, 36, and 37.

Upper genital tract infection related to delivery, induced abortion, or IUD insertion also may lead to infertility and ectopic pregnancy. These infections may be due to underlying STDs that are not detected prior to the procedure, poor technique among health care providers (particularly in the case of clandestine abortion), or both. In several African hospitals, postpartum RTIs are responsible for 14–30 percent of maternal mortality.[3] In a population of over 1,000 pregnant Nairobi women with a 21 percent prevalence of chlamydia and a 7 percent prevalence of gonorrhea, one fifth developed upper tract infection following vaginal delivery, a rate roughly 10 times that in industrialized settings.[3,35] In this hospital-based population, over 90 percent of whom had received at least some prenatal care, 35 percent of the postpartum infectious morbidity was attributable to STDs. Among the majority of Third World women, who neither obtain prenatal services nor deliver in hospitals, it is likely that the overall incidence of postpartum RTIs is even greater, since both the prevalence of STDs and the incidence of iatrogenic infection may well be higher.

A landmark World Health Organization (WHO) study of infertile couples conducted in 33 centers in 25 developing and industrialized countries between 1979 and 1984 raises additional issues about the relative contributions of childbirth and abortion to infertility.[36,37] In all sites, history of STDs and pregnancy complications played a role in infertility; however, in Africa and Latin America, number of live births was a more important predictor of bilateral tubal occlusion than number of previous abortions, while in Asia and in industrialized countries, the opposite was true. Furthermore, in the first two regions, STD history was a more important determinant of infertility than any type of pregnancy-related problem. From the data collected, it was impossible to ascertain the impact of specific STDs, or delivery and abortion practices, on upper tract infection and its sequelae for each region. In addition, biases may have resulted from regional differences in the availability and utilization of health care services. Nevertheless, the data suggest that STDs, unsafe obstetric practices, and clandestine abortion may contribute differentially in various parts of the world, and they highlight the importance of these issues in women's reproductive health.

Cervical Cancer. The third of the common complications of RTIs, cervical cancer, like ectopic pregnancy, frequently results in death. Cervical cancer is the most common cancer in women in the Third World, where over three quarters of all cases of the disease occur.[3,38] Because of limited human and financial resources for cervical cytological screening (Papanicolaou smears), as many as 80 percent of diagnosed cases are detected in advanced stages in which treatment, even if available, has a markedly reduced likelihood of success.[39] Many more cases are never diagnosed at all. In fact, one estimate suggests that in some regions, 3–5 percent of adult female deaths are due to this disease.[40] Although HPV infection alone is probably not sufficient for the development of cervical cancer, it appears to be strongly associated with an increased risk of cervical neoplasia,[41] as well as being the cause of genital warts. For example, in a large case-control study conducted in Latin America, HPV infection was linked with a 4–9-fold increased risk of invasive cervical cancer, depending upon viral type.[42] Many questions about the mechanisms by which HPV causes cervical cancer remain unanswered, but available evidence clearly suggests that HPV infection plays a major role in cervical cancer throughout the world.

Adverse Outcomes of Pregnancy. In addition to ectopic pregnancy, poor pregnancy outcomes that are linked to RTIs include fetal wastage (spontaneous abortion or stillbirth), low birth weight (due to either premature delivery or intrauterine growth retardation), and congenital or perinatal infection (including potentially blinding eye infections, infant pneumonias, and mental retardation) (Table 3). The impact of RTIs on pregnancy depends upon the organism involved, the chronicity of infection, and the stage of gestation during which the woman becomes infected.[4,43–48] In general, acute infections appear to be more likely than chronic RTIs to result in adverse infant outcomes. Because it is easier to study congenital infections than fetal wastage or low birth weight, data are most reliable in this area. Particularly in developing countries, information on the other two outcomes may be extremely difficult to obtain and heavily confounded by competing risk factors. Nevertheless, policymakers and health care professionals concerned about child survival must address these infections because of emerging data on the role of RTIs in fetal wastage and low birth weight; the clear-cut relationships between RTIs and congenital or perinatal infections; the high incidence of death among low-birth-weight or blind Third World infants; and the availability of inexpensive, efficacious interventions for several RTIs in pregnancy.

HIV Transmission. Table 4 shows the degree to which RTIs facilitate transmission of HIV. Data supporting genital ulcer disease (GUD) as a risk factor for HIV transmission are currently most compelling. However, several well-designed, prospective studies that adjust for sexual behavior now suggest that nonulcerative STDs also promote HIV transmission, and that both types of STDs increase the risk of transmission at least 3–5-fold.[5,6] Indeed, if the latter syndromes do facilitate HIV transmission, the proportion of HIV infection attributable to the nonulcerative STDs will far outweigh that due to GUD, because in most populations, diseases such as chlamydia, gonorrhea, and trichomoniasis are far more common than genital ulcers. Furthermore, preliminary data suggest that at the

Table 3. Proportion of Pregnant Women Experiencing Adverse Outcomes

Maternal diagnosis	Fetal wastage	Low birth weight or prematurity	Congenital or perinatal infection
Chlamydia	?rare	10–30%	40–70%
Gonorrhea	?rare	11–25%	30–68%
Early syphilis	20–25%	15–50%	40–70%
Genital herpes Primary Recurrent	7–54% ?rare	30–35% ?rare	30–50% 0.4–8%
Bacterial vaginosis	?rare	10–25%	Rare
Trichomoniasis	?rare	11–15%	Rare
No RTI	4–10%	2–12%	NA

Source: reference 15.

community level, HIV infection may increase the prevalence of some STDs (e.g., genital ulcers). If coinfection with HIV prolongs or augments the infectiousness of individuals with STDs, and if the same STDs facilitate transmission of HIV, these infections may greatly amplify one another. This "epidemiological synergy" may well help account for the explosive growth of the HIV pandemic in some Third World populations.[6] Obviously, in these communities, effective STD control programs will be essential to HIV prevention.

In summary, the morbidity associated with RTIs is substantial in any context; it is particularly so in the Third World, because of cultural factors, lack of access to care, coexisting diseases, and antibiotic resistance patterns. Despite the widespread impression that RTIs are not fatal, six of the seven complications discussed above frequently result in death in the Third World. Infertility, ectopic pregnancy, cervical cancer, fetal wastage, low birth weight, congenital infection, and HIV infection cannot be considered minor health problems.

Socioeconomic Costs of RTIs

In comparison to the biomedical costs of RTIs, the socioeconomic costs are much less well studied. Assessment of some costs is relatively straightforward. The direct costs of diagnosis and treatment of uncomplicated RTIs clearly are substantially lower than those for sequelae. In addition, several analyses demonstrate that the major factor driving clinical management costs is the price of diagnostic tests, rather than the price of antimicrobial agents.[4,12,49]

Other costs are difficult to quantify. For example, what is the true impact of RTI-related infertility or adverse outcomes of pregnancy, when a woman's self-image and status within her family and community are tied to her roles as wife and mother? Undoubtedly, in many cases, it goes far beyond the physical discomfort of gonorrhea or PID. But how

Table 4. Role of STDs in HIV Transmission

Syndrome	Risk estimate	
	Median	Range
Genital ulcers	4.7	3.3–18.2
Syphilis	3.0	2.0–9.9
Genital herpes	3.3	1.9–8.5
Chlamydial infection	4.5	3.2–5.7
Gonorrhea	4.7	3.5–8.9
Trichomoniasis	2.7	?
Anogenital warts	3.7	?

Source: reference 6.

should costs, such as family disruption, abandonment, divorce, or social ostracism be factored into the cost-benefit equation in attempting to set health priorities? What value should be given to the ongoing societal burden of congenitally or perinatally infected individuals who are permanently disabled?

Mead Over and Peter Piot recently completed one of the first systematic evaluations of the public health and socioeconomic impact of STDs in the developing world.[12] To compare the health impact of various diseases, they used the concept of age-adjusted "healthy life years lost per capita per year" (HLYL), the product of "healthy life years lost per case" and "cases per capita per year." The analysis revealed that STDs (including HIV, syphilis, chancroid, chlamydia, and gonorrhea) are responsible for approximately 15 percent of the disease burden in urban areas with high STD prevalence (i.e., greater than 5 percent prevalence of gonorrhea among sexually active adults or greater than 10 percent seroprevalence of syphilis among pregnant women). This model suggests that in high-prevalence communities, STDs rank third after measles and malaria among common Third World diseases in their public health and socioeconomic impact. When *productive* HLYL are calculated, STDs are second only to measles in their health burden. These calculations may, in fact, underestimate the impact of STDs both because they appear to minimize the incidence of chlamydia in women and because they do not include a role for STDs in competing outcomes such as prematurity and congenital malformations.

PROGRAM AND POLICY IMPLICATIONS

Interdependence of RTI Prevention Initiatives

We believe that the lack of effective, coordinated efforts among initiatives for the health of women and their children, and for the prevention of STDs and HIV, represents an extreme example of programmatic tunnel vision—an increasing embarrassment in light of modern, holistic concepts of public health. The theme of this book is that intersectoral investment in STD control and prevention of RTI morbidity will synergistically improve the return on existing health initiatives that concern family planning, safe motherhood and women's health, child survival, and HIV prevention. A convergence of these interests during the AIDS era calls for integrated programs, integrated research and training, and a strengthened infrastructure for STD control. We will examine the premise that integrated programs will be synergistic. A 1990 WHO consultative group, convened to consider the case for closer integration of AIDS and STD control programs at the national level, and developed two criteria for assessing the potential synergy of integrated public health programs: conceptual over-lap/strategic interdependence and critical mass/cost-effectiveness.[16]

Conceptual Overlap and Strategic Interdependence. Where there is epidemiological, clinical, scientific, or other overlap in problem formulation, and similarity or interdependence of strategies for interventions, coordinated planning leads to conceptually balanced and technically sound approaches that also best serve women's needs. This book presents a strong case for conceptual overlap and strategic interdependence among programs for family planning, safe motherhood and women's health, child survival, HIV prevention, and prevention of other STDs. A number of complementary interventions that could be pursued have been summarized in Table 5.

Principal areas of conceptual overlap promote the concept of reproductive health. The movement toward a reproductive health framework emerges from the fact that the major RTI complications (other than HIV infection) involve the female reproductive tract and the newborn infant. In addition, the term "reproductive health" connotes a more positive goal than the term "STD control" (analogous to choosing the term "family planning" rather than the term "population control"), and encompasses the related health objectives and initiatives. Similarly, in family planning programs, the reproductive health concept encourages the inclusion of RTI prevention and control to ensure contraceptive safety, to prevent infertility, and to increase contraceptive acceptance and continuation.

Table 5. Overview of Complementary RTI Interventions, by
Reproductive Health and Development Initiative

| Initiative | Existing programs | Complementary RTI interventions | | Priority research areas for future RTI interventions |
		Currently feasible	Available in five years*	
Child survival	Antenatal care Safe delivery MCH services EPI Diarrheal disease and acute respiratory infection control	Antenatal testing for syphilis Ophthalmia neonatorum prophylaxis at birth Screening for asymptomatic GUD Syndromic diagnosis/therapy of symptomatic cervicovaginal infection and PID Counseling about condoms, partner notification, and RTI reduction Training traditional birth attendants and antenatal and MCH health care workers about RTIs Development of tailored RTI management guidelines	Antenatal screening for gonorrhea, chlamydia, bacterial vaginosis, and trichomoniasis using simple, inexpensive tests	Development of short-course, inexpensive antimicrobials that are safe during pregnancy Development of simple, inexpensive RTI diagnostics Elucidation of the impact of RTIs on prematurity and intrauterine growth retardation Surveillance of sexual and health care behaviors, RTI prevalence, and antibiotic resistance
Family planning	Contraceptive services Pregnancy termination services	Syndromic diagnosis/therapy of symptomatic cervicovaginal infection and PID Screening for GUD with testing for syphilis Pap smear screening for cervical cancer Counseling about condoms, partner notification, and RTI reduction Training family planning workers about RTIs Development of tailored RTI management guidelines Use of medical abortifacients with low risk of RTIs (e.g., RU-486)	Screening for gonorrhea, chlamydia, bacterial vaginosis, and trichomoniasis using simple, inexpensive tests Recommendations for antibiotic prophylaxis of IUD insertion and pregnancy termination	Development of simple, inexpensive RTI diagnostics Evaluation of antibiotic prophylaxis for transcervical procedures Development of female-controlled contraceptives that protect against RTIs Surveillance of sexual and health care behaviors, RTI prevalence, and antibiotic resistance Evaluation of downstaging for cervical cancer

Table 5 continues on next page.

Table 5. Overview of Complementary RTI Interventions, by
Reproductive Health and Development Initiative (continued)

Initiative	Existing programs	Complementary RTI interventions		Priority research areas for future RTI interventions
		Currently feasible	Available in five years*	
HIV control	AIDS care Counseling about condoms, partner notification, and RTI reduction	Syndromic diagnosis/ therapy of symptom- atic cervicovaginal infection and urethritis Short-course therapy for chlamydia Screening for GUD with testing for syphilis Pap smear screening for cervical cancer Development of tailored RTI management guidelines	Screening for gonorrhea, chlamydia, bacterial vaginosis, and trichomoniasis using simple, inexpensive tests Effective RTI treatment regimens for HIV-positive individuals	Development of simple, inexpensive RTI diagnostics Development of female-controlled contraceptives that protect against RTIs Surveillance of sexual and health care behaviors, RTI prevalence, and antibiotic resistance Development and evaluation of effective RTI treatment regimens for HIV-positive individuals
Safe motherhood/ women's health	Antenatal care Safe delivery MCH services	Screening for GUD; antenatal syphilis testing Syndromic diagnosis/ therapy of symptom- atic cervicovaginal infection and PID Pap smear screening for cervical cancer Counseling about condoms, partner notification, and RTI reduction Training traditional birth attendants, antenatal and MCH health care workers about RTIs Development of tailored RTI management guidelines Use of medical abortifacients with low risk of RTIs (e.g., RU-486)	Screening for gonorrhea, chlamydia, bacterial vaginosis, and trichomoniasis using simple, inexpensive tests	Development of simple, inexpensive RTI diagnostics Development of female-controlled contraceptives that protect against RTIs Development of short-course, inexpensive antimicrobials that are safe during pregnancy Development of improved detection and treatment for HIV infection and cervical cancer Surveillance of sexual and health care behaviors, RTI prevalence, and antibiotic resistance

*Assumes increased targeted support for expedited development.

There are many areas of strategic interdependence between initiatives concerned with RTI morbidity, including:

1. *Family planning.* RTIs may decrease acceptance and continuation of contraceptive methods in two ways: directly, when the contraceptive user believes that the symptoms of infection are a contraceptive side effect; and indirectly, by creating a fear of limiting or delaying fertility in the face of frequent complications of RTIs, which prevent healthy childbearing. In either case, one might argue that rather than stigmatizing family planning programs, care for RTIs may well be essential to their success.[2,12] Conversely, effective family planning is important in preventing RTI morbidity because the current epidemic of sexually transmitted infection, including HIV infection, is fueled by rapid growth in the absolute number and the relative proportion of adolescents and young adults in the total population. Hence, effective family planning can play a significant role in eventually stemming the epidemic spread of STDs. The synergy between RTI prevention and control and family planning provides a compelling argument for their integration.

2. *Gender-specific access.* In general, family planning, antenatal care, and maternal health programs deal with women and ignore STDs. STD programs in developing countries deal primarily with men and ignore other services, such as family planning. A strong potential exists here for synergistic and interdependent strategies.

3. *Condom strategies.* Currently, some AIDS programs promote condom use for HIV prevention; some family planning programs promote condoms only as a second-choice method and in some cases only during midcycle for contraception (as opposed to consistent use for both contraception and STD/HIV prevention); and some STD programs fail to promote condoms at all. Clearly, in those developing countries where family planning and STD/HIV prevention are equally important goals, there is a need for a well-articulated and widely disseminated consensus on condom promotion strategies.

Critical Mass and Cost-effectiveness. When components of separate programs are ineffective because of limited financial or human resources, integrated programs, coordinated allocation of resources, and concerted action can achieve a "critical mass" of resources and improve effectiveness. Furthermore, when separate programs are duplicative or competitive, integrated ones are likely to be more cost-effective. A strong case for combined programs for STD and HIV prevention has been made by the 1990 WHO Consultative Group.[16] There appears to be considerable potential for increasing the effectiveness of other reproductive health programs by integrating elements to prevent RTI morbidity, such as health education, clinic personnel and facilities, diagnostic reagents and laboratories, medication and treatment guidelines, and training.

Interventions to Prevent RTI Morbidity in Women and Infants

We will examine interventions that fall into two general categories: those that represent simple, inexpensive, and proven-effective strategies in preventing RTIs or RTI sequelae at the *individual level,* and those based on theoretically cost-effective strategies to prevent RTI morbidity by lowering the overall incidence of STDs at the *population level.*

Individual- vs. Population-level Interventions. Family planning and MCH interventions generally involve prevention of pregnancy or disease in the individual served and are designed to reach the largest possible number of women. Interventions used in STD and HIV prevention have, by comparison, generally been designed to benefit the population as a whole. Specifically, the latter have frequently focused on so-called core groups of high-frequency transmitters in an effort to lower the overall incidence of RTI morbidity in the population by reducing the level of STDs in people with large numbers of sex partners. While such efforts are essential, the authors of the following chapters recognize the importance of reaching individual women in the general population, both to ensure the health and well-being of individual women and to generate the synergistic efforts described above. This perspective creates significant program and policy choices.

For example, one might initially think that the most direct way to reduce RTI morbidity in women would be to develop interventions that are directed principally toward female populations. However, such interventions at the individual level are most easily directed at the postadolescent subset of health-conscious and relatively affluent women, who have greatest access to health care. These initiatives may therefore be an extremely inefficient strategy for reducing the RTI morbidity of all women and children. Instead, a population-oriented strategy that combines biomedical and behavioral interventions for both men and women, particularly those who are high-frequency transmitters of STDs, is likely to be the most efficient approach to reducing RTI morbidity in women and infants. Other interventions directed at individual women or infants are complementary and cost-effective and can be recommended now. Even for these interventions, however, strategies that include the male partner are often essential.

Individual-level Interventions. A working group was convened by the WHO in Geneva in 1988 to examine cost-effective interventions to reduce maternal and infant infectious morbidity. The group concluded that five cost-effective interventions are available, of which the first four concern infectious morbidity related to RTIs.[50] The five interventions are as follows (not necessarily in order of priority): prophylaxis against gonococcal ophthalmia neonatorum (eye infections in the newborn); prenatal screening and treatment for maternal syphilis; training of traditional birth attendants (TBAs); hepatitis B immunization of infants; and immunization of mothers with tetanus toxoid to prevent neonatal tetanus. Because strategies for universal infant immunization for prevention of hepatitis B and maternal immunization for prevention of neonatal tetanus have been formulated and are being increasingly implemented, we will focus on the first three interventions.

1. Prophylaxis against gonococcal ophthalmia neonatorum. Gonococcal eye infection of the newborn occurs in about 40 percent of infants born to infected mothers and can result in blindness. Credé prophylaxis, consisting of application of silver nitrate drops in the newborn's eyes promptly after delivery, is one of the oldest preventive health measures, and is considered to be over 90 percent effective. Application of tetracycline or erythromycin into the newborn's eyes is also considered to be highly effective for preventing newborn gonococcal conjunctivitis, and may have advantages over silver nitrate in the developing country setting.

The cost per case of gonococcal conjunctivitis prevented depends upon the prevalence of gonorrhea in pregnant women. As discussed by Peter Piot and Jane Rowley,[49] the cost of prophylaxis is lower than the cost of treating cases of gonococcal conjunctivitis when the prevalence of prenatal gonorrhea is 6 percent or greater. However, this does not take into consideration the severity of the complication of neonatal gonococcal eye infection, blindness. When the prevention of blindness is considered, routine ophthalmic prophylaxis is justified at much lower prevalences of gonorrhea. Therefore, this inexpensive intervention should be implemented throughout Sub-Saharan Africa, Latin America, Oceania, and in most Asian countries.

A principal need for research in this area is to evaluate the potential for training TBAs to administer ophthalmic prophylaxis, and to evaluate the impact of this intervention.

2. Prenatal screening for syphilis. Syphilis during pregnancy may result not only in potentially severe morbidity for the woman, but also in spontaneous abortion, stillbirth, or, in the majority of infants, fatal or disabling congenital infection. Prevention usually depends on screening maternal blood specimens drawn using needles and syringes, and involves relatively simple laboratory technology. Screening is most effective when it occurs as early as possible in pregnancy and is repeated later in pregnancy, and when all infected mothers are promptly treated. As reviewed by Piot and Rowley,[49] the cost of screening per complication prevented is relatively low, especially in developing countries, where the prevalence of prenatal syphilis is high. Routine prenatal screening for syphilis provides an opportunity to identify women who are (and whose partners are) in need of treatment. It also represents one of the most useful surveillance methods to assess the magnitude of STD morbidity in the general population and to evaluate the effectiveness of AIDS and STD prevention and control programs.

The greatest research need in this area is probably for the development and evaluation of tests that can be performed on blood obtained by finger stick. This would obviate the need for drawing blood using needles and syringes, and for separation of serum from red blood cells by centrifugation. Equally important in the AIDS era, it could reduce the risk of needle stick accidents. The tests should be rapid, to permit immediate treatment. A second need is for demonstration projects to show the feasibility, cost, and benefit of prenatal syphilis testing in several of the least developed and developing countries.

3. Training of TBAs. As of 1984, only about half of all births in Sub-Saharan Africa and Asia were attended by trained personnel (Figure 3). There is evidence from ecological studies that infant mortality is lower when births are attended by TBAs who have received training. No data are available on whether TBAs could be trained to give prenatal or perinatal care that would reduce RTI-related morbidity for mothers or infants. Is it feasible to add materials for ophthalmia prophylaxis to TBA birth kits? Does TBA training reduce the rate of postpartum RTIs caused by "endogenous" vaginal or other microorganisms? What is the potential role of TBAs in monitoring infection or postpartum febrile morbidity, and in initiating antibiotic therapy or referral by management algorithms? Could a simple technology be developed to allow testing of cord blood for syphilis antibody outside the clinic setting?

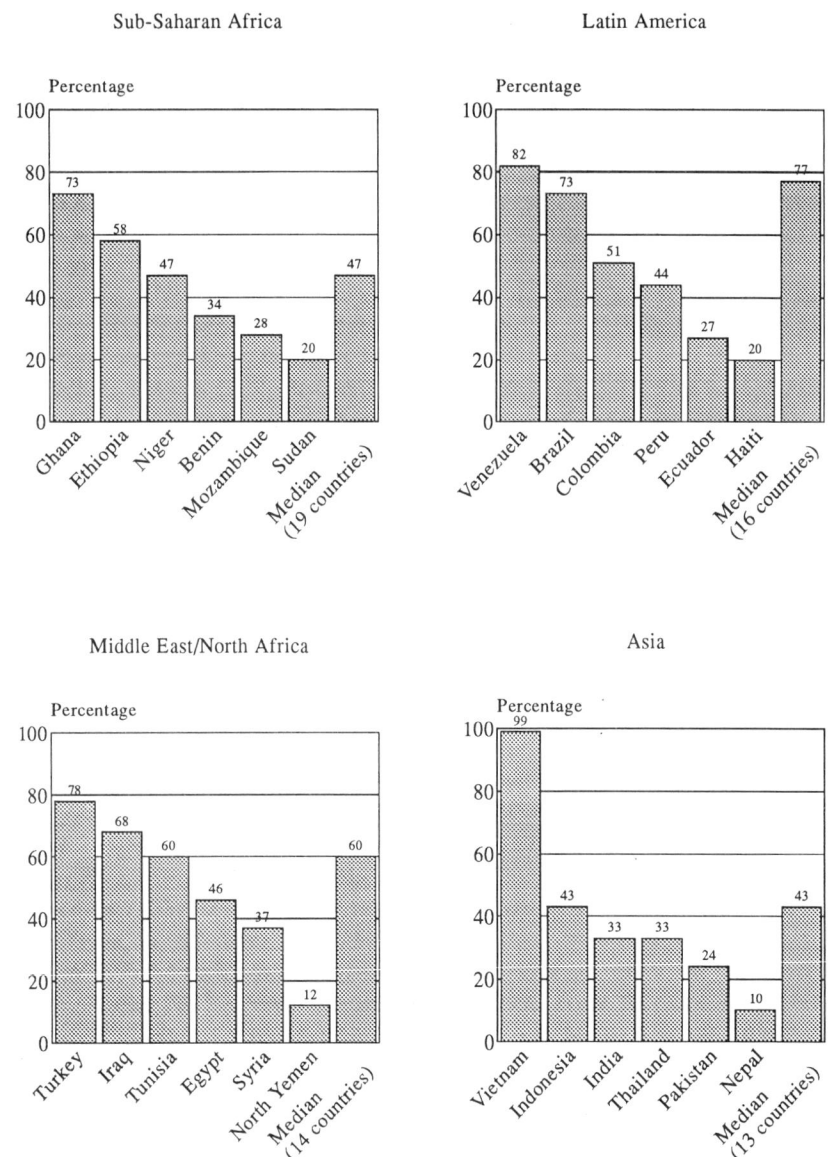

Sources: reference 61.

**Figure 3. Percentage of Births
Attended by Trained Personnel, 1984**

4. *Early detection and treatment of RTIs.* Early detection and treatment of RTIs can prevent complications or minimize the severity of long-term sequelae of complications that do arise. This is termed "secondary prevention." Strategies for secondary prevention of complications or late sequelae differ for the acute and the chronic STDs. Certain STDs—gonorrhea, for example—have a short incubation period (the interval between acquisition of infection and development of acute symptoms). Assuming that the time between appearance of acute symptoms of gonorrhea and the development of complications such as PID is short—and there is some evidence for this[24]—then symptoms would have to be recognized very promptly to result in treatment and prevention of complications. The detection of symptomatic disease, termed "diagnosis" (as opposed to "screening," which detects asymptomatic infection), can be based on recognition of syndromes—such as, with gonorrhea, vaginal or urethral discharge.

Unfortunately, diagnosis of symptomatic gonorrhea in women is not very useful, for two reasons. Many women with gonorrhea never develop any symptoms. And even the early, acute manifestations of gonorrhea are often vague and nonspecific in women. Therefore, even in industrialized countries, early recognition of symptoms and signs of gonorrhea in women has been a relatively ineffective strategy for preventing development of PID.

In contrast, gonorrhea usually produces obvious, acute symptoms in men. Consequently, its early recognition in men provides an opportunity to notify their partners to whom they may have passed on the infection—usually regular female partners. Treatment of incubating or early gonorrhea in exposed female partners of men with the disease is an important—if underrated and underutilized—strategy for preventing PID in exposed *individual* women. Thus, although it is paradoxical and counterintuitive, for preventing gonococcal PID, early diagnosis of gonorrhea in men, followed by partner notification, could be more effective than early detection of symptomatic gonorrhea in women.

For certain chronic RTIs, on the other hand, the interval from initial infection of the female reproductive tract to development of complications is quite long—often years. Examples include infections with HPV, HIV, and syphilis. With each of these chronic STDs, there may be no intervening symptoms to call attention to the infection. For these infections, strategies for preventing complications in individual women can be based upon screening for chronic, subclinical infection (as opposed to diagnosis and treatment of syndromes produced by acute symptomatic infection). For example, if cervical dysplasia represents a step in the progression from cervical HPV infection to cervical cancer, then Pap smear screening and treatment for cervical dysplasia currently represents such a strategy.

Chlamydial infection of the cervix may represent an intermediate case. The course of infection is less acute than that of gonorrhea, and less chronic than that of the postulated HPV–dysplasia–cancer time frame. The evolution of tubal damage caused by chlamydial infection may be more chronic than is the case with gonococcal disease. Thus, strategies for preventing infertility caused by chlamydial infection could include all of the options discussed above: early diagnosis and treatment of early symptoms, treatment of exposed female partners of men with acute infections, and screening for subclinical chlamydial disease.

In summary, cost-effective interventions for prevention of RTI-related morbidity at the individual level clearly include neonatal ocular prophylaxis for prevention of gonococcal eye infections and prenatal screening for syphilis. Training of TBAs to use ocular prophylaxis and to recognize and help manage postpartum febrile morbidity warrants evaluation. Early detection and treatment of RTIs at the individual level can be based upon early diagnosis of acute syndromes (where, paradoxically, recognition of the more obvious syndromes in men may provide the most practical access to recently infected women), and on screening for detection of chronic subclinical infection.

The development of simple and inexpensive diagnostic tests may contribute most to improved screening in women, since early detection of acute infection would no longer be limited to testing the minority of women whose symptoms lead them to seek medical consultation. The greatest contribution of improved diagnostic tests for certain diseases (e.g., gonococcal and chlamydial infection) could be in interventions that are directed at the population or societal level.

Population-level Interventions. R. Anderson and R. May have shown that during the early period of a sexually transmitted epidemic, the rate of spread of infection within the population (the reproductive rate) is the product of three variables: the average efficiency of sexual transmission of the infection; the average duration of infectiousness of an infected person; and the sum of the average rate of partner change and the variance in rate of partner change, divided by the average rate of partner change.[51] The last term estimates the probability of exposure to STDs within the population. This model is useful in identifying the most important intervention targets designed to most efficiently slow the spread of STDs and reduce the overall levels of infection in the population.

In general, the *efficiency of transmission* of an STD can be lowered by condom use, by avoidance of the sexual practices that most efficiently transmit the infection (e.g., receptive anorectal intercourse for HIV and hepatitis B virus), and by eliminating risk factors that increase the efficiency of transmission (e.g., by aggressively controlling STDs that increase transmission of HIV). Reduction in the *duration of infectiousness*, the traditional goal of biomedical interventions used to control curable STDs, can be accomplished by early detection (diagnostic testing, screening, and partner notification), followed by treatment. Reduction in *rates of partner change* or in *numbers of high-risk partners* (those who themselves have many partners) can be attempted through behavioral interventions.

Health education is a key approach to changing all the parameters affecting the rate of spread: to reduce the rate of sexual partner change, the efficiency of transmission (via condom promotion and prevention of risky sexual practices), and the duration of infectiousness (by promoting effective health-care-seeking behavior and effective health care delivery).

Each of these interventions can be deployed widely to cover the entire population at risk, or can be concentrated on core groups of high-frequency transmitters. The potential feasibility and utility of *wide coverage* vs. *focused concentration* of interventions in a particular population depends upon the epidemiology of sexual behavior and of STDs in that population. In populations where a small number of easily identified individuals form a high proportion of sexual partnerships, interventions focused on these individuals should have the greatest cost-effectiveness. Such interventions could be much more cost-effective in lowering the incidence of STDs in the population, and thus in reducing the overall morbidity of STD-related RTIs, than interventions designed to cover all individuals within the population.[49]

Formal behavioral surveys, ethnographic research, and STD surveillance can help determine where and how to best focus public health core-group interventions. However, general patterns of high-risk sexual behavior and predominant patterns of STD epidemiology are now widely recognized in many developing countries, and could be used without further delay to initiate focused interventions. Given the almost total lack of STD interventions in most developing countries, initiating basic intervention strategies where these are lacking certainly need not await extensive ethnographic research; formal studies of knowledge, attitudes, behaviors, and practices; and comprehensive countrywide STD surveillance.

On the basis of the above considerations, a format for classifying and prioritizing STD interventions at the population level is presented in Table 6. Elsewhere in this volume, Allan Ronald and Sevgi Aral present a detailed and thoughtful assessment of these and other interventions, and of the health systems and health policy changes needed to effect such interventions.[8] Behavioral interventions through health education and counseling are essential for each of the interventions, as shown in Table 6. These interventions can involve mass communications, and can be directed at the individual, at specific groups, or at the entire population.

In general, during the AIDS era, the emphasis in developing countries has been on use of mass communications for HIV prevention, with coverage of the general population. The messages have usually encouraged fewer partners, promoted use of condoms, and addressed humanistic concerns. Behavioral interventions that focus on individuals or groups at high risk have been much more limited, and interventions generally have not specifically addressed prevention of RTI-related morbidity other than HIV infection. Efforts to promote health-care seeking for STD treatment or to otherwise provide early detection of STDs have been negligible.

FUTURE DIRECTIONS

Persistent Dilemmas

Several issues concerning RTI prevention and control interventions remain to be addressed. As discussed above and described more fully in the following chapters, a number of dilemmas that face women, scientists, health care providers, and policymakers have hampered progress in the past. Recognition of these dilemmas is probably the first step toward their resolution.

Several dilemmas crosscut the reproductive health and development initiatives. First, Third World women's gender roles often jeopardize their health by placing them at risk of RTIs; HIV infection and other STDs, pregnancy-related infection, or contraceptive-related infection. Second, STDs occur predominantly in resource-poor settings, in which intervention is usually most difficult. Third, while interventions focused on "core groups of high-frequency transmitters" are most cost-effective in reducing the level of STDs in a population,[1,49] such approaches are frequently viewed as stigmatizing and, from the individual's perspective, do not directly address the needs of many women. Fourth, several aspects of development, such as prolonged spousal separations, may catalyze "risk situations." Finally, the dichotomy of male-oriented HIV and STD programs vs. female-oriented MCH and family planning programs ignores the reality that RTIs affect the health of couples.

**Table 6. Population-level STD Interventions Targeting
the Three Determinants of STD Spread***

Determinant of spread and objective of intervention	Focused intervention for core groups	Widespread intervention for general coverage
Efficiency of transmission		
Condom promotion	*Encourage condom use by clients of prostitutes*	Change norms: condom use by youth, nonmonogamous adults
Avoiding risky practices	Encourage avoidance of unprotected anorectal sex	Encourage adolescent women (who have cervical ectopy) to defer sexual debut
Reducing risk factors for transmission	*Control STDs in prostitutes, to lower HIV transmission*	? Promote male circumcision where GUD and HIV are hyperendemic
Duration of infectiousness		
Early detection	*Promote early health-care seeking and regular periodic screening for syphilis and gonorrhea*	*Implement guidelines and training for syndromic diagnosis and treatment; partner notification; and neonatal screening through integrated programs in family planning and MCH clinics and TBAs*
Effective treatment	? Periodic mass treatment	*Implement treatment guidelines, drug supply system*
Frequency of exposure		
Decreasing rates of partner change	Counsel patients with STDs to change behavior	Implement health and family life education in schools, use mass communication
Avoiding risky partners	Counsel men with STDs to avoid risky partners	Difficult without stigmatizing

* Italics show high-priority population-level interventions not yet widely endorsed, funded, or implemented for prevention of RTIs in women.

Additional dilemmas are more specific to individual programs. Women attending family planning clinics currently must choose between methods that are highly effective in preventing pregnancy, but offer little protection against infection, and methods that optimize protection against infection, but require cooperation by men or are less reliable in pregancy prevention.[7] On the other hand, women who want to become pregnant but wish to protect themselves against RTIs are confronted by the biological reality that virucidal or bactericidal agents will probably also adversely affect sperm. Perhaps most disturbing, MCH programs continue to focus on women almost exclusively as mothers, while ignoring their health needs as individuals in their own right.[4,52]

Programmatic Challenges and Research Implications

In summary, RTIs are among the most challenging problems facing the international health community. They occur most frequently in populations that are difficult to reach, and are intertwined with gender roles and sexuality, issues that may be difficult to confront. Yet, RTIs are a frequent source of severe morbidity among Third World women. As a result of economic and cultural factors, both the prevalence of these infections and the incidence of their sequelae appear to be greater in many developing country populations than in comparable settings in industrialized countries. Limited data also suggest that the socioeconomic costs of RTIs are substantial. Furthermore, from a programmatic perspective, because of the impact of RTIs on reproductive health and HIV transmission, it is likely that interventions to prevent and control these diseases will synergistically promote family planning, child survival, safe motherhood, and HIV prevention programs.

This book, and the conference out of which it grew, attempt to take a crucial first step in addressing RTIs by confronting several difficult issues. On the basis of feasibility, acceptability, and cost-effectiveness, which interventions should receive highest priority at the individual level and at the population level? How effective are core-group interventions in decreasing RTI morbidity in the general population? Given cost-effectiveness, ethical, and programmatic considerations, what should be the balance of resources committed to interventions focused on core groups vs. those focused on segments of the general population? What is the role of "quick" interventions, such as "mass treatment" of core-group members, as strategies to reduce the overall RTI incidence in the population? Does this represent an approach that could complement more gradual strengthening of health care infrastructure?

In developing countries where genital ulcer diseases are highly endemic, should highest priority in STD control programs be given to these syndromes, which are probably the most susceptible of all STDs to conventional control measures, including health education, early detection, and effective treatment? Or should equal emphasis be given to the generally more common discharge syndromes, such as gonorrhea and chlamydial infection, which have such severe consequences for the health of women and infants? How might RTI interventions promote the goals of existing health programs, such as those focusing on family planning, child survival, safe motherhood, and HIV prevention? Conversely, what is the role of these critical health and development initiatives in achieving STD control and prevention of RTI-related morbidity? What strategies are likely to be most effective in integrating RTI prevention with these programs?

Finally, what information is most urgently needed to guide rational program and policy decisions, and to facilitate rapid development of future interventions? How can productive research efforts best be launched within developing countries to provide this site-specific information? Where do RTIs belong on the international health agenda? And, of course, what is the next step, who should take it, and how?

The chapters that follow attempt to answer these critical questions by presenting state-of-the-art reviews of the biomedical, programmatic, and socioeconomic impact of RTIs in the Third World, and by examining a broad range of potential interventions. The rich discussion of the conference is crystallized in the summary recommendations that appear in the appendix at the end of the volume.

REFERENCES

1. Brunham RC, Embree JE. Sexually transmitted diseases: current and future dimensions of the problem in the third world. In: Germain A, Holmes KK, Piot P, Wasserheit JN, eds. Reproductive tract infections: global impact and priorities for women's health, New York: Plenum Press, 1992:35–58.
2. Wasserheit JN. The significance and scope of reproductive tract infections among third world women. Int J Gynecol Obstet 1989; Suppl 3:145–68.
3. Meheus AZ. Women's health and reproductive tract infections: the challenges posed by pelvic inflammatory disease, infertility, ectopic pregnancy, and cervical cancer. In: Germain A, Holmes KK, Piot P, Wasserheit JN, eds. Reproductive tract infections: global impact and priorities for women's health, New York: Plenum Press, 1992:61–91.
4. Schulz KF, Schulte J, Berman S. Maternal health and child survival: opportunities to protect both women and children from the adverse consequences of RTIs. In: Germain A, Holmes KK, Piot P, Wasserheit JN, eds. Reproductive tract infections: global impact and priorities for women's health, New York: Plenum Press, 1992:145–82.
5. Laga M. HIV prevention: the need for complementary STD control. In: Germain A, Holmes KK, Piot P, Wasserheit JN, eds. Reproductive tract infections: global impact and priorities for women's health, New York: Plenum Press, 1992:131–44.
6. Wasserheit JN. Epidemiological synergy: interrelationships between HIV infection and other STDs. In: Chen L, Sepulveda J, Segal S, eds. AIDS and women's health: science for policy and action, New York: Plenum Press, 1992 (in press).
7. Cates W Jr, Stone KM. Family planning: the responsibility to prevent both pregnancy and reproductive tract infection. In: Germain A, Holmes KK, Piot P, Wasserheit JN, eds. Reproductive tract infections: global impact and priorities for women's health, New York: Plenum Press, 1992:93–129.
8. Ronald A, Aral SO. Assessment and prioritization of actions to prevent and control reproductive tract infections in the third world. In: Germain A, Holmes KK, Piot P, Wasserheit JN, eds. Reproductive tract infections: global impact and priorities for women's health, New York: Plenum Press, 1992:199–226.
9. Boyd W, Moran JS. The state of STD control programs in less-developed countries: lessons from ten consultancies. USAID AIDS Prevention Conference, Abstract, Virginia, November 1991.
10. World Bank. Population change and economic development, New York: Oxford University Press, 1985:1–193.
11. World Health Organization. Economically active population estimates and projections 1950–2025, third edition, volume 5 (world summary), Geneva: International Labour Office.

12. Over M, Piot P. HIV infection and other sexually transmitted diseases.
    In: Jamison DT, Mosley WH, eds. Disease control priorities in developing
    countries, New York: Oxford University Press for the World Bank, 1992 (in
    press).

13. Jejeebhoy SJ. Women's status and fertility: successive cross-sectional evidence from
    Tamil Nadu, India, 1970–80. Stud Fam Plann 1991; 22:217–30.

14. World Health Organization. Women's health and development: progress report by
    the director-general. Forty-fourth World Health Assembly, Document No.
    A44/15, Geneva, April 4, 1991.

15. Wasserheit JN, Hitchcock PJ. Future directions in sexually transmitted disease
    research. In: Quinn T., ed. Advances in host defense mechanisms. Volume 8:
    immunopathogenesis of sexually transmitted diseases, New York: Raven Press,
    1992 (in press).

16. World Health Organization. Report of the AIDS/STD Task Force.

17. Wasserheit JN, Aral SO, Holmes KK, Hitchcock PJ, eds. Research issues in human
    behavior and sexually transmitted diseases in the AIDS era, Washington DC:
    American Society for Microbiology, 1991.

18. Hitchcock PJ, Wasserheit JN, Harris JR, Holmes KK. Sexually transmitted diseases
    in the AIDS era: development of STD diagnostics for resource-limited settings
    is a global priority. Sex Transm Dis 1991; 18:133–5.

19. Jones RB. New treatments for Chlamydia trachomatis. Am J Obstet Gynecol 1991;
    164:1789–93.

20. Johnson RB. The role of azalide antibiotics in the treatment of chlamydia.
    Am J Obstet Gynecol 1991; 164:1794–6.

21. Stamm WE, Holmes KK. Chlamydia trachomatis infections of the adult.
    In: Holmes KK, Mårdh P-A, Sparling PF et al., eds. Sexually transmitted
    diseases, second edition, New York: McGraw-Hill, 1990:181–93.

22. Jones RB, Wasserheit JN. Introduction to the biology and natural history of sexually
    transmitted diseases. In: Wasserheit JN, Aral SO, Holmes KK, Hitchcock PJ,
    eds. Research issues in human behavior and sexually transmitted diseases in the
    AIDS era, Washington DC: American Society for Microbiology, 1991:11–37.

23. Weström L. Incidence, prevalence, and trends of acute pelvic inflammatory disease
    and its consequences in industrialized countries. Am J Obstet Gynecol 1980;
    138:880–92.

24. Platt R, Rice PA, McCormack WM. Risk of acquiring gonorrhea and prevalence of
    abnormal adnexal findings among women recently exposed to gonorrhea.
    JAMA 1983; 250:3205–9.

25. Stamm WE, Guinan ME, Johnson CE. Effect of treatment regimens for Neisseria
    gonorrhoeae on simultaneous infection with Chlamydia trachomatis. N Engl J
    Med 1984; 310:545–9.

26. Weström L, Mårdh P-A. Salpingitis. In: Holmes KK, Mårdh P-A, Sparling PF et al.,
    eds. Sexually transmitted diseases, New York: McGraw-Hill, 1984:615–32.

27. Belsey MA. The epidemiology of infertility: a review with particular reference to
    sub-saharan Africa. Bull WHO 1976; 54:319–41.

28. Frank O. Infertility in sub–saharan Africa. Center for Policy Studies working paper
    no. 97, New York: Population Council, 1983:1–107.

29. Rosenberg MJ, Schulz KF, Burton N. Sexually transmitted diseases in sub-saharan
    Africa. Lancet 1986; 2:152–3.

30. Sherris JD, Fox G. Infertility and sexually transmitted disease: a public health challenge. Popul Rep 1983; L-11:113–51.
31. Mtimavalye LA, Belsey MA. Infertility and sexually transmitted disease: major problems in maternal and child health and family planning. International Conference on Better Health for Women and Children through Family Planning 1987, Nairobi, WHO document MCH/BH/87.1:1–25.
32. Weström L. Effect of acute pelvic inflammatory disease on fertility. Am J Obstet Gynecol 1975; 121:707–13.
33. Weström L, Bengtsson LPH, Mårdh P-A. Incidence, trends and risks of ectopic pregnancy in a population of women. Br Med J 1981; 282:15–18.
34. CDC. Ectopic pregnancy surveillance, United States, 1970–1987. MMWR 1990; 39(SS-4):9–17.
35. Plummer FA, Laga M, Brunham RC et al. Postpartum upper genital tract infections in Nairobi, Kenya: epidemiology, etiology, and risk factors. J Infect Dis 1987; 156:92–8.
36. Cates W, Farley TMM, Rowe PJ. Worldwide patterns of infertility: is Africa different? Lancet 1985; 2:596–8.
37. World Health Organization Task Force on the Diagnosis and Treatment of Infertility. Infections, pregnancies, and infertility: perspectives on prevention. Fertil Steril 1987; 47:964–8.
38. Stanley K, Stjernsward J, Koroltchouk V. Women and cancer. World Health Stat Q 1987; 267–78.
39. Luthra UK, Roy M, Sehgal A. Clinical downstaging of uterine cervix by paramedical personnel. Lancet 1988; 1:1401.
40. WHO Meeting. Control of cancer of the cervix uteri. Bull WHO 1986; 64:607–18.
41. Franco EL. Viral etiology of cervical cancer: a critique of the evidence. J Infect Dis 1991; 13:1195–1206.
42. Reeves WC, Brinton LA, Garcia M et al. Human papillomavirus infection and cervical cancer in Latin America. N Engl J Med 1989; 320:1437–41.
43. Cates W Jr, Alexander ER. Sexually transmitted diseases and the fetus. In: Kundsin RB, Falk L, Hipp SS, eds. Impact on the fetus of parental sexually transmitted disease. Annals of the New York Academy of Sciences, volume 549, New York: New York Academy of Sciences, 1988:1–16.
44. Brunham RC, Holmes KK, Embree JE. Sexually transmitted diseases in pregnancy. In: Holmes KK, Mårdh P-A, Sparling PF et al., eds. Sexually transmitted diseases, second edition, New York: McGraw-Hill, 1990:771–801.
45. Nugent R, Martin D, Cotch MF, Rettig P. Chlamydial infection and adverse pregnancy outcome: interim results from a multicenter prospective study. In: Bowie WR, Caldwell HD, Jones RP et al., eds. Chlamydial infections: proceedings of the seventh international symposium on human chlamydial infections, New York: Cambridge University Press, 1990:344–7.
46. Cotch MF for the Vaginal Infections and Prematurity Study Group. Carriage of Trichomonas vaginalis is associated with adverse pregnancy outcome. ICAAC, Atlanta 1990; Abstract 681.
47. Elliott B, Brunham RC, Laga M et al. Maternal gonococcal infection as a preventable risk factor for low birth weight. J Infect Dis 1990; 161:531–6.
48. Datta P, Laga M, Plummer A et al. Infection and disease after perinatal exposure to Chlamydia trachomatis in Nairobi, Kenya. J Infect Dis 1988; 158:524–8.

49. Piot P, Rowley J. Resources needed for the control of reproductive tract infections.
    In: Germain A, Holmes KK, Piot P, Wasserheit JN, eds. Reproductive tract
    infections: global impact and priorities for women's health, New York: Plenum
    Press, 1992:227–49.
50. World Health Organization. Report of the consultation on maternal and newborn
    infections, Geneva: World Health Organization, 1992 (in press).
51. May R, Anderson R. Transmission dynamics of HIV infection. Nature 1987;
    326:137–42.
52. Rosenfield A, Maine D. Maternal mortality—a neglected tragedy: where is the "M"
    in MCH. Lancet 1985; 2:83–5.
53. Maggwa ABN, Ngugi EN. Reproductive tract infections in Kenya: insights for action
    from research. In: Germain A, Holmes KK, Piot P, Wasserheit JN, eds.
    Reproductive tract infections: global impact and priorities for women's health,
    New York: Plenum Press, 1992:275–95.
54. Adekunle AO, Ladipo OA. Reproductive tract infections in Nigeria: profound
    challenges for a fragile health infrastructure. In: Germain A, Holmes KK,
    Piot P, Wasserheit JN, eds. Reproductive tract infections: global impact and
    priorities for women's health, New York: Plenum Press, 1992:297–316.
55. Faúndes A, Tanaka CA. Reproductive tract infections in Brazil: solutions in a
    difficult economic climate. In: Germain A, Holmes KK, Piot P, Wasserheit JN,
    eds. Reproductive tract infections: global impact and priorities for women's
    health, New York: Plenum Press, 1992:253–73.
56. Luthra UK, Saxena BN. Reproductive tract infections in India: the need for
    comprehensive reproductive health policy and programs. In: Germain A,
    Holmes KK, Piot P, Wasserheit JN, eds. Reproductive tract infections: global
    impact and priorities for women's health, New York: Plenum Press,
    1992:317–42.
57. Luyeye M, Gerniers M, Lebughe N et al. Prevalence et facteurs de risque pour les
    MST chez les femmes enceintes dans les soins de santé primaires a Kinshasa.
    Fifth International Conference on AIDS in Africa, Abstract No. T.P.C.8,
    Kinshasa, 1990.
58. World Health Organization. Global epidemiology of STD. Presented at the meeting
    on STD as Cofactors of AIDS, January 4–6, 1989.
59. Ndoye I, Coordinator, Project SIDA, Dakar, Senegal. Personal communication.
60. Susanti I, WKBT Clinic Director, Denpasar, Indonesian Planned Parenthood
    Association. Personal communication.
61. Center for Population and Family Health. Family planning and child survival: 100
    developing countries. Ross JA, Rich M, Molzah JP, Pensak M, eds. New York:
    Columbia University, 1988; 12.

SEXUALLY TRANSMITTED DISEASES: CURRENT AND FUTURE DIMENSIONS OF THE PROBLEM IN THE THIRD WORLD

Robert C. Brunham, M.D.
Professor and Head
Department of Medical Microbiology

Joanne E. Embree, M.D., FRCP(C)
Assistant Professor
Departments of Pediatric Child Health
and Medical Microbiology

University of Manitoba
730 William Avenue
Winnipeg, Manitoba
Canada R3E OW3

INTRODUCTION

Reproductive tract infections (RTIs) have been broadly defined to include sexually transmitted infections and infections that are nonsexually transmitted, including endogenous infections, caused by an overgrowth of organisms that are normally present in the reproductive tract (such as bacterial vaginosis and vulvovaginal candidiasis) and iatrogenic infections, caused by improperly performed procedures (such as unsafe abortion, poor delivery practices, pelvic examinations, and IUD insertions).[1] Although this definition has comprehensive appeal, this discussion will center on sexually transmitted RTIs. This narrower focus is deliberately chosen because the majority of RTIs are sexually transmitted, surveillance data are usually not available for nonsexually transmitted RTIs, and epidemiological forces that determine transmission are better understood for sexually transmitted than nonsexually transmitted RTIs. Among the nonsexually transmitted RTIs, incidence data are partially available on the frequency of and mortality associated with unsafe abortion.[2] These data suggest that worldwide, 40–60 million abortions take place annually, and up to 200,000 maternal deaths occur because of bleeding or infection complicating unsafe abortion. Over 98 percent of these deaths occur in the developing world. Clearly, unsafe abortion is a great neglected problem of health care in developing countries and benefits by separate consideration.

This paper will provide an overview of STDs in developing countries, with an emphasis on these illnesses in women, since women appear to experience the impact of STDs more harshly than men.[3-13] Women seem to be more susceptible to acquiring infection, and are more likely to experience complications arising from the primary infection. This skewed emphasis also reflects in part the greater abundance of epidemiological data regarding the prevalence of STDs in women than in men. Where available, the more limited data on the prevalence of STDs among high-risk men will be provided.

This paper has three components. First, a summary of STD prevalence rates among defined populations of women at varying risk of STDs will be provided, along with an estimate of the impact of maternal STDs on maternal and child health. These data are obtained from a search of the literature, and from a summary of a series of studies on pregnancy-associated STDs at a maternity hospital in Nairobi, Kenya. The potential demographic effect of human immunodeficiency virus (HIV) and gonococcal infections on population growth rates will be discussed as examples to show some of the possible demographic consequences of STDs. The demographic consequences of control of gonococcal infection vividly illustrate the important impact of STDs on human reproduction and serve to emphasize the rationale for linking STD control to family planning services if developing countries are to achieve "sustainable health." Second, a conceptual model of the transmission dynamics of STDs will be described in order to rationalize the projected changes in STD rates. Third, the implications of the information summarized in the paper will be discussed in terms of future research needs.

SEXUALLY TRANSMITTED PATHOGENS AS AGENTS OF DISEASE

A large variety of microorganisms can produce RTIs, including some agents that constitute the normal microbial flora of reproductive tract mucosal surfaces. The most prevalent and pathogenic agents are the sexually transmitted pathogens. Table 1 shows eight major STD pathogens producing RTIs. The four principal bacterial pathogens are *Neisseria gonorrhoeae*, *Chlamydia trachomatis*, *Treponema pallidum*, and *Haemophilus ducreyi*; the four most significant viral agents are HIV, human papilloma virus (HPV), herpes simplex type 2 (HSV-2), and hepatitis B virus (HBV).

Until recently, STDs were recognized primarily to produce acute illnesses, such as genital discharges and genital ulcers. Recent epidemiological investigations have elucidated a wider spectrum of diseases due to STDs. This spectrum includes a variety of pregnancy-associated conditions and chronic diseases, such as infertility, genital cancers and AIDS.

REPRODUCTIVE IMPACT OF STDs

We have been interested in the impact that maternal STDs have on reproduction in developing countries, and have collaborated with the University of Nairobi in research on this subject using both cohort and case-control studies conducted at one large maternity hospital in Nairobi. This hospital delivers approximately 25,000 women per year (about 2 percent of all births per year in Kenya) and is a low-risk birthing center. Among women

Table 1. Major STD Microbial Agents and the Conditions They Produce

Agent	Acute disease	Pregnancy-associated condition	Chronic conditions
Neisseria gonorrhoeae	Urethritis Cervicitis Salpingitis	Prematurity Septic abortion Ophthalmia Postpartum endometritis	Infertility Ectopic pregnancy
Chlamydia trachomatis	Urethritis Cervicitis Salpingitis	Ophthalmia Pneumonia Postpartum endometritis	Infertility Ectopic pregnancy

Treponema pallidum	Primary and
	  secondary syphilis
		Spontaneous
		  abortion
		Stillbirth
		Congenital syphilis
			Neurosyphilis
			Cardiovascular
			  syphilis
			Gumma

Haemophilus ducreyi	Genital ulcer	None known	?Impotence
HIV	Mononucleosis syndrome	Prematurity Stillbirth Perinatal HIV	AIDS
HPV	Genital warts	Laryngeal papillomatosis	Genital cancer
HSV-2	Genital ulcer	Neonatal HSV Prematurity	?Genital cancer
HBV	Acute hepatitis	Perinatal HBV	Chronic hepatitis Cirrhosis Hepatoma Vasculitis

delivering at this center, 5 percent have low-birth-weight babies, 2 percent have stillbirths, 20 percent develop postpartum infection, and 20 percent have newborns who develop ophthalmia neonatorum.

The prevalence rates of *Neisseria gonorrhoeae, Chlamydia trachomatis, Treponema pallidum,* and HIV observed at this hospital are as shown in Table 2. The relationship of these STDs to adverse pregnancy outcomes (expressed as odds ratios or etiologic percent) is also shown in the table. Clearly, these STDs are moderately or strongly associated with these adverse pregnancy outcomes.

Assuming that the prevalence rates of these STD agents and the incidence rates of disease observed at this hospital are generalizable to all of Kenya, the absolute magnitude

Table 2. Prevalence of Selected STDs and Their Effect on
Pregnancy-Associated Conditions at One Maternity Hospital in Nairobi

Disease	Prevalence	Stillbirth*	Prematurity*	Postpartum pelvic inflammatory disease*	Ophthalmia neonatorum†	Perinatal AIDS‡
Neisseria gonorrhoeae	6%	—	2.9	4.4	42%	na
Chlamydia trachomatis	7%	—	—	1.4	31%	na
Treponema pallidum	3%	5.3	—	na	na	na
HIV	3%	2.7	2.1	—	na	33%

* Odds ratio.
† Etiologic percent.
‡ Percent transmission.
Note: na = not applicable; — = no significant association.
Source: references 7, 14, 15, and 16.

of their impact for this medically developing country is substantial. Like many other developing countries, Kenya has a growing population. The crude population size in 1987 was 23.5 million, and the crude birthrate per capita was 0.0540. Thus, approximately 1.2 million live births occurred that year. Some 10 percent of all births were adversely affected by maternal STD; over 22,000 infants died or sustained permanent disabling sequelae:

1. An estimated 50,000 infants developed gonococcal ophthalmia neonatorum, of whom 10,000 developed corneal ulceration and were at risk for blindness.
2. Some 40,000 infants developed chlamydial ophthalmia, and 10,000 infants acquired chlamydial pneumonia.
3. About 80,000 mothers developed postpartum pelvic infection due to gonococcal or chlamydial infection, and 8,000–16,000 of these mothers became infertile because of this infection.
4. Approximately 10,000 neonates were born prematurely because of gonococcal infection; 1,500 infant deaths were due to prematurity.
5. An estimated 4,000 stillbirths occurred because of maternal syphilis; 10,000 live-born infants acquired congenital syphilis.
6. Approximately 10,000 infants developed perinatal HIV.

Clearly, these estimates emphasize that STDs are major determinants of perinatal, neonatal, and maternal morbidity rates. Other studies have shown that mortality related to reproductive tract disease can be substantial for women in the developing world. A particularly elegant study conducted in Abidjan, Ivory Coast, concluded that "28 percent of adult female deaths and 34 percent of adult female years of productive life lost were due to AIDS, pregnancy related conditions, or induced abortions, illustrating how reproductive health dominates the lives and deaths of women in this city."[17] Given the large impact that reproductive health has on women, further examination of these issues in terms of their relationship to RTIs in general and STDs in particular is indicated.

STDs are likely having demographic effects in many areas of the developing world. This is a dimension of the burden of RTIs that is poorly appreciated at present. In general, infectious diseases reduce population growth rates by causing premature death prior to reproduction, by indirectly reducing reproductive competitiveness, or by directly diminishing reproductive capacity. The potential demographic consequences of an STD in developing countries are best estimated for HIV. A mathematical model that combined the demography of a developing country population having a positive net growth rate with the currently known epidemiological characteristics of heterosexual HIV transmission suggested that HIV is capable of changing population growth rates from positive to negative values over a period of several decades.[18] The principal determinants of this effect were the result of perinatal transmission of HIV and the loss of women in the reproductive age groups. Emerging epidemiological data are beginning to confirm predictions of this model. AIDS was found to be the leading cause of death and years of potential life lost in adult men in Abidjan.[17] It was the second leading cause of death and premature mortality for women, after deaths related to pregnancy and abortion.

Because most other STDs are nonfatal, they are unlikely to have the same degree of demographic impact as HIV. Nonetheless, gonococcal and chlamydial infections may exert significant population biologic effects through their effects on fertility. In population terms, infertility of individuals is equivalent to premature death. In social terms, infertility for women often means isolation and loss of status. *Neisseria gonorrhoeae* and *Chlamydia trachomatis* produce infertility mainly in women by creating tubal occlusion. Data show that lower genital tract infection with *Neisseria gonorrhoeae* is more prevalent among women from Sub-Saharan Africa than among those from other developing countries.[1] Tubal occlusion as a cause of infertility is also greater in Africa than in other areas of the world[19] (Figure 1). Additionally, epidemiological data reported by H. B. Griffiths and colleagues and modified by D. G. Muir and M. A. Belsey,[12] documented an important negative correlation (r=0.64) between the incidence of gonococcal infection and population fertility rates among 14 districts in Uganda. High rates of gonorrhea reduced fertility rates by approximately half.

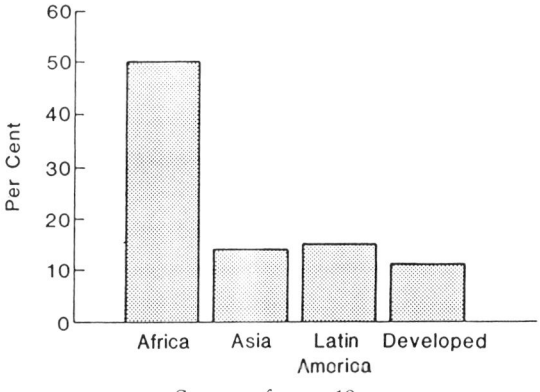

Source: reference 19.

Figure 1. Percentage of Cases of Fallopian Tubal Occlusion Reported As the Cause of Infertility, Africa, Asia, Latin America, and Developed Countries

We believe STDs are underestimated as determinants of population growth. Available data and mathematical models suggest they have profound demographic effect. The relationship of gonococcal infection (and likely chlamydial infection) to fertility rates and thus to population growth is exceedingly important to clarify. Perhaps more evidently here than elsewhere, linkage of STD control to family planning programs will be important, since rapid population growth in many developing countries is forecasted to exceed available social and economic resources. Future studies should focus on precisely delineating the population biologic effects of STDs and other RTIs.

PREVALENCE ESTIMATES OF STDs IN DEVELOPING COUNTRIES

The incidence and prevalence of STDs are major proximate determinants of the magnitude of the problem of RTIs. We review published studies in the English language available in the *Index Medicus* from 1970 to December 1990 that reported the prevalence of STDs among population samples from developing countries to illustrate the epidemiological characteristics of STD distribution and prevalence. The data analysis covered only those studies that reported the sampling method, included more than 100 subjects (exceptions were made for review of data on prevalence rates involving commercial sex workers (CSWs)), and used acceptable microbiologic techniques. Results from these studies are listed in Tables 3 and 4 by author, country, risk strata, STD sampled, and prevalence rate. In general, these reports show that rates are higher among CSWs, STD clinic attendees, and men in the military than among women attending antenatal clinics or family planning clinics, or among men and women sampled in community surveys. STD rates among women from the general population (as measured by studies of asymptomatic pregnant women attending antenatal clinics) are higher in Africa than elsewhere in the developing world. Among CSWs, STD rates are inversely correlated with socioeconomic status. Finally, serosurveys disclose higher STD exposure rates than do culture surveys in all groups sampled.

Prevalence of STDs among High-risk Groups

The extremely high prevalence rate of STDs among female CSWs, military personnel, and other groups, such as long-distance truck drivers has been repeatedly observed in studies from different geographic areas (Table 3). In these high-risk populations, the prevalence of gonorrhea is as high as 50 percent, the prevalence of chancroid is up to 12 percent, and the prevalence of syphilis ranges from 7 percent for acute or early syphilis to 23 percent for previous syphilis exposure; isolation rates of *Chlamydia trachomatis* range from 2 percent to 25 percent, and *Trichomonas vaginalis* is detected in 4–20 percent of women studied.

Studies of CSWs in Nairobi have shown the important effect of socioeconomic level on STD prevalence rates. Upper-socioeconomic-strata CSWs had lower STD rates than did lower-socioeconomic-strata workers.[22] This effect may be due to both the lower number of sexual partners for upper-socioeconomic-strata CSWs and the lower prevalence of STDs among their clients. Additionally, better education among upper-socioeconomic-strata CSWs may increase awareness of STDs, implementation of risk reduction methods, and access to diagnostic and treatment services. For lower-socioeconomic-strata workers, limited financial resources among the women and their clients may affect the use of condoms, since

Table 3. STD Prevalences in High-risk Populations

Study	Country	Risk group	STD	Prevalence	
Reeves, 1987[20]	Panama	CSWs	Neisseria gonorrhoeae	12/39	(31%)
			Syphilis (RPR)*	8/35	(23%)
			Chlamydia trachomatis	1/38	(3%)
			HSV	0/38	
		CSWs	Neisseria gonorrhoeae	100/956	(10%)
			Syphilis (RPR)*	31/455	(7%)
			Chlamydia trachomatis	15/920	(2%)
			HSV	9/974	(1%)
Khoo, 1977[21]	Singapore	CSWs	Neisseria gonorrhoeae	14/200	(7%)
D'Costa, 1985[22]	Kenya	CSWs:			
		Upper socio-	Neisseria gonorrhoeae	11/71	(16%)
		economic strata	Genital ulcers	2/71	(3%)
		Middle socio-	Neisseria gonorrhoeae	14/51	(28%)
		economic strata	Genital ulcers	6/51	(12%)
		Lower socio-	Neisseria gonorrhoeae	32/71	(45%)
		economic strata	Genital ulcers	6/71	(8%)
Simonsen, 1990[23]	Kenya	CSWs:			
		Lower socio-	HIV	259/418	(62%)
		economic strata	Haemophilus ducreyi (HIV+)	42/259	(16%)
			Haemophilus ducreyi (HIV-)	12/159	(7%)
			Neisseria gonorrhoeae	211/418	(50%)
			Chlamydia trachomatis	105/418	(25%)
			Genital warts	13/418	(3%)
			Syphilis (RPR + TPHA)*†	133/418	(32%)
Omer, 1985[24]	Sudan	Females, STD clinic	Trichomonas vaginalis	25/123	(20%)
Odongo, 1977[25]	Uganda	Females, STD clinic	Trichomonas vaginalis	244/1,757	(14%)
Kibukamusoke, 1965[26]	Uganda	Patients, STD clinic	Neisseria gonorrhoeae	665/1,000	(66%)
			Syphilis	41/1,000	(4%)
			Lymphogranuloma venereum	36/1,000	(3.6%)
			Chancroid	99/1,000	(10%)
Kuvanont, 1988[27]	Thailand	Males, military, STD clinic	Neisseria gonorrhoeae	61/150	(41%)
			Chlamydia trachomatis	20/150	(13%)
			HSV	5/150	(3%)
		Males, nonmilitary, STD clinic	Neisseria gonorrhoeae	67/275	(24%)
			Chlamydia trachomatis	39/275	(14%)
			HSV	0	
Ballard, 1981[28]	South Africa	Females, STD clinic	Neisseria gonorrhoeae	18/135	(13%)
Ratnam, 1980[29]	Zambia	Females, STD clinic	Neisseria gonorrhoeae	190/1,000	(19%)

Table continues on next page.

Table 3. STD Prevalences in High-risk Populations (continued)

Study	Country	Risk group	STD	Prevalence	
Shadid, 1983[30]	Costa Rica	Females, STD clinic	Neisseria gonorrhoeae	243/1,427	(17%)
Osoba, 1972[31]	Nigeria	Females, STD clinic	Neisseria gonorrhoeae	147/442	(33%)
			Trichomonas vaginalis	15/442	(4%)
		Males, STD clinic	Neisseria gonorrhoeae	38/228	(17%)
			Trichomonas vaginalis	44/228	(19%)
Mabey, 1982[32]	Gambia	Females, STD clinic	Chlamydia trachomatis	12/78	(15%)

* RPR = rapid plasma reagin.
† TPHA = treponema pallidum haemagglinntination.

condom cost relative to the cost of sex may be significant (up to 20 percent of the charge for the CSW's service). At least two studies, in Kenya and in Panama, have reported the potentially important observation that gonococcal prevalence rates are inversely correlated with the duration of commercial sex.[20,33] This may reflect increased awareness of STDs (and hence implementation of risk reduction) or the development of partial immunity in CSWs who practice for extended periods of time.

Studies in Kenya of CSW cohorts have quantified the important role that commercial sex plays in the transmission of *Neisseria gonorrhoeae*, *Haemophilus ducreyi*, and HIV.[22,33,34] More than 60 percent of men with gonococcal urethritis or chancroid who attended an urban STD clinic reported commercial sex exposure as their source of infection. The role of commercial sex in the spread and maintenance of syphilis and chlamydia within populations has not been well studied, but is likely to be substantial as well.

The behavior of STD pathogens appears to be highly dynamic among CSWs. This ecologic instability is apparent in the rapid fluxes in gonococcal serovars, in the rapid intragerieric and intergeneric spread of antimicrobial resistance plasmids among genital pathogens, and in the rapid spread of newly introduced STD pathogens. This was most vividly seen in the explosive spread of HIV-1 among members of a specific urban cluster of CSWs in Nairobi.[23,35,36] These women were initially recruits in the early 1980s for the study of gonococcal epidemiology, and they have been closely followed since that time. In 1981, no woman was identified as seropositive for HIV; by 1985, 63 percent were HIV-seropositive. Seroconversion to HIV-1 was observed to occur very rapidly among new seronegative recruits to the CSW cohort.

Effect of HIV among High-Risk Groups on the Epidemiology and Natural History of Conventional STDs. Since entering this group of CSWs, HIV has been exerting a destabilizing influence on the epidemiology of conventional STDs because the immunosuppression associated with HIV infection affects STD transmission determinants and response to treatment. In addition, STD-related RTIs (and perhaps other RTIs) are having a destabilizing impact on the epidemiology of HIV by facilitating heterosexual transmission.[37] This effect is most pronounced among highly sexually active individuals because of the high prevalence of concurrent infection. Clearly, the interactive and synergistic effects of HIV on conventional STDs will amplify their impact at the population level and make projections of the incidence of STDs more difficult. Additionally, uncontrolled RTIs and STDs will exacerbate the spread of HIV.

Prevalence of STDs among Low-risk Groups

Prevalence rates of STDs among low-risk groups are shown in Table 4. In general, data are much less available and are especially deficient from developing countries outside Sub-Saharan Africa. Nonetheless, they are remarkable in showing unexpectedly high prevalence rates in women thought to be at low risk for STDs. Asymptomatic women attending antenatal clinics are an important sentinel population for determining population prevalence of STD and for use in comparison of different geographic areas, and many

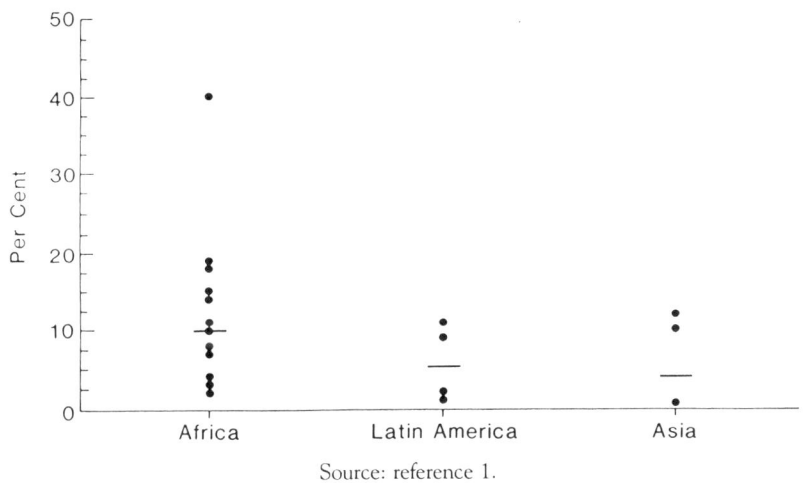

Source: reference 1.

Figure 2. Prevalence Rates of *Neisseria gonorrhoeae* Infection Among Asymptomatic Pregnant Women

studies have reported results among such women. Analysis of gonococcal prevalence rates among asymptomatic pregnant women dramatically illustrates that rates are highest in Sub-Saharan Africa and lower in Latin America and Asia (Figure 2). Data from 12 studies from Africa, four from Latin America, and three from Asia show that prevalence rates are 2–3 times as high among pregnant women in Africa as elsewhere. Although substantial geographic variation in the data is apparent, the paucity of data from Latin America, Asia, and the Middle East is troublesome. Additional studies in these areas should be a priority. This knowledge is of importance, since the absolute numbers of affected individuals may be even larger in these areas than in Africa because of their larger populations.

Table 4. STD Prevalences in Low-risk Populations

Study	Country	Risk group	STD	Prevalence	
Arya, 1973[38]	Uganda	Teso males	Neisseria gonorrhoeae	24/251	(10%)
		Teso females	Neisseria gonorrhoeae	50/231	(22%)
		Ankole males	Neisseria gonorrhoeae	7/166	(4%)
		Ankole females	Neisseria gonorrhoeae	4/168	(2%)
Bang, 1988[39]	India	Rural females	Neisseria gonorrhoeae	2/650	(0.3%)
			Trichomonas vaginalis	67/558	(12%)
Wasserheit, 1989[40]	Bangladesh	Rural females	Neisseria gonorrhoeae	2/472	(0.4%)
			Chlamydia trachomatis	9/472	(2%)
			Trichomonas vaginalis	23/472	(5%)
Ratnam, 1982[41]	Zambia	Antenatal patients	Syphilis	25/202	(12%)
		Women delivering	Syphilis	30/464	(7%)
Nasah, 1980[42]	Cameroun	Antenatal patients	Neisseria gonorrhoeae	106/720	(15%)
			Trichomonas vaginalis	140/720	(19%)
Galega, 1984[6]	Cameroun	Women delivering	Neisseria gonorrhoeae	40/296	(14%)
Mabey, 1985[13]	Gambia	Antenatal patients	Chlamydia (ab)	13/37	(35%)
			Gonococcus (ab)	8-10/37	(22-27%)
O'Farrell, 1989[43]	South Africa	Antenatal patients	Neisseria gonorrhoeae	11/193	(6%)
			Chlamydia trachomatis	22/193	(11%)
			Trichomonas vaginalis	95/193	(49%)
			HIV	0	
			Syphilis	23/193	(12%)
Weissenberger, 1977[34]	South Africa	Antenatal patients	Neisseria gonorrhoeae	1/50	(2%)
Elliott, 1989[15]	Kenya	Delivery:			
		Low birth weight	Neisseria gonorrhoeae	18/160	(11%)
			Neisseria gonorrhoeae	6/159	(4%)
		Normal birth weight	Chlamydia trachomatis	42/284	(15%)
			Syphilis	16/290	(5%)
			HIV	9/194	(5%)
Osoba, 1972[31]	Nigeria	Antenatal patients	Neisseria gonorrhoeae	7/208	(3%)
Gyaneshwar, 1987[45]	Fiji	Antenatal patients	Neisseria gonorrhoeae	10/430	(2%)
			Syphilis	39/430	(9%)
			Chlamydia trachomatis	110/430	(26%)
			Trichomonas vaginalis	26/430	(6%)
Gini, 1989[46]	Nigeria	Antenatal patients	Syphilis	103/29,083	(0.3%)
Laga, 1986[14]	Kenya	Women delivering	Neisseria gonorrhoeae	72/1,019	(7%)
			Chlamydia trachomatis	295/1,019	(29%)
Donoso, 1984[47]	Chile	Antenatal patients	Neisseria gonorrhoeae	5/256	(2%)
Nasah, 1980[42]	Cameroun	Family planning clinic clients	Neisseria gonorrhoeae:		
			Symptomatic	17/81	(21%)
			Asymptomatic	1/53	(2%)
			Trichomonas vaginalis	10/134	(7%)

Table continues on next page.

Table 4. STD Prevalences in Low-risk Populations (continued)

Study	Country	Risk group	STD	Prevalence	
Hopcraft, 1973[48]	Kenya	Family planning clinic clients	Neisseria gonorrhoeae Trichomonas vaginalis	30/200 46/178	(15%) (25%)
Weissenberger, 1977[44]	South Africa	Family planning clinic clients	Neisseria gonorrhoeae	12/100	(12%)
Nsofor, 1989[49]	Nigeria	Family planning clinic clients	Neisseria gonorrhoeae Trichomonas vaginalis Syphilis	5/150 7/150 27/150	(3%) (5%) (18%)

Determinants of geographic variation in prevalence rates of STDs are poorly described. Variation may be related to cultural and social differences, including sexual behavior, and the availability of health services for diagnosis, management, and prevention of RTIs. For instance, in Africa, polygamy may be an important factor in determining the prevalence of STDs. One particularly well done study[10] determined the point prevalence of gonococcal infection among a random sample of rural men and women in eastern Uganda. Some 10 percent of 251 men and 22 percent of 231 women were found to have gonococcal infection. Among men, older age and polyamy were significantly correlated with an increased risk of gonorrhea. Among women, younger age, polygamy, and pregnancy were significantly associated with an increased risk of infection. Since levels of polygamy may be 10 times higher in Sub-Saharan Africa than elsewhere, with 20–50 percent of wives in polygamous marriages, polygamy may contribute to the higher STD prevalence rates observed in Africa.[50] However, other social factors are of even greater importance, since this study also reported significantly different prevalence rates for gonorrhea in two communities with identical levels of polygamy. The role of sexual behavior and the existence of discreet subgroups of individuals with a high prevalence of STDs in determining population prevalence of STDs will be discussed in a subsequent section.

Serosurveys for Antibodies to STD Pathogens among Selected Populations

In general, serosurveys are an excellent tool for determining the levels of STD transmission, especially in endemic circumstances. Most of these studies have been conducted in Africa as either population studies or surveys of individuals attending antenatal or family planning clinics. Such surveys also show remarkably high prevalence rates for STD exposure among individuals who would be considered to be at relatively low risk in the developed world. In the largest of these studies, STD seroprevalence results were reported on 2,111 Ethiopian women: 58 percent had antibodies to Neisseria gonorrhoeae, 52 percent to Chlamydia trachomatis, 38 percent to HSV-2, and 43 percent to Treponema pallidum.[51] The risk of having antibodies to an STD pathogen was strongly correlated with onset of sexual activity at an early age (especially before menarche).

Except for syphilis serology, such studies are, however, difficult to interpret because of the nonstandardized or cross-reacting nature of serologic tests for antibodies to Neisseria gonorrhoeae, Haemophilus ducreyi, Chlamydia trachomatis, and HSV. Nevertheless, syphilis seroprevalence surveys do offer a standardized methodology to evaluate population morbidity and geographic and temporal trends. Comparison of syphilis seroprevalence surveys among women attending antenatal clinics in Africa shows astounding results (Table

5). The median seroprevalence rate was 9 percent (2–33 percent in 12 countries). These rates are 100–1,000 times those observed in developed countries. Two recent studies of syphilis in pregnancy from developing countries are noteworthy. In a study conducted in Zambia, A. V. Ratnam and colleagues[41] reported the prevalence of syphilis in three populations of women: 202 pregnant women at the time of their first prenatal visit; 340 women whose pregnancy ended in spontaneous abortion (prior to 20 weeks' gestation) or stillbirth (after 20 weeks' gestation); and 464 women in labor. Reactive serologic tests were found in 13 percent of antenatal patients, 10 percent of women who had spontaneous abortions, 42 percent of women who had stillbirths, and 7 percent of women admitted for delivery. *Treponema pallidum* infection was strongly associated with in utero fetal death. This study shows that population selection has an important effect on the observed association between an STD and an adverse pregnancy outcome. S. K. Hira and colleagues,[52] also from Zambia, noted that 57 percent of untreated syphilitic pregnancies had adverse outcomes, but that on-site screening for and treatment of syphilis among antenatal clinic attendees reduced adverse outcomes by almost two thirds. The cost per adverse reproductive outcome prevented was only US$12.00. This study was exemplary in devising a culturally and politically acceptable intervention program that was cost effective.

Given these data, the weight of epidemiological data affirm that RTIs, especially those due to STDs, are a major health problem for women in the developing world. The mortality caused by RTIs in total (postabortal and puerperal sepsis, fetal and perinatal death) is clearly very high in developing countries. The impact of RTIs on transmission of HIV and the morbidity and mortality of HIV itself add further to the health impact of these infections. The additional morbidity attributable to RTIs, including infertility in women and gonococcal ophthalmia neonatorum, are of special interest in developing countries because of the cultural importance of childbearing and the inadequacy of services for the treatment of gonococcal ophthalmia.

A substantial amount of theoretical work has been applied to elucidating the epidemiological principles of sexually transmitted RTIs, because of the great importance of this class of diseases, especially in relation to AIDS. This work is reviewed because of its relevance in providing an explanation for the epidemiological characteristics of STDs, in suggesting areas for further research, and in clarifying control strategies.

A GENERAL MODEL OF THE EPIDEMIOLOGY OF STDs

Although STDs vary greatly in the clinical aspects of the diseases they produce, they do have a common epidemiological paradigm.[53] A consideration of STD epidemiology using this paradigm facilitates understanding of the differences in prevalence rates observed between developed and developing countries. The paradigm also helps in projecting incidence estimates and in formulating control programs.

J. Yorke and H. Heathcote,[54] and R. Anderson and R. May[55,56] developed models for STD epidemiology that define the importance of core groups in maintaining STD endemicity and that quantify transmission parameters. The essential concept in these models is the reproductive rate (R_o) of the infection. R_o is defined as the number of secondary infections that a spreader produces in a fully susceptible population. For STD transmission, R_o is determined by three variables. These are the effective average rate at

Table 5. Syphilis Seroprevalence in Antenatal Clinics in Africa

Country	Prevalence (%)
Kenya	3.0
Ethiopia	16.9
Gambia	11.0
Malawi	13.7
Mozambique	6.3
Nigeria	2.1
Somalia	3.0
South Africa	20.8
Swaziland	33.3
Tanzania	16.4
Zambia	12.5
Zaire	2.0

Sources: references 1, 16, and 40–45.

which new sexual partners are acquired (c), the average probability that infection is transmitted from an infected person to a susceptible individual (B), and the average duration of infectivity (D). Transmission dynamics are approximated by the following formula:

$$R_o = BcD$$

The principal determinant of STD spread in a population is the rate at which new sexual relationships occur in that population, rather than the more complicated measure of number of sexual exposures per new partnership. Empiric observations on sexual transmission of HIV suggest that the number of exposures to one infected partner may be less important than any exposure to any infected sexual partner in determining transmission.[57] For most individuals in a population, the rate at which new sexual partners are acquired is substantially lower than the rate at which immune responses or medical interventions eliminate or reduce infectivity of an STD pathogen. Thus, effective transmission for STD agents occurs only among individuals with higher-than-average rates of sexual partner change. Sexual activity (defined as the number of partners per unit of time) varies greatly among individuals, and variance in activity greatly exceeds the mean level. A minor component of the population with high levels of sexual activity is found within the tail of the probability distribution curve of sexual activity. Within this small subset of the population are found individuals who appear to be central to STD persistence and who determine STD transmission dynamics because only they maintain partner change rates sufficient to regularly acquire and transmit infection.

In order to reflect the disproportionate role played by highly sexually active individuals in transmission dynamics, the parameter c, previously defined as the average rate at which new sexual partners are acquired, can be defined by the mean of the population (m) plus the ratio of the variance (σ^2) to the mean:

$$c = m + \frac{\sigma^2}{m}$$

This precise mathematical definition of c implies that the reproductive rate of an STD is determined not only by the average number of new sexual partners acquired per unit of time for the population as a whole, but also by the variance in this number within the population. The greater the variance, the higher the reproductive rate. A particularly illustrative example used by Anderson and May to depict the importance of variability in sexual activity is as follows. (The example is deliberately nonrealistic and is meant to characterize the importance of the relationship.) Thus, consider a population in which all males are identically heterosexually active, with an average of three new female sexual partners per year. Females, on the other hand, are assumed to be more heterogeneous in sexual behavior; 90 percent have one new sexual partner per year, and 10 percent have an average of 21 new partners annually (the latter may be, for example, CSWs). Within this hypothetically closed population, both males and females must have the same average number of new sexual partners per year, three. For males, the epidemiologically relevant parameter c is equal to 3 per year, since $m = 3$ and $\sigma^2 = 0$. For females, c is equal to 16 per year, since $m = 3$ but $\sigma^2 = 40$. The overall effect of heterogeneity in sexual behavior is as if females on average acquired new sexual partners at a rate five times that of males. This, in part, explains why CSWs have such a dramatic effect on the reproductive and general health of women who are not within the high sexual activity classes.

The mathematical models explicitly show that the extent of sexual contact among individuals of differing sexual activity classes has a marked influence on the population prevalence of STD. When individuals are classified on the basis of the number of new partners acquired per unit of time, extreme patterns of like-with-like pairing ("assortive mixing") have been shown to generate the most rapid early growth of the epidemic; the extreme pattern of like-with-unlike pairing ("disassortive mixing"), by contrast, generates a larger epidemic over a longer time period.[58] Furthermore, it has been estimated with these mathematical models that the differing age and gender mixing patterns have strong demographic impact. When older men with STDs are sexual partners of younger women, the demographic impact is greatest because infections in younger women maximally reduce reproduction.

Despite the central importance of sexual behavior in determining the epidemiology of STDs, surprisingly little is known about the quantitative aspects of sexual behavior at the population level. This is especially true for almost all areas of the developing world. Reliable data collected through probability sampling would improve accurate forecasting of the magnitude of the problem of STDs and other RTIs. The essential information needed is an estimate of the rate of change of sexual partners, its variance, and the extent of mixing among sexual activity classes.

Anderson and May[55] reviewed over 100 published and unpublished studies that recorded the number of sexual partners per time unit. After pooling the data and constructing a log-log plot (variance y-axis, mean x-axis), the authors noted an interesting general relation between the mean (m) and variance (σ^2) of sexual behavior, which was expressible in the form of a power law:

$$\sigma^2 = am^b$$

The coefficients were estimated by regression techniques as $a = 0.555$ and $b = 3.231$. The finding of this relationship allows c to be expressed in terms of the mean as follows:

$$c = m + am^{b-1}$$

Of possible importance is that this power law was derived from studies performed in different geographic areas with different ethnic groups, suggesting that this relationship may be generalizable across cultures. Why there should be such a tight relation between the two statistics is unclear, but it does suggest that one can derive a great deal of information about the distribution of sexual behavior in a population simply by knowing its mean.

Available data also suggest that sexual behavior is significantly age-related. The 1985 General Social Survey in the United States observed a striking correlation of high sexual partner acquisition rates with younger age among the sexually active population.[59] E.Konings and colleagues[60] used random sampling to characterize sexual behavior among rural residents in Tanzania. Again, sexual behavior was observed to be an age-dependent variable. Age at onset of sexual activity in this sample averaged 15 years for men and 14 for women. Onset of sexual activity was followed by a latent period of relative sexual inactivity. At approximately age 20, the rate of sexual partner acquisition began to increase in both men and women, peaking at about age 30 for women and age 40 for men. Age-specific attack rates of pelvic inflammatory disease (PID) strongly resemble age-dependent sexual partner change rates and substantiate the epidemiological importance of the latter.[61]

The Urban Focus of STDs

Urbanization is a major demographic trend in developing countries. The proportion of the population in urban centers in Sub-Saharan Africa doubled between 1965 and 1988, from 14 percent to 28 percent. Cities are growing faster in Sub-Saharan Africa than elsewhere in the developing world. This trend is of significance to the epidemiology of STDs, since it is accompanied by large-scale migration, especially of men, and is correlated with higher rates of STDs in urban than rural areas. This was strikingly seen in the Rwandan HIV Seroprevalence Study, where the seropositivity rate recorded among urban dwellers (17.8 percent) was about 14 times that among rural residents (1.3 percent).[62] Interestingly, STDs often maintain low endemicity in rural settings, but exhibit rapid changes in the urban environment.[63] The influence of the urban environment on STD epidemiology is paradoxical, as STDs are classically thought of as "density-independent" infectious diseases. We consider that at least three factors may account for the clustering of STDs in urban areas.

The population structure in urban and rural areas can differ dramatically. Figure 3a shows the age structure for Kenya, by urban-rural residence, as revealed in the 1975–85 census data. Urban areas have a disproportionately large population between the ages of 20 and 45 years (42 percent, compared with 26 percent in rural areas). Since sexual behavior is age-dependent, with partner change rates greatest between ages 20 and 30, a population with age structure biased to overrepresent individuals in these age classes may exhibit higher STD transmission rates.

In addition to differences in age structures between urban and rural areas, profound differences in the male-to-female sex ratio may also exist. Using the Kenyan census data (1975–85), Figure 3b shows this ratio for rural and urban environments across age classes. The urban environment shows a marked inequality in the sex ratio, which is greatest during the reproductive years and at its peak is biased 2:1 in favor of men. This disproportionate density of sexually active men likely alters the dynamics of sexual behavior, possibly through the use of commercial sex and thereby favoring the spread of STDs.

Another major factor serving to concentrate STDs in an urban environment is the preferential occurrence of commercial sex there. As previously described, one study[22] reported that over two thirds of men with STDs seen at an STD clinic in Nairobi claimed that contact with a CSW was their infection source. Despite the potential importance of commercial sex in STD transmission, few data are available regarding distribution of CSWs in different societies, in different environments, and over time. Nor are there accurate data to estimate the magnitude of the role of commercial sex in STD transmission in different areas and in relation to specific STDs. Answers to these and related questions are needed in order to evaluate the role of commercial sex in maintaining STD endemicity. Delineating the quantitative role of CSWs in STD transmission is important because if their role is as large as some observers believe, control strategies targeting them may be relatively easily implemented.

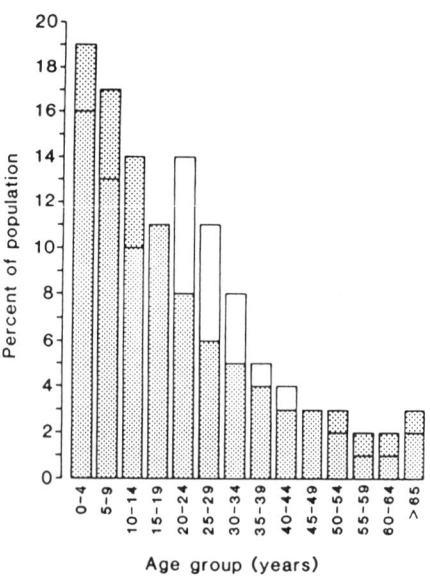

Source: based on 1975–85 Census data.

Figure 3a. Age Structure of the Kenyan Population for
Urban (clear) and Rural (shaded) Areas

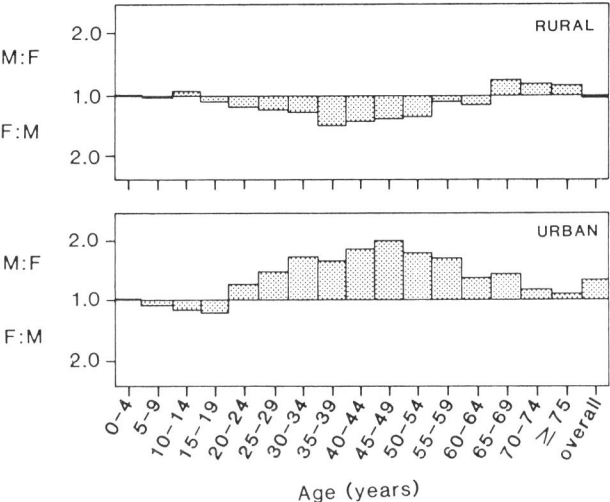

Source: based on 1975–85 Census data.

**Figure 3b. Male-to-Female Sex Ratios in Kenya,
Rural and Urban Areas**

Recognition of urban clustering of STDs may be of importance in rationalizing the distribution of resources for control programs. Limited geographic foci may improve program feasibility.

The Core Group Concept in STD Epidemiology

It seems as if each STD pathogen requires a critical rate of sexual partner change (defined by the parameter c) in order to persist in a population, and the required threshold level of sexual partner change rate is often in excess of the mean rate found in the population. Using rough approximations of values for B and D (which are in large measure determined by biologic properties of the organism and the host) for various STD agents, values of c can be derived to define subgroups with sufficient sex partner change rates to permit maintenance of an STD pathogen at an endemic level (Table 6). Estimated values of c vary from 4 for *Chlamydia trachomatis* to 15 for *Haemophilus ducreyi*. When an STD is introduced into a subgroup with homogeneous sexual mixing rates above this threshold level, the STD is predicted to persist. In this sense, the threshold value of c is akin to the threshold population size necessary to sustain persistence of rapidly immunizing infectious diseases such as measles, chicken pox, whooping cough, and pertussis.

Social factors are of paramount importance in clustering a critical number of individuals within a population to form a mixing subset that exceeds the threshold value of c. The urban environment provides the geographic context for clustering of sexually active persons and may also produce changes in sexual behavior through crowding, poverty, loneliness, and alienation. Aggregation of individuals exceeding threshold values of sexual behavior results in the formation of STD "core" groups. Characteristics of individuals within

Table 6. Estimates of Key Epidemiological Parameters Necessary
to Sustain Transmission of Five STDs (c = 1/BD)

STD	Duration of infectiousness (years)	Transmission efficiency	Effective sex partner change rate per year
Neisseria gonorrhoeae			
No control	0.5	0.5	4
Control	0.15	0.5	13
Chlamydia trachomatis	1.25	0.2	4
Treponema pallidum			
No control	0.5	0.3	7
Control	0.25	0.3	13
HIV			
African parameters	2.0	0.1	5
American parameters	8.0	0.01	13
Haemophilus ducreyi	0.8	0.8	15

Source: reference 53.

the core seem to be highly society-specific. For instance, in one urban center in the United States, characteristics of core group members included minority ethnicity, young age, and low socioeconomic status; members often engaged in illicit drug use and commercial sex.[64] In developing countries, characteristics are less well known, but the core group seems to include CSWs and their clients. Long-distance truck drivers, military personnel, and single migrant male workers entering cities may also belong to the core.

The core appears to be highly dynamic, changing its characteristics over short periods of time. This is due in part to the usual transient nature of a particular individual's residence within the core and the need for a constant crop of new members to enter the core in order to sustain its dynamics. The core may grow or shrink in response not only to the number of individuals involved, but also to changes in the transmissibility of STD pathogens, changes in health-care-seeking behavior, and alterations in the availability of health care. For example, the presence of control programs dramatically changes estimated values of c for Neisseria gonorrhoeae and Treponema pallidum (Table 6). Presumably, changes in the value of c are accompanied by changes in the size of the core group. The core group concept has major implications for STD control programs. If core group members can be identified and kept free of STDs, infection should eventually disappear from the entire population, according to predictions based upon these mathematical models.

Given this theoretic understanding of the epidemiology of STDs, we conclude that forces are at play in much of the developing world to increase rates of STDs and consequent reproductive tract disease. Although the direction of change in STD rates in developing countries, particularly in Sub-Saharan Africa, seems clear, the absolute magnitude is uncertain. For other developing countries, STD prevalence rates (where known) are lower than in Sub-Saharan Africa, but similar social and economic factors are present. Thus, even within these regions, STD rates will likely increase. Furthermore, since populations are larger in developing regions outside Sub-Saharan Africa, the absolute case numbers may be even greater in these regions than in Africa.

To summarize, factors favoring increasing STD incidence and prevalence in developing countries include the following:

1. High birthrate and relatively large proportion of the population in sexually active age groups
2. Urbanization, male migration, and changing social structures
3. Poverty and sexual inequality fostering commercial sex
4. Social upheaval, including war
5. Absence of medical service for diagnosis and treatment of STDs
6. HIV infection and its destabilizing influence on conventional STD epidemiology

IMPLICATIONS AND FUTURE NEEDS

The data reviewed in this article show that STDs cause significant reproductive tract morbidity, especially in conjunction with pregnancy, and likely exert growth-reducing forces at a population level. Furthermore, STDs may substantially contribute to the exceptional reproductive mortality that women face in the developing world. Comparative data suggest that STDs are a greater burden in developing than developed countries and that the ill effects seem greatest in Sub-Saharan Africa.

Recent progress in theory formulation for infectious disease transmission has resulted in the development of simple models of STD epidemiology. Successful transmission of an STD pathogen in a population is seen to depend on three factors: its transmissibility; the duration of time that the infectious agent continues to be shed in a contagious form from an infected host; and the average rate of sexual partner change in the population. Each STD requires a critical rate of sexual partner change in order to persist, and this rate is found within only a small subset of the entire population. These small groups are termed core groups (usually found in cities), and they act as the reservoir for the STD for the entire population. All models of STD epidemiology strongly emphasize the role of sexual behavior in regulating STD transmission. Despite the obvious importance of sexual behavior, this is the variable about which least is known. Crude data suggest that great heterogeneity in sexual behavior exists across and within cultures. Heterogeneity in rates of sexual partner change within developing countries appears similar in magnitude to that recorded in developed countries, where average behavior is related to variability in behavior by the power law $\sigma^2 = am^b$. The uniformity in this pattern across societies is an observation requiring explanation. It may be linked to a set of basic transcultural rules governing pair formation and dissolution. In addition to partner change rates, the important processes that determine the pattern of STD transmission are those governing sexual mixing within and between population strata. These strata include sexual activity classes, age classes, and spatial location classes (urban versus rural). Information on many of these processes is scant at present. Data from at least three recent sexual surveys[65] (two conducted in developed countries and one conducted in a developing county) show that sexual behavior is highly age-dependent. Because population structures are vastly different between urban and rural areas of a developing country, the association of sexual behavior with age may in part explain the high prevalence of STDs in urban centers in developing countries. The unbalanced sex ratio in some urban areas may likewise be important. The occurrence of commercial sex core groups in urban centers is also thought to be of great significance in community persistence of STDs, although an estimation of their role in quantitatively determining STD transmission has thus far escaped calculation.

On the basis of data summarized in this paper and the ideas engendered by them, the following are identified as priority areas for future research on assessing the reproductive and general health impact of STDs in developing countries:

1. Improved surveillance for both STD-related diseases and selected STD agents is needed to track temporal and geographic trends. Because of economic restrictions, it is appropriate to collect such data from sentinel populations. We recommend random or cluster sampling of pregnant women attending antenatal clinics, women attending family planning clinics, men in the military, and CSWs. Women should have cervical cultures collected for *Neisseria gonorrhoeae* and *Chlamydia trachomatis* testing, and serology for *Treponema pallidum* and HIV. Men should have first-void urine samples collected for pyuria (to detect urethritis) and serology for *Treponema pallidum* and HIV.

2. STD clinics should be strengthened to improve their treatment and diagnostic services, and data on attendance at these clinics should be used to track temporal and regional trends in the incidence of gonococcal infection, syphilis, chancroid, HIV infection, and PID. Antimicrobial resistance patterns of *Neisseria gonorrhoeae* and *Haemophilus ducreyi* should be determined at periodic intervals in samples collected from patients attending these clinics. Since many women with STDs and other RTIs seek assistance through family planning, maternal-child health, or primary care clinics, linkage of STD services with these programs would be of benefit.

3. The pregnancy impact of STDs needs to be studied in additional geographic areas and in rural areas to determine if the magnitude of the effect observed in Nairobi is generalizable. Particular attention should be paid to gonococcal ophthalmia neonatorum, prematurity and pregnancy wastage, HIV, and syphilis in pregnancy.

4. Better data on sexual behavior and its relationship to STD incidence and prevalence are essential to understanding transmission dynamics, plotting spread, and devising control programs. Few data are available from developing countries. Theoretical considerations suggest that STD spread in a population is dependent on average rate of change of sexual partners, on the variance of this rate across the population, and on the mixing patterns across sexual activity classes. Probability sampling of subjects in a variety of geographic areas, including both rural and urban sites, should assist in determining the generalizability of the power law relating variance to the mean. Number of sexual partners per unit time should be enumerated. Mixing patterns will be difficult, if not impossible, to discern, and emphasis should be placed on defining frequency of contact with CSWs. The relationships of sexual partner change rate and commercial sex exposure to age should be determined.

5. Better empiric data linking sexual behavior to incidence and prevalence measures of STDs are needed. Therefore, sex behavior surveys should be linked to serosurveys for

syphilis and HIV antibodies (possibly HBV, HSV-2, *Chlamydia trachomatis*, and *Haemophilus ducreyi* could also be included), and to cervical tests for *Neisseria gonorrhoeae* and *Chlamydia trachomatis* in women and first-void pyuria and *Neisseria gonorrhoeae/Chlamydia trachomatis* antigen testing in men. Both common sense and mathematical models suggest that measures of STD incidence should correlate with sexual behavior rate measurements. Cumulative lifetime partners should also correlate with prevalence markers of STD exposure (e.g., HSV-2, *Treponema pallidum*, HIV serology). In addition to focusing on risk groups, these studies should enumerate the importance of STDs among males and females in the general population. Linkage of STD rates to demographic measurements such as fertility rates should be undertaken.

Information in these areas can assist in defining the regional magnitude of the problem of RTIs especially in relation to competing concerns within and outside the medical arena; in estimating future trends; in providing an early warning system as important changes occur; and in suggesting control strategies. STDs have a positive track record of responsiveness to control initiatives, and focused efforts can be designed to maximize the cost-benefit ratio. In particular, STD control programs seem to have had important influences on the transmission dynamics of chancroid, syphilis, and, to a lesser extent, gonorrhea. Provision of diagnostic and treatment services seems to have been the key element in these programs. Economic analysis can assist politicians in balancing needs in this area with the many competing needs elsewhere.

REFERENCES

1. Wasserheit JN. The significance and scope of reproductive tract infections among Third World women. Int J Gynecol Obstet 1989; Suppl 3:145–68.
2. Germain A. The Christopher Tietze International Symposium: an overview. Int J Gynecol Obstet 1989; Suppl 3:1–8.
3. Schulz KF, Cates W Jr, O'Mara PR. Pregnancy loss, infant death, and suffering: legacy of syphilis and gonorrhoea in Africa. Genitourin Med 1987; 63:320–5.
4. Perine PL, Duncan ME, Krause DW, Awoke S. Pelvic inflammatory disease and puerperal sepsis in Ethiopia. Am J Obstet Gynecol 1980; 138:969–73.
5. Rosenfield A. Maternal mortality in developing countries: an ongoing but neglected "epidemic." JAMA 1989; 262:376–9.
6. Galega FP, Heymann DL, Nasah BT. Gonococcal ophthalmia neonatorum: the case for prophylaxis in tropical Africa. Bull WHO 1984; 62:95–8.
7. Plummer FA, Laga M, Brunham RC et al. Postpartum upper genital tract infections in Nairobi, Kenya: epidemiology, etiology and risk factors. J Infect Dis 1987; 156:92–8.
8. Temmerman M, Laga M, Ndinya-Achola JO et al. Microbial aetiology and diagnostic criteria of postpartum endometritis in Nairobi, Kenya. Genitourin Med 1988; 64:172–5.
9. Belsey MA. The epidemiology of infertility: a review with particular reference to Sub-Saharan Africa. Bull WHO 1976; 54:319–41.
10. Arya OP, Taber SR, Nsanze H. Gonorrhea and female infertility in rural Uganda. Am J Obstet Gynecol 1980; 138:929–32.

11. Van Roosmalen J. Perinatal mortality in rural Tanzania. Br J Obstet Gynecol 1989; 96:827–34.
12. Muir DG, Belsey MA. Pelvic inflammatory disease and its consequences in the developing world. Am J Obstet Gynecol 1980; 138:913–28.
13. Mabey DCW, Ogbaselassie G, Robertson JN, Heckels JE, Ward ME. Tubal infertility in the Gambia: chlamydial and gonococcal serology in women with tubal occlusion compared with pregnant controls. Bull WHO 1985; 63:1107–13.
14. Laga M, Nsanze H, Brunham RC et al. Epidemiology of ophthalmia neonatorum in Kenya. Lancet 1986; 2:1145–8.
15. Elliott B, Brunham RC, Laga M et al. Maternal gonococcal infection as a preventable risk factor for low birth weight. J Infect Dis 1990; 161:531–6.
16. Temmerman M, Plummer F, Mirza N et al. Infection with HIV as a risk factor for adverse obstetrical outcome. AIDS 1990; 4:1087–93.
17. De Cock K, Barrere B, Diaby L et al. AIDS—the leading cause of adult death in the West African city of Abidjan, Ivory Coast. Science 1990; 249:793–6.
18. Anderson RM, May RM, McLean AR. Possible demographic consequences of AIDS in developing countries. Nature 1988; 332:228–34.
19. Cates W Jr., Farley TMM, Rowe PJ. Worldwide patterns of infertility: is Africa different? Lancet 1985; 1:596–8.
20. Reeves WC, Quiroz E. Prevalence of sexually transmitted diseases in high-risk women in the Republic of Panama. Sex Transm Dis 1987; 14:69–74.
21. Khoo R et al. A study of sexually transmitted diseases in 200 prostitutes in Singapore. Asian J Infect Dis 1977; 1:77.
22. D'Costa LJ, Plummer FA, Bowmer I et al. Prostitutes are a major reservoir of sexually transmitted diseases in Nairobi, Kenya. Sex Transm Dis 1985; 12:64–7.
23. Simonsen JN, Plummer FA, Ngugi EN et al. HIV infection among lower socioeconomic strata prostitutes in Nairobi. AIDS 1990; 4:139–44.
24. Omer E-F, Catterall RD, Ali MH, El-Naeem HA, Erwa HH. Vaginal trichomoniasis at a sexually transmitted disease clinic at Khartoum. Trop Doctor 1985; 15:170–2.
25. Odongo EAI. The role of the venereal disease laboratory, Mulago Hospital, Kampala, in the diagnosis of sexually transmitted diseases in Uganda. East Afr Med J 1977; 54:385–92.
26. Kibukamusoke JW. Venereal disease in East Africa. Trans Roy Soc Trop Med Hyg 1965; 59:642–8.
27. Kuvanont K, Chitwarakorn A, Rochananond C et al. Etiology of urethritis in Thai men. Sex Transm Dis 1989; 16:137–40.
28. Ballard RC, Fehler HG, Duncan MO et al. Urethritis and associated infections in Johannesburg: the role of Chlamydia trachomatis. S Afr J Sex Transm Dis 1981; 1:24.
29. Ratnam AV, Din SN, Chatterjee TK. Gonococcal infection in women with pelvic inflammatory disease in Lusaka, Zambia. Am J Obstet Gynecol 1980; 138:965–8.
30. Shadid CM, Garrido JG. Diagnostico de Neisseria gonorrhoeae en la mujer mediante el examen de varias regiones anatomicas. Bol Sanit Panam 1983; 94:47–53.
31. Osoba AO. Epidemiology of urethritis in Ibadan. Br J Vener Dis 1972; 48:116–20.
32. Mabey DCW, Whittle HC. Genital and neonatal chlamydial infection in a trachoma endemic area. Lancet 1982; 2:300–1.

33. Plummer FA, Simonsen JN, Chubb H et al. Epidemiological evidence for the development of serovar specific immunity after gonococcal infection. J Clin Invest 1989; 83:1472–6.

34. Plummer FA, D'Costa LJ, Nsanze H, Dylewski J, Karasira P, Ronald AR. Epidemiology of chancroid and Haemophilus ducreyi in Nairobi, Kenya. Lancet 1983; 2:1293–5.

35. Kreiss JK, Koech D, Plummer FA et al. AIDS virus infection in Nairobi prostitutes: extension of the epidemic to East Africa. N Engl J Med 1986; 314:414–8.

36. Piot P, Plummer FA, Rey M-A et al. Retrospective seroepidemiology of AIDS virus infection in Nairobi populations. J Infect Dis 1987; 155:1108–12.

37. Pepin J, Plummer FA, Brunham RC, Piot P, Cameron DW, Ronald AR. The interaction of HIV and other sexually transmitted diseases: An opportunity for intervention. AIDS 1989; 3:3–9.

38. Arya OP, Nsanzumuhire H, Taber SR. Clinical, cultural and demographic aspects of gonorrhoea in a rural community in Uganda. Bull WHO 1973; 49:587–95.

39. Bang R. An approach to the gynecological problems of rural women: epidemiologicalal study and intervention through primary health care. First annual meeting, Community Epidemiology/Health Management Network, Kon Kaen, Thailand, February 1–4, 1988. Quoted in: Wasserheit JN. The significance and scope of reproductive tract infections among Third World women. Int J Gynecol Obstet 1989; Suppl 3:145–68.

40. Wasserheit JN, Harris JR, Chokraborty J et al. Reproductive tract infections in a family planning population in rural Bangladesh: a neglected opportunity to promote MCH-FP programs. Stud Fam Plann 1989; 20:69–80.

41. Ratnam AV, Din SN, Hira SK et al. Syphilis in pregnant women in Zambia. Br J Vener Dis 1982; 58:355–8.

42. Nasah BT, Nguematcha R, Eyong M, Godwin S. Gonorrhea, trichomonas and candida among gravid and nongravid women in Cameroon. Int J Gynecol Obstet 1980; 18:48–52.

43. O'Farrell NO, Hoosen AA, Kharsany BM, Van den Ende J. Sexually transmitted pathogens in pregnant women in a rural South African community. Genitourin Med 1989; 65:276–80.

44. Weissenberger R, Robertson A, Holland S et al. The incidence of gonorrhoea in urban Rhodesian black women. S Afr Med J 1977; 52:119.

45. Gyaneshwar R, Nsanze H, Singh KP, Pillay S, Seruvatu I. The prevalence of sexually transmitted disease agents in pregnant women in Suva. Aust NZ J Obstet Gynecol 1987; 27:213–5.

46. Gini PC, Chukudebelu WO, Njoku-Obi AN. Antenatal screening for syphilis at the University of Nigeria Teaching Hospital, Enugu, Nigeria—a six year survey. Int J Gynecol Obstet 1989; 29:321–4.

47. Donoso E, Vera E, Villaseca P et al. Infection gonococica en el embarzo. Rev Chil Obstet Ginecol 1984; 49:84–7.

48. Hopcraft M, Verhagen AR, Ngigi S, Haga ACA. Genital infections in developing countries: experience in a family planning clinic. Bull WHO 1973; 48:581–6.

49. Nsofor BI, Bello CSS, Ekwempu CC. Sexually transmitted disease among women attending a family planning clinic in Zaria, Nigeria. Int J Gynecol Obstet 1989; 28:365–7.

50. Caldwell J, Caldwell P. High fertility in Sub-Saharan Africa. Scientific American 1990; May:118–25.
51. Duncan ME, Tibaux G, Pelzer A et al. First coitus before menarche and risk of sexually transmitted disease. Lancet 1990; 2:338–40.
52. Hira SK, Bhat GJ, Chikamata DM et al. Syphilis intervention in pregnancy: Zambian demonstration project. Genitourin Med 1990; 66:159–64.
53. Brunham RC, Plummer FA. A general model of sexually transmitted disease epidemiology and its implications for control. Med Clin N Amer 1991; 74:1339–52.
54. Yorke JA, Heathcote HW, Nold A. Dynamics and control of the transmission of gonorrhea. Sex Transm Dis 1978; 5:51–7.
55. Anderson RM, May RM. Transmission dynamics of HIV infection. Nature 1987; 26:137–142.
56. Anderson RM, May RM. Epidemiologicalal parameters of HIV transmission. Nature 1988; 333:514–9.
57. Peterman TA, Stoneburner RL, Allen JR, Jaffe HW, Curran JW. Risk of HIV transmission from heterosexual adults with transfusion-associated infection. JAMA 1988; 259:55–9.
58. Gupta S, Anderson RM, May RM. Networks of sexual contacts: implications for the pattern of spread of HIV. AIDS 1989; 3:807–17.
59. CDC. Number of sex partners and potential risk of sexual exposure to human immunodeficiency virus. MMWR 1988; 37:565–8.
60. Konings E, Ph.D. student, pure and applied biology, Imperial College. Personal communication, February 1991.
61. Muir DG, Belsey M. Pelvic inflammatory disease and its consequences in the developing world. Am J Obstet Gynecol 1980; 138:913–28.
62. Rwandan HIV Seroprevalence Group. Nationwide community-based serological survey of HIV-1 and other human retrovirus infections in a central African country. Lancet 1989; 1:941–3.
63. Nzilambi N, DeCock FM, Forthal DN et al. The prevalence of infection with human immunodeficiency virus over a ten-year period in rural Zaire. N Engl J Med 1988; 318:276–9.
64. Handsfield HH, Rice RJ, Roberts MC, Holmes KK. Localized outbreak of penicillinase-producing Neiserria gonorrhoeae: paradigm for introduction and spread of gonorrhea in a community. JAMA 1989; 261:2357–61.
65. Anderson RM, May RM, Boily MC, Garnett GP, Rowley JT. The spread of HIV-1 in Africa: sexual contact patterns and the predicted demographic impact of AIDS. Nature 1991; 352:581–9.

PART II
PROGRAMMATIC ISSUES

WOMEN'S HEALTH: IMPORTANCE OF REPRODUCTIVE TRACT INFECTIONS, PELVIC INFLAMMATORY DISEASE AND CERVICAL CANCER

Dr. André Meheus, M.D., D.P.H., Ph.D.
Programme of Sexually Transmitted Diseases
World Health Organization
1211 Geneva 27, Switzerland

INTRODUCTION

Upper reproductive tract infections and their consequences are major health problems for women worldwide, particularly in resource-poor settings. The syndrome of pelvic inflammatory disease (PID) is mostly due to sexually transmitted infections that start in the lower reproductive tract and ascend into the upper reproductive tract. Cervical cancer is also usually the result of sexually transmitted infection, and human papilloma virus (HPV) appears to be the causal agent. These conditions can be effectively controlled and prevented by relatively simple and inexpensive methods, and what is needed now is the commitment of human and financial resources for activities to prevent and treat reproductive tract infections.

PID

The cervix of the uterus separates the lower reproductive tract (vagina) from the upper reproductive tract (uterine cavity, fallopian tubes) and functions as a fairly effective barrier, impeding the entry of potentially pathogenic agents from the vagina and the cervical area to the upper reproductive tract and peritoneal cavity. Most PID, or upper reproductive tract infection in women, is due to infections that start in the lower reproductive tract (e.g., gonococcal or chlamydial cervicitis and bacterial vaginosis (BV)), and frequently results in severe, irreversible sequelae, particularly infertility, ectopic pregnancy, and chronic pelvic pain (Figure 1). Dilatation of the uterine cervix, by instruments (e.g., for induced abortion) or any other mechanical means (e.g., during spontaneous abortion, stillbirth, or childbirth), facilitates the entry and spread of pathogens into the upper reproductive tract; leading thereby to sepsis, PID, and subsequent partial or total occlusion of the fallopian tubes due to postinflammatory scarring. Partial occlusion of the fallopian tubes can result in ectopic pregnancy, and total occlusion may result in infertility.

Reproductive Tract Infections, Edited by A. Germain *et al.*
Plenum Press, New York, 1992

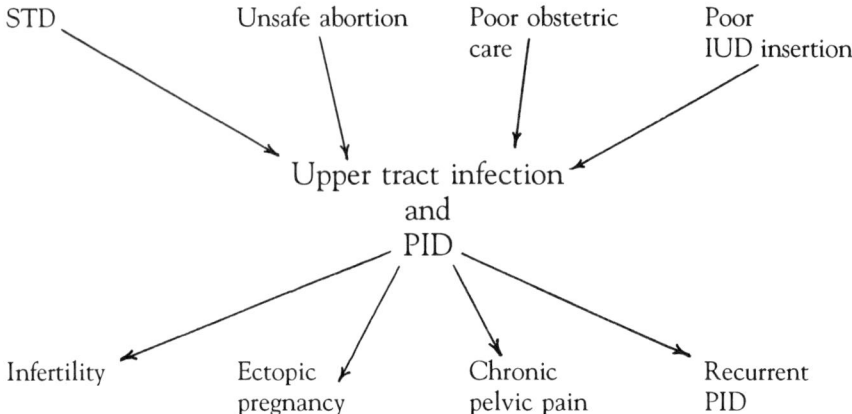

Figure 1. Spectrum of Reproductive Tract Infections in Women

PID Risk

The incidence of PID in women with lower reproductive tract infections, shown in Table 1, has been estimated from studies in industrialized countries, but these data can be applied to other settings. PID occurs in 8–10 percent of women with untreated chlamydial cervicitis[1] and in 8–20 percent of women with untreated gonococcal cervicitis.[2] Chlamydial and gonococcal lower genital tract infections are at least 10 times as common in Southern countries as in industrialized regions. The health problem posed by PID in these countries is therefore tremendous. Among women with untreated chlamydial cervicitis who have abortions, 10–23 percent develop PID.[3,4,5] Among women with untreated gonococcal cervicitis who have abortions, approximately 15 percent develop postabortion endometritis, three times the proportion among women with negative gonococcal cultures.[6]

Table 1. Proportion of Women with Lower Tract Infection Who Develop PID

Lower tract infection	Without instrumentation (%)	With abortion (%)
Chlamydial cervicitis	8–10	10–23
Gonococcal cervicitis	8–20	± 15
BV	?	?

Source: references 1–8.

The incidence of PID in women with untreated BV has not been quantified. But the polymicrobial flora recovered from peritoneal fluid and tubal specimens of women with PID often include organisms characteristic of BV.[7,8] This finding indicates that BV may be an antecedent of pelvic infection. PID due to BV-associated organisms would usually occur when host defenses have been impaired by infection with more aggressive cervical pathogens, by prior PID or by iatrogenic infections from transcervical procedures (e.g., poorly performed abortion or IUD insertion).

Extent of the Problem

Studies on PID in the developing world are limited to hospitalized women, and this introduces a number of biases related mainly to patient selection and availability of laboratory facilities. Women who have had a delivery, abortion, or IUD insertion at a health service might be more likely than others to consult for PID; hospitalization practices for PID might be very different according to health care provider; the extent of self-treatment with antibiotics might strongly influence PID symptoms and hospitalization patterns. Because chlamydial infection is often asymptomatic, this etiology may be underrepresented in hospital cases. Furthermore, PID etiology is largely dependent on the spectrum of laboratory tests available. Available data suggest that a substantial proportion of gynecologic admissions in much of the developing world is related to PID.[11] African studies indicate that 17–40 percent of gynecologic admissions are related to pelvic infection.[12-17] In Southeast Asia, the range is 15–37 percent; in India, it is 3–10 percent.

The spectrum of precipitating causes of PID seems to vary from region to region. In Sub-Saharan Africa, spontaneous PID accounts for approximately 70 percent of admissions for pelvic infections; the remaining cases are associated more often with childbirth than with abortion. The etiology of PID in Africa is incomplete because of lack of laboratory facilities, but gonococcus is implicated in 25–50 percent of cases, and *Chlamydia trachomatis* is probably at least as frequently implicated.[15,18] Case-control studies on chlamydial and gonococcal antibodies indicate that both infections must play a major role in the development of PID in Africa.[18,19,20] In Southeast Asia, postabortion infection seems to be the dominant cause of PID, having accounted for 65–86 percent of hospitalized cases. By contrast, in Pakistan, 72 percent of PID cases were related to childbirth, 23 percent followed abortion, and 5 percent were classified as spontaneous. Postpartum infection was also more common than postabortion infection in Cuba.[21]

Postpartum Infection and Sepsis

Endometritis (infection of the lining of the uterus) is the most common maternal postpartum infection. It can be divided into early infection, which has its onset within 48 hours following delivery, and late infection, occurring from two days to two weeks after delivery. Cesarean section greatly increases the risk of an early postpartum infection. In developed countries, most postpartum infections are related to cesarean section; no fewer than 20–55 percent of women who undergo cesarean section will develop (early) postpartum endometritis, compared with 2–5 percent of those who have vaginal deliveries.[22] The high infection rate following cesarean section is probably the result of direct uterine contamination by organisms in the amniotic cavity. Cesarean sections are not performed very often in most of the developing world, but the procedure is very common in the urban areas of Latin America and results in many complications.

Postpartum infection is rare if delivery is spontaneous and normal, and if nothing is introduced in the vagina during labor. However, it accounts for up to 30 percent of maternal deaths in Southern countries,[23] and also contributes to a large proportion of secondary infertility in those who survive. Furthermore, postpartum upper reproductive tract infections after vaginal delivery are approximately 10 times more common in developing countries than in developed countries.[15] A major cause of infection is the entry of germs into the genital tract through the use of unwashed hands and unsterilized instruments during delivery. The introduction of foreign objects such as leaves, earth, or cow dung into the birth canal by untrained birth attendants, who believe these objects are beneficial, is also a common cause of infection. Additionally, women who remain undelivered 12 hours after rupture of the membranes are at serious risk of infection; almost 100 percent of women still in labor after 24 hours are likely to develop infections.

In several African hospitals, postpartum infection accounted for 14–30 percent of maternal mortality.[24-27] Among 1,013 women who delivered vaginally in Nairobi, Kenya, approximately 20 percent developed postpartum upper reproductive tract infection, and 35 percent of these cases were associated with gonococcal or chlamydial infection;[15] the prevalences of gonococcal and chlamydial infection in that population were 7 percent and 21 percent, respectively. At a referral hospital at Harare, Zimbabwe, puerperal sepsis accounted for over 15 percent of admissions.[28]

The prevalence of specific upper genital tract infections varies geographically. In Africa, between 3 percent and 18 percent of antenatal clients are infected by gonococci. The level of chlamydial infections now exceeds this level. A majority of postpartum ascending infections are caused by these pathogens and BV-associated bacteria.[29,30,31] By comparison, a study in India indicated that 86 percent of postpartum infections studied were caused by staphylococcal or fecal bacteria; no gonococci were found.[33] It should be stressed that the most efficacious, least expensive treatment to prevent these upper reproductive tract infections and their devastating sequelae—infertility and ectopic pregnancy—is the timely diagnosis and treatment of all lower tract syndromes.[32]

Postabortal Infection and Sepsis

The risk of developing ascending reproductive tract infection with sepsis, pelvic inflammation, and tubal damage is substantial in women who have improperly performed abortions. Like women in developed countries,[34] those in Southern countries undergoing spontaneous or induced abortion are more frequently infected with sexually transmitted diseases (STDs) than are their antenatal counterparts.[35,36] Thus, in addition to the risk of infection from improper surgery, women are at risk of ascending lower tract infections and are likely to develop postabortal sepsis. The infection rate with *Neisseria gonorrhoeae* and *Chlamydia trachomatis* among females with postabortal sepsis was about three times the level observed in uncomplicated deliveries in Zimbabwe.[24]

Where induced abortions are legally restricted, or where they are legal but not widely provided in public health facilities, they are performed clandestinely, usually with a minimum of sanitary precautions. In Lagos, Nigeria, for example, fewer than half the abortions done for adolescents were performed by physicians.[37] The consequences of clandestine abortion are severe. In one study in Ibadan, Nigeria, it was found that the risk of secondary infertility for women with previous abortions was 3.6 times that among women who had not yet had an abortion.[38] Such situations are even more significant given the immense demand for abortion services in Africa, as revealed by various studies. In Ibadan, among 841 unmarried women 14–25 years old, 183 out of 203 first pregnancies were terminated by induced abortion.[39] Among 950 secondary school students 12–20 years old, more than 100 pregnancies occurred, and all of these women obtained abortions so they could continue their schooling.[37] In Monrovia, Liberia, among 748 unmarried young women 14–21 years old, 278 experienced at least one pregnancy, and 151 of these pregnancies ended in abortion.[40]

There are no accurate worldwide figures for induced abortion, as many people involved in the activity wish to keep it secret. However, estimates are that 40–60 million women a year seek termination of an unwanted pregnancy, which means 30–45 abortions occur per 1,000 women of reproductive age. Abortion mortality worldwide is estimated at 100,000–200,000 women per year. Therefore, the complications of unsafe abortions are a leading cause of maternal death, accounting for at least 7–29 percent of maternal deaths in the developing world,[23] and an even higher percentage in some countries.

SEQUELAE OF PID

The frequent and usually irreversible complications of PID are major health problems. In nonpregnant women, these complications include infertility, ectopic pregnancy, chronic pelvic pain, and recurrent infection, conditions due to tubal scarring during healing of the acute infection. The social, psychological, and health consequences of these sequelae provide strong justification for allocation of resources to the control of reproductive tract infections (RTIs).

In industrialized countries, the overall incidence of infertility after PID is 15–25 percent, but becomes as high as 50–60 percent after a third episode.[2] Ectopic pregnancy is 6–10 times more frequent in women who have had PID than among those who have never had upper reproductive tract infection. Chronic pelvic pain and recurrent infection develop in approximately 20 percent of women who have had PID. In developing countries, treatment for PID is usually delayed, inadequate, or totally unavailable. Therefore, the incidence of PID sequelae is much higher than in industrialized countries. Data from the preantibiotic era, when post-PID infertility occurred in 60–70 percent of cases, are probably very relevant to the current situation in most developing countries.[9]

Chronic pelvic pain is perhaps the most debilitating of the PID sequelae. The pain waxes and wanes, but is often so severe that it interferes with daily activities. This sequela is attributed to extratubal scarring and is often associated with infertility.[10] Recurrent PID, which is difficult to distinguish from chronic pelvic pain, occurs in one quarter of women because of damage to normal tubal clearance mechanisms, incomplete treatment of sex partners or unchanged sexual behavioral patterns. Endogenous vaginal bacteria, such as BV-associated organisms, are often involved in recurrent PID.

PID-related Infertility

The link between PID and infertility, predominantly tubal infertility, is clearly established in numerous studies worldwide. The most reliable data come from Sweden,[41] but some studies are also available from Southern countries. In a recent study in Zimbabwe, women who had PID, were infertile, or had an ectopic pregnancy as a result of tubal pathology were significantly more likely than pregnant controls to report a history of PID (see Table 2).[20]

Several risk factors have a bearing on whether PID results in tubal occlusion. The most important variable is previous episodes of PID, but age and severity of PID, as judged by laparoscopy, also influence fertility outcome (see Table 3).[9] Regarding microbial etiology, PID due to either *Neisseria gonorrhoeae* or *Chlamydia trachomatis* has been causally related to infertility.[42] Some studies indicate that *Chlamydia trachomatis* may carry a worse fertility prognosis than other organisms, because it causes more severe subclinical tubal inflammation, and chlamydial PID is thus more chronic, leading to more tubal damage. In both

Table 2. PID and Its Sequelae among Various Groups of Women, Zimbabwe

Group	Number	Mean age	History of PID	
			Mild (%)	Severe (%)
Pregnant women (at term)	104	26.6	12	1
Women with PID	66	26.9	65†	12*
Women with ectopic pregnancy/tubal pathology	39	28.9 ·	65†	22†
Women with ectopic pregnancy/normal tubes	21	27.6	6	0
Infertile women/ tubal pathology	135	28.4	81†	3
Infertile women/ normal tubes	92	27.1	30	0

*p <.01 compared with pregnant women.
†p <.001 compared with pregnant women.
Source: reference 20.

developed and developing countries, serologic studies have uniformly associated evidence of past chlamydial or gonococcal infection with tubal occlusion. Fertility prognosis after PID is only marginally improved by adequate therapy. If therapy is inadequate, the prognosis is, of course, worse. The bottom line is that in order to have a significant impact upon infertility, PID must be prevented, in part by improved access to adequate services for management of cervical infections.

Table 3. Prevalence of Tubal Infertility after PID, by Number and
Severity of Episodes, according to Age, Lund, Sweden, 1960–1979

Number and severity of episodes of PID	% with tubal infertility	
	Age 15–24	Age 23–34
None	0	0
One (average)	9	19
One (mild)	4	8
One (moderate)	11	22
One (severe)	27	40
Two	21	31
Three or more	52	60

Source: reference 9.

Extent of Infertility

The popular definition of infertility, which is also the one most often used by demographers, is "childlessness." However, a couple may not have a living child because of infertility, or because of pregnancy wastage, or because of infant or child mortality. For public health purposes, we should distinguish between infertility (inability to conceive) and pregnancy wastage, because the etiology is different. In addition, a nearly irreducible core of involuntary infertility is related to chromosomal, congenital, or endocrinological abnormalities affecting both men and women. This core is generally estimated at 5 percent of all couples, and African countries are far above this level. Thus, acquired infertility, which is of infectious origin, is very common.

Table 4 shows the rate of childlessness for 22 African countries ranked according to their population size and the shortfall in total fertility due to childlessness.[43] For Gabon, childlessness is as high as 32 percent, Congo and Zaire have a level of 21 percent, and several other countries are above the 10 percent level. Especially high rates of infertility are found in the countries of the so-called infertility belt, which extends from Gabon in the west to southwestern Sudan in the east.

Infertility overall is sometimes divided into primary infertility (i.e., the couple is unable to conceive) and secondary infertility (i.e., the women has had a pregnancy, but has been unable to conceive in the last two years). Secondary infertility in particular is a good indicator of tubal blockage due to PID. The World Health Organization (WHO) has undertaken epidemiological studies at the community level to determine the amount and type of infertility.[44] Table 5 shows the results of these investigations.

Table 4. Population Size, Infertility, and Fertility Shortfall,
22 Countries of Sub-Saharan Africa

Country	1980 population (millions)	Percentage of women childless*	Shortfall in total fertility caused by infertility (births per woman)†
Nigeria	90.0	8	.6
Zaire	28.3	21	1.9
Sudan	18.4	9	.6
Tanzania	17.9	10	.8
Kenya	15.9	7	.4
Ghana	11.7	3	0.0
Mozambique	19.5	14	1.2
Cameroun	8.4	15	1.3
Ivory Coast	8.0	10	.8
Angola	7.1	12	.9
Mali	6.9	8	.5
Burkina Faso	6.9	6	.3
Zambia	5.8	14	1.2
Senegal	5.7	4	.1
Niger	5.3	9	.6
Guinea	5.0	6	.3
Chad	4.5	11	.9
Burundi	4.1	3	0.0
Central African Republic	2.3	17	1.6
Congo	1.5	21	1.9
Lesotho	1.3	4	.1
Gabon	.5	32	3.2
Weighted mean, all countries	270.0	10	.8

*Women aged 45–49, or closest age group.
†The mean total fertility rate for these countries is 7.3 births per woman. The shortfall represents the difference between each country's total fertility rate and the mean.
Source: reference 43.

Table 5. Primary and Secondary Infertility, WHO Community Surveys

Country	Primary infertility (%)		Secondary infertility (%)	
	Urban	Rural	Urban	Rural
Benin	3	3	11	9
Cameroun	—	12	—	33
Tanzania	5	4	20	19
India (Chandigarh)	2	4	6	7
Thailand	3	2	14	12

Source: reference 44.

In all five countries surveyed, secondary infertility is more prevalent than primary infertility. For nearly all countries, there is practically no difference between urban and rural areas. Among countries, however, there is a considerable difference in the amount of infertility. Very low proportions of couples in Chandigarh, India, are infertile. On the other hand, in Cameroun, primary infertility is at 12 percent and secondary infertility is at 33 percent.

WHO undertook a multicenter study to determine the pattern of diagnostic category in patients presenting at gynecologic clinics.[45] When diagnostic categories that are infection-related—such as bilateral tubal occlusion, pelvic adhesions, and acquired tubal abnormality—were grouped, 66 percent of infertility in Africa was infection-related, compared with 34 percent in Asia and 31 percent in industrialized countries.

Apart from the medical consequences, the social and psychological impacts of infertility may be far more devastating in developing than in industrialized countries. In many countries, a woman who fails to produce children faces divorce and social ostracism. Thus, infertility is not just a personal tragedy for the woman, but it reduces her status to one of social outcast. In order to survive, many infertile women turn to commercial sex. This, in turn, increases transmission of sexually transmitted infections and the risk of infertility in the community. Adequate STD control could effectively break this vicious circle.

PID and Ectopic Pregnancy

A predisposing factor in the genesis of ectopic pregnancy is any condition that retards or prevents migration of the fertilized ovum to the uterus. Important risk factors for ectopic pregnancy in the industrialized world are a history of infertility, a history of PID, prior tubal surgery, and current IUD use.[46,47,48] The relationship between PID and ectopic pregnancy has been explored in studies carried out in the industrialized world. These have revealed a significant correlation between ectopic pregnancy and markers for sexually transmitted infections.[49-52] An STD most likely predisposes a woman to subsequent ectopic pregnancy in that as a mono-organism lower tract infection it can ascend, creating a multiorganism upper tract infection that scars the intraluminal tubal space and the surrounding area. In

Sweden, the risk of an ectopic pregnancy is 6–10 times greater among women who have had PID than among women without a history of pelvic infection; the first conception following PID leads to an extrauterine pregnancy in approximately 6 percent of women.[1,10,53]

The situation in the developing world is even more serious as postinfectious ectopic pregnancy has been shown to occur more frequently there than in industrialized countries.[14] As in the industrialized world, a large proportion of ectopic pregnancies are the result of previous RTIs. In Zimbabwe, women with ectopic pregnancy and tubal abnormalities were found to have significantly higher levels of antibodies against Chlamydia trachomatis (26 percent) than pregnant controls (7 percent) and women with ectopic pregnancy but no tubal abnormalities (5 percent). The prevalence of gonococcal antibodies was six times higher among women with ectopic pregnancy and tubal disease (33 percent) than in the control group.[20] Some 80 percent of women with ectopic pregnancies in Trinidad had histological evidence of chronic PID.[54] A study in Gabon showed evidence of acute or chronic tubal infection in 25 percent of women with ectopic pregnancies.[55] In a South African hospital, 41 percent of 100 consecutive ectopic pregnancy cases showed signs of prior PID,[56] while in a study in Nigeria, 58 percent of women with an ectopic pregnancy showed signs of pelvic inflammation.[57]

Extent of the Problem

Population-based incidence rates for ectopic pregnancy are rarely available for developing countries. Available data come from hospital-based reports by diagnostic category; consequently, they are as much a function of the infrastructure in a country and the utilization of health services as of the incidence of ectopic pregnancy. Reports on ectopic pregnancy use several measures to indicate its frequency: the ratio of ectopic pregnancies to normal deliveries, the rate of ectopics per 1,000 live births, and such cases as a proportion of all gynecologic admissions.

Table 6 shows the ratio of ectopic pregnancies to normal deliveries in eight countries. The ratio in the United States has increased from 1:208 in 1970, when monitoring of ectopic pregnancy trends began, to 1:43 in 1987.[58] Potential reasons given for this increase are heightened awareness, improved diagnostic technology, and increased occurrence of PID resulting from STDs. In Benin City, Nigeria, the ratio increased from 1:58 to 1:43 between 1973 and 1979.[60]

Table 7 presents ectopic pregnancy rates from hospital-based studies in the developing world. In Africa, the rate ranges from 3.2 to 32.2 ectopic pregnancies per 1,000 live births; in Asia, the rate ranges from 2.1 to 23.2 per 1,000 live births. The proportion of all gynecologic admissions represented by ectopic pregnancies varied from 0.3 percent to 1 percent in India and was 1.4 percent in Zambia and 0.9 percent in Australia.[14]

Impact of Ectopic Pregnancy

In the developed world, ectopic pregnancy is one of the most important causes of maternal mortality. In the United States, it is one of the two leading causes of maternal deaths.[58] In the developing world, where pregnancy, abortion, and delivery services are still poor, and where ectopic pregnancies and deaths from them are very poorly measured, the full impact of ectopic pregnancy is difficult to assess. However, limited data do suggest that it is a serious health problem, especially where women do not have easy access to routine as well as emergency medical care. Table 8 shows maternal mortality due to ectopic pregnancy per 1,000 live births, based on hospital studies.

The impact of ectopic pregnancy is also shown by the large proportion of women who suffer either from repeat ectopic pregnancies or from infertility subsequent to an ectopic

Table 6. Ratio of Ectopic Pregnancies to Normal Deliveries

Country	Ratio
Gabon (Libreville)[55]	1:62
Greenland[59]	1:42
Nigeria (Benin City)[60]	1:43
South Africa (Edenvale)[56]	1:66
Sweden[14]	1:133
Trinidad[54]	1:110
Uganda (Kampala)[14]	1:91
United States[58]	1:43

pregnancy. In Finland, the risk of recurrent ectopic pregnancy was shown to be 20 percent, and 15 percent of women who had had an ectopic pregnancy subsequently failed to conceive.[62] In Gabon, a 30 percent recurrent ectopic pregnancy rate was found.[55] In Nigeria, a 14 percent recurrent ectopic pregnancy rate was found, along with a 37 percent subsequent secondary infertility rate.[63] A repeat ectopic pregnancy clearly elevates the risk for maternal mortality, but increased awareness and medical attention could result in both primary and secondary prevention.

Table 7. Numbers and Rates of Ectopic Pregnancy

Country	Date	Number	Ectopic pregnancies per 1,000 live births
Africa			
Ghana	1963–67	965	32.2
Kenya	1967–68	119	7.6
Lesotho	1980	12	4.8
Nigeria	1973–76	68	17.1
Nigeria	1978–79	251	10.3
South Africa	1985	350	19.9
Tanzania	1971–77	251	10.3
Tunisia	1978	104	3.2
Uganda	1965	144	10.1
Asia			
China	1977–81	102	23.2
Hong Kong	1946–53	210	4.7
Hong Kong	1956–59	332	10.2
India	1979–84	125	2.9
India	1967–71	12	2.1
India	1964–73	500	4.4
Malaysia	1961–63	100	4.7
Thailand	1962–75	1,455	6.7
Singapore	1975–80	121	3.7
Singapore	1972–77	148	2.9
Middle East			
Iran	1969–75	96	2.9
Jordan	1976–82	75	6.2
Saudi Arabia	1973–79	68	2.4
Saudi Arabia	1978–79	0	0.0
Caribbean			
Jamaica	1954–61	438	35.7

Source: reference 61.

Table 8. Maternal Mortality due to Ectopic Pregnancy

Country	Date	Number of ectopic pregnancy deaths	Total number of maternal deaths	Ectopic pregnancy deaths per 1,000 live births
Africa				
Gabon (Libreville)	1984–68	5	34	0.22
Ghana (Accra)	1963–67	27	325	0.77
Kenya (Nairobi)	1972–77	5	75	0.24
Malawi (Linongwe)	1985	3	87	0.37
Nigeria (Ilesha)	1958–70	2	133	0.14
Nigeria (Benin City)	1970–71	1	30	0.14
Nigeria (Zaria)	1976–79	1	92	0.04
Nigeria (Ibadan)	1962–71	6	183	0.27
South Africa (National S.)	1980–82	5	660	0.01
Sudan (Omdurman)	1980–85	1	102	0.04
Sudan (Khartoum)	1976–81	1	12	0.13
Tanzania (Moshi)	1971–77	4	80	0.16
Tanzania (National S.)	1983	1	85	0.01
Zimbabwe (Salisbury)	1972–73	1	73	0.03
Zambia (Lusaka)	1982–83	4	64	0.08
Asia				
Bangladesh (Dhaka)	1967–68	1	41	0.19
China (Shanghai)	1978–84	11	390	0.01
China (Beijing)	1974–78	3	38	0.04
China (Beijing)	1979–83	1	46	0.01
China (Provinces)	1984	23	1,211	0.01
Taiwan (Taipei)	1981–84	16	259	0.01
India (National S.)	1978–81	83	4,703	0.13
Malaysia (National S.)	1978–81	5	930	0.01
Thailand (Provinces)	1973–77	6	212	0.02
Thailand (Provinces)	1979	15	240	0.10
Vietnam (National S.)	1984–85	8	227	0.36
Yemen, Dem. (Abood)	1982–86	1	60	0.04

Table continues on next page

Table 8. Maternal Mortality due to Ectopic Pregnancy (continued)

Country	Date	Number of ectopic pregnancy deaths	Total number of maternal deaths	Ectopic pregnancy deaths per 1,000 live births
Latin America and Caribbean				
Colombia (San Vincente)	1963–67	1	50	0.13
Colombia (Medellin)	1968–72	0	54	0.00
Colombia (Bogota)	1971–73	1	209	0.02
Cuba (National S.)	1985–87	18	258	0.07
Jamaica (National S.)	1981–83	20	181	0.11
Puerto Rico (National S.)	1978–79	3	75	0.02
Venezuela (Maracaibo)	1961–67	1	84	0.02
Oceania				
Fiji (National S.)	1969–76	5	164	0.03
Papua New Guinea (Goroka)	1964–73	1	142	0.17

Source: reference 61.

PID: PROGRAM, POLICY, AND RESEARCH

Prevention, in principle, is better than treatment and essential for infertility, chronic pelvic pain, or ectopic pregnancy because treatment is expensive and often not successful. In order to control PID, sexually transmitted infections, poor obstetric care, and unsafe abortion must be addressed.

Program Recommendations and Policy Implications

Programs to combat the above health problems are not easy to implement, for several reasons. First, they require political support, which is often difficult to obtain. Second, such programs compete for funding with prevention and control programs for other epidemic and endemic diseases, such as tropical diseases and tuberculosis. Third, programs require information that is often unavailable, on the magnitude and distribution of the health problem. These obstacles have been somewhat reduced, at least in the case of sexually transmitted infections, by the advent of the human immunodeficiency virus (HIV). Public health programs that can play a role in preventing upper reproductive tract infections and their sequelae include the following:

1. *STD/HIV education programs:* to inform the public about STDs, including information on HIV, avoiding infection, identifying infection, and seeking adequate care when infected
2. *Clinical STD services:* to provide services for prevention, detection, and comprehensive treatment management of persons with sexually transmitted infections

3.   *Obstetric care services:* to train traditional and other birth attendants to reduce
        the risk of infection, and to recognize when to refer, along with enhanced
        support for pregnancy and delivery care at all levels of the health system
4.   *Family planning programs:* to provide safe and appropriate contraceptive services
        (including IUD insertion) and promotion of contraceptive methods that
        protect against infection (especially condoms)
5.   *Safe abortion services:* to provide services for safe termination of pregnancy
        carried out by qualified personnel under aseptic conditions

STD/HIV Education Programs. Health promotion activities are crucial in any
STD/HIV prevention and control program, and involve a number of objectives: informing
the public about STDs, how they are transmitted, and their long-term effects (especially
PID and its sequelae); promoting primary preventive sexual behaviors (stable monogamy;
reduction of number of sex partners; safe sex practices; use of barrier contraceptive methods,
including condoms, diaphragms, and spermicides; sexual abstinence); informing people
where to go for appropriate STD treatment and making sure that all partners, especially
men, understand the importance of notifying sexual partners about the need for treatment.

The growing importance of incurable viral STDs, particularly HIV infection, has
tremendously increased the importance of health education in changing behaviors toward
safer sex practices. Major efforts must be directed toward groups at particularly high risk,
including adolescents, STD patients and their contacts, commercial sex workers (CSWs)
and their clients, the military, students, long-distance truck drivers, and other migrant
labor. (See "Assessment and Prioritization of Actions to Prevent and Control Reproductive
Tract Infections in the Third World," by A. Ronald and S. O. Aral in this volume
regarding RTI interventions.) Methods of communication such as mass media, manuals for
primary and secondary schools, posters, and leaflets are important. However, since many
children drop out of school and adult illiteracy might be high (especially among women),
other methods of communication must also be used, such as radio messages, meetings,
discussions, drama, songs, and pictures. Religious and cultural sensitivities should be
considered, and both the groups of concern and community leaders should be involved in
the development of the messages.

Although the rapid spread of HIV infection has made the need to change sexual
behavior urgent,[64] skepticism prevails on the possibility of doing so, and to date results have
been mixed. For instance, among community leaders in Uganda, group health education
did not increase condom acceptability, which remained at about 40 percent. By contrast,
among military populations in Central Africa, STD/AIDS education was successful in
increasing condom use, which in turn led to decreased STD prevalence. Condom use also
increased significantly among CSWs in Nairobi following a health promotion and condom
distribution program.

Primary prevention of STDs is especially important, in order to decrease the risk of
STD acquisition during pregnancy. Health education and information concerning the
consequences of STDs in pregnancy should be directed to the community as a whole, with
special emphasis on those who are sexually active. Men should be made fully aware of their
role in protecting both nonpregnant and pregnant women against the risk of STDs. At the
first prenatal visit, the health worker should identify whether the pregnant woman is at
increased risk for having or acquiring an STD. A standard history on sexual behavior and
sexually transmitted diseases should be obtained, together with information on age,
socioeconomic status, marital status, health-care-seeking behavior, ethnicity, and so forth.

The information thus obtained should be used in counseling on how to avoid an STD. Women identified as being at higher risk are furthermore a priority group for screening for STDs.

Clinical STD Services/Prevention and Treatment. Adequate clinical management of STD cases encompasses detecting or ruling out disease, administering treatment if necessary, counseling the patient to prevent STDs by changing risky sexual behavior, advising the patient to comply with treatment, ensuring that the patient's sex partners are treated, and screening for other STD (including HIV) infection. While most of these services could be provided in primary health care settings—including maternal-child health (MCH) and family planning clinics—they are generally provided only in specialized clinics, which tend to be few, underfunded, and of limited quality. In most developing countries, STD referral is a severe problem. Therefore, practical, useful guidelines for simplified approaches to STD control, such as simple management protocols, are of utmost importance. Figure 2 outlines a protocol for managing lower abdominal pain.[65]

Counseling should be provided to individual STD patients and their partners. By definition, persons with an STD are at high risk for repeat infections and HIV because of their own or their partners' sexual behavior. Counseling should offer health education about lowering the risks of acquisition and transmission of STDs in a one-on-one, judgmental, confidential setting. This may also be a useful opportunity to provide other information on relevant topics, such as family planning. In addition, treatment of the sexual partners of STD-infected individuals is central to STD prevention and control. Such treatment not only prevents reinfection by their regular sexual partners, but also reduces the likelihood of further STD transmission throughout the population.

The ratio of male to female STD patients in curative services ranges from 2:1 to 10:1. Women are underrepresented among STD patients because the infection is less often symptomatic in them than in males. Furthermore, many psychological, cultural, and other barriers prevent women from using STD clinical services. For this reason, STD programs must actively reach out to women in order to control STDs in female populations, and health services for women—such as MCH and family planning services—should include STD prevention and control.

Clinical STD Services/Early Detection of STDs. Detection programs for STDs are usually designed to reach asymptomatic individuals. Therefore, laboratory tests should be available in sufficient quantity and must be checked regularly for quality of performance. Cost-effectiveness and possible operational problems should be evaluated before the introduction of routine STD detection programs. Cost-effectiveness of the detection program can be increased by concentrating on high-risk individuals, who can be identified on the basis of symptoms, clinical signs such as cervicitis, or an epidemiological risk profile. Among pregnant women in Nairobi, for example, risk factors for gonorrhea were being single and residing in a particular area of town.

Under certain circumstances—such as high prevalence of an STD, insufficient or nonexistent laboratory facilities, and highly mobile populations—mass treatment (i.e., treatment without diagnosis) of high-risk groups could be considered. Occasional or more regular mass treatment of CSWs for a number of STDs is done in some countries, but the strategy remains controversial, owing to insufficient data on its impact.

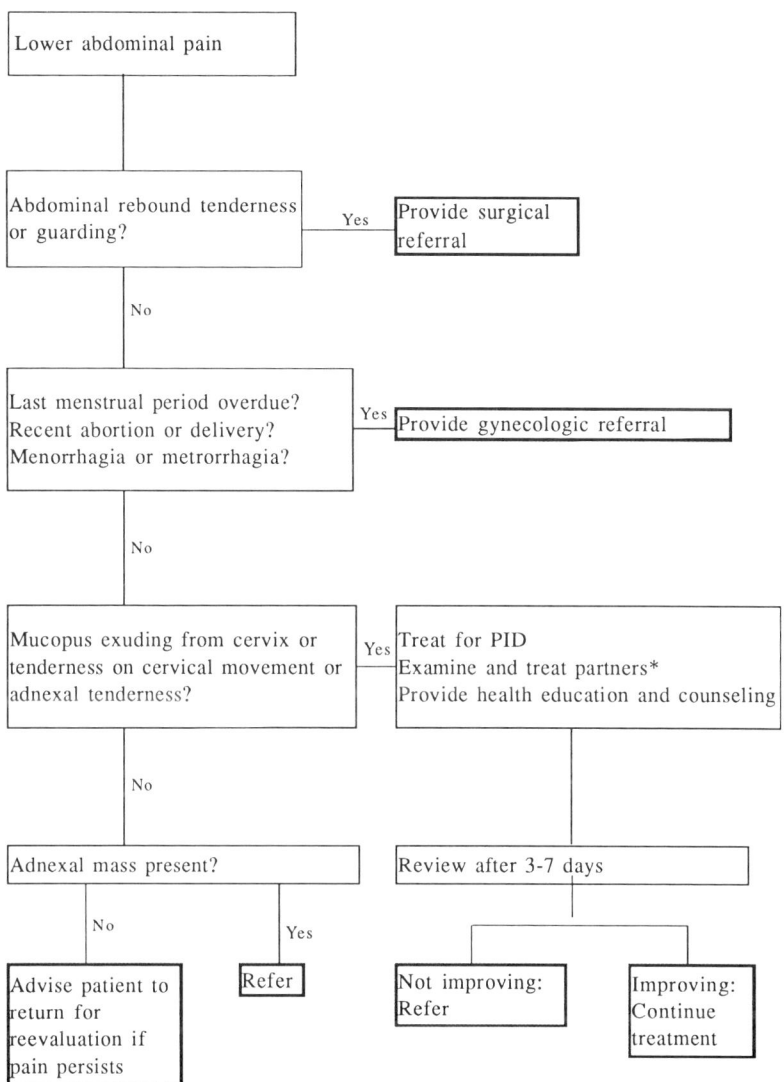

*In the absence of a confirmed diagnosis, the decision to notify partners should take into account local cultural and epidemiological factors.
Source: reference 65.

**Figure 2. Protocol for Managing Lower Abdominal Pain
(speculum and bimanual examination possible,
with or without microscopy)**

Obstetric care, family planning, and safe abortion services. Recommendations for these programs are covered extensively in "Family Planning: the Responsibility to Prevent Both Pregnancy and Reproductive Tract Infections," by W. Cates and K. M. Stone, and in "Maternal Health and Child Survival: Opportunities to Protect Both Women and Children from the Adverse Consequences of Reproductive Tract Infections," by K. F. Schulz, J. M. Schulte, and S. M. Berman, in this volume.

Research Needs

Further research on RTIs is urgently needed.[66] Research priorities must include both clinical and programmatic aspects of these infections, particularly in geographic areas in which data are currently lacking. Research should be designed to define the magnitude, microbiological spectrum, and epidemiology of RTIs in developing countries. Initially, this will require funding for the development of local clinical and laboratory resources so that reliable data can be collected to establish the incidence and prevalence of different types of RTIs and their effects on reproductive health.

As a large proportion of PID, infertility, and ectopic pregnancies can be attributed to previous RTIs, it follows that prevention and control of such infections is essential, and operations research is therefore needed to establish the best ways to combat them. Applied research is needed to develop simple, inexpensive methodologies to identify women who are at high risk of developing upper reproductive tract infection and who may require prophylactic treatment prior to delivery or induced abortion. Prophylactic intervention to reduce antepartum carriage of potential pathogens might well reduce the risk of sepsis following delivery.

Furthermore, research should be undertaken to develop techniques to diagnose ectopic pregnancies early and effectively, and interventions that guarantee, to the greatest degree possible, future fertility. The potential for fertility-sparing interventions will be greatly increased when early diagnosis is possible.

CERVICAL CANCER

Epidemiological studies, combined with recent biotechnological assessments, strongly suggest that cervical cancer is usually the result of a sexually transmitted infection, and HPV appears to be the causal agent. Carcinoma of the cervix is a major public health problem throughout the world. It is the second most common malignancy in women worldwide and the leading cancer in women in developing countries, where approximately 77 percent of the world's 460,000 new cases are found each year (see Table 9).[67,68] Within the developing world, highest incidence appears to cluster in Eastern and Middle Africa, the Caribbean, tropical South America, and parts of Asia (see Table 10).[69]

Cervical cancer is almost always fatal if it is not detected until an advanced, symptomatic stage. If detected early, it is nearly always curable by surgery or radiotherapy. Unfortunately, in the developing world, early detection is rare, and many women die needlessly. For example, malignant tumors are responsible for 25 percent of all deaths among women in Latin America; of those deaths, almost one fifth are due to cervical cancer.[70]

In contrast to most other cancers, which are frequent in older age groups, invasive cervical cancer is not more common among those over 50 years of age; this disease is thus an important cause of premature death.[71] All too often, it strikes down the mother in a family with many children in a poor socioeconomic situation, causing hardship far beyond its effects on the woman herself.

Cervical Cancer Risk

Infectious Etiology. Ever since it was noted more than one century ago that Catholic nuns were at very low risk for cervical cancer, it has been hypothesized that the disease might be caused by a sexually transmitted infectious agent. Numerous epidemiological

Table 9. Estimated Annual New Cases of Cervical Cancer, by Region

Region	New cases (x 1,000)
Africa	37
Latin America	44
China	132
India and other Asia	142
Subtotal: developing regions	354
Industrialized regions	105
Total: worldwide	459

Source: reference 67 and 68.

studies have been conducted on the frequency of cervical cancer in population groups with high or low risk of sexually transmitted infections to see if a relationship between such infections and cervical cancer or its precursor lesion could be found.

Studies in groups at high risk of sexually transmitted infections, for instance, showed that the prevalence of abnormal cervical smears is considerably higher in women seen at an STD clinic than in those presenting at a family planning clinic.[72] Mortality due to cervical cancer in England and Wales showed a decrease in women born between 1881 and 1911, but an increase in those born between 1911 and 1926. This difference might be due

Table 10. Estimated Crude Incidence Rate of Cervical Cancer,
Number of New Cases, and Relative Frequency in
Developing Countries, by Area, 1980

Area	Incidence (per 100,000 women)	New cases (x 1,000)	Relative frequency (% of all cancers in women)
Eastern Africa	23.3	16.8	31
Middle Africa	23.2	6.1	22
Northern Africa	15.1	8.1	18
Southern Africa	15.7	2.6	21
Western Africa	14.0	10.2	24
Caribbean	23.5	3.5	20
Central America	20.0	9.2	25
Temperate South America	22.9	4.9	10
Tropical South America	31.7	31.3	20
China	27.4	132.3	25
Other East Asia	33.0	10.4	29
Southeastern Asia	22.3	40.4	25
Southern Asia	19.9	91.2	25
Western Asia	4.0	1.9	5
Melanesia	25.9	0.5	27
Micronesia/Polynesia	15.4	0.1	18
Total developing areas		369.5	
Total worldwide		465.6	

Source: reference 69.

to more unstable sexual relations in the latter group of women, who reached adult age during World War II.[73] In populations at low risk of STDs, the prevalence of abnormal cervical smears is lower in lesbian women than in bisexual women, and the frequency of abnormal smears increases as bisexual women have more heterosexual experience.[74] The low incidence of cervical cancer in a number of religious groups, including Old Order Amish, Mormons, Seventh Day Adventists, and Orthodox Jews, has been attributed to their strictly monogamous marriages.[75-78]

HPV Infection. The evidence supporting a causal role for HPV in cervical cancer comes from multiple sources. DNA hybridization studies have shown that there are more than 50 types of HPV in humans.[79] HPV 6 and 11 are associated with genital warts and with mild premalignant cervical abnormalities called dysplasia.[80,81] HPV 16 and 18 are consistently associated with invasive cervical, vulvar, penile, and anal cancer, and with high grades of dysplasia.[81,82,83] HPV proteins have been found in a large proportion of biopsy specimens containing early malignant changes (cervical intraepithelial neoplasia).[84] About 10 percent of benign warts contain sequences of HPV 16 and 18, and some cancers contain sequences of HPV 11, 31, 33, and 35. Other nontyped HPV strains have also been found in some cervical cancers.[85]

The association found between HPV 16 and 18 and genito-anal cancer has been so consistent that these viruses are often called oncogenic types. Controversy remains, however. Although 5–20 percent of the adult population, both males and females, probably harbor HPV on the genital mucosa, and a large proportion of this is HPV 16 and 18, only a small fraction of infected people develop cervical or other genito-anal cancer. Furthermore, it is not well understood how an infection contracted most often in early adulthood leads to cervical cancer 10, 20, or 30 years later. The current consensus is that the progression of HPV-associated lesions into carcinomas most likely involves the activation or inactivation of some as yet unknown genes, possibly under the influence of cofactors such as tobacco smoking, other genital infections, and immunologic and other poorly understood factors.[86]

Infectious Agents Other than HPV. In most studies, a history of any sexually transmitted infection is associated with increased risk for cervical cancer, but such infections may simply be a proxy indicator for HPV infection or high-risk sexual behavior. During the past 20 years, much effort has gone into assessing herpes simplex virus type 2 (HSV-2) as a potential oncogenic virus for the cervix uteri. The suggestion that HSV-2 might play a role in cervical cancer was based mainly on serological studies showing a higher rate of antibodies to HSV in cervical cancer patients than in control groups. It is doubtful that HSV-2 by itself causes cancer. Rather, the virus may act as an initiator or promoter in the presence of another factor (the so-called hit-and-run hypothesis).[87,89] Chlamydial infections also have been shown to be associated with cervical cancer,[90] but an oncogenic role remains unproven.

Other Factors

Sexual and Contraceptive Behaviors. Various indicators of sexual activity have long been associated with cervical cancer. Early reports tended to emphasize marital status and reproductive history; in the early 1970s, the total number of sexual partners and age at first intercourse were identified as better indices.[91] Subsequently, it has been shown that number of sexual partners is the major independent risk factor for cervical cancer, whereas age at first intercourse is a confounder.[92–96]

The hypothesis that cervical cancer is an STD was reinforced by the finding that women who use barrier contraceptives have a much lower risk of cervical cancer[96,97,98] than

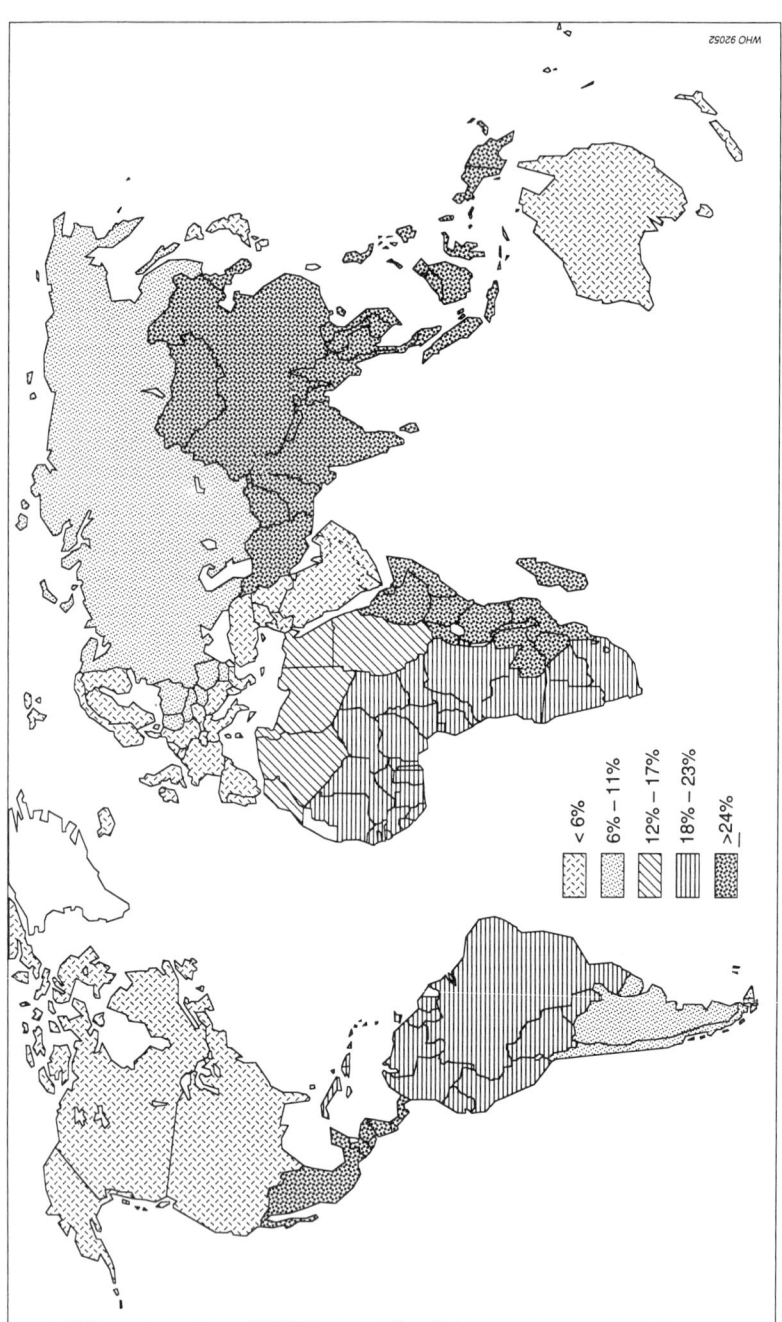

Note: The designations employed and the presentation of material on this map do not imply the expression of any opinion whatsoever on the part of the World Health Organization concerning the legal status of any country, territory, city, or area or of its authorities, or concerning the delimitation of its frontiers or boundries.
Source: reference 69.

Figure 3. Cervical Cancer as a Percentage of All Cancers in Women, 1980

Legend:
< 6%
6% – 11%
12% – 17%
18% – 23%
>24%

those who do not. In the United States, for example, Jewish women use the diaphragm as a contraceptive more frequently than other groups, which may explain their lower incidence of cervical cancer.[99] The protective effect of the diaphragm could be due to reduced exposure of the cervix to infectious agents or could reflect concurrent use of spermicides, which have antiviral properties.[100]

Studies on oral contraception and cervical neoplasia have in general been reassuring, but recent investigations show some evidence of an increased risk, particularly in long-term users.[101,102] Conclusions, however, are difficult because of the large number of confounding variables, especially sexual behavior.[103] While extensive evidence of the importance of women's sexual behavior in the etiology of cervical cancer exists, men's sexual behavior is also important. For example, some populations (e.g., in Latin America) have a high incidence of cervical cancer despite the fact that women have few sexual contacts.[104] Furthermore, husbands of women with cervical cancer have reported significantly more sexual partners and histories of sexually transmitted infection than husbands of women without the disease.[93,105,106]

Male Circumcision. Geographic differences in incidence and particularly the finding that the disease is rare in Jewish populations have led to the conclusion that circumcision of males, which enhances genital hygiene, protects women against cervical cancer.[107,108] A recent study from Denmark showed that wives of circumcised men had one third the risk for cervical cancer.[105] This conclusion, however, has been contradicted by data from different parts of the world: in Africa, incidence of cervical cancer is uniformly high, irrespective of differences in circumcision practices.[109,110] In Lebanon, incidence is comparable in circumcised Muslims and noncircumcised Christians.[111] In Fiji, incidence in native Fijians and Muslim Indians who are circumcised is comparable to that in Hindu Indians who are not.[112] The question therefore remains open.

Cigarette Smoking. In the last 15 years, cigarette smoking has emerged as an important etiologic factor for both preinvasive and invasive cervical cancer.[113] The excess risk for smokers is about twofold, with the highest risk generally found in long-term or heavy smokers. Studies have demonstrated the existence of high levels of tobacco-related carcinogens in the cervical mucus of smokers.[114] Furthermore, cigarette smoking could be a cofactor in the carcinogenicity of HPV.[87]

Reproductive and Immunological Factors. Evidence is growing that multiparity may increase the risk for cervical cancer.[115,116] Explanations for this effect could be cervical trauma during parturition and hormonal or nutritional influences of pregnancy. High rates of HPV have been found in pregnant women, and these are probably related to the effect of immunosuppression on viral activity.[117] HIV infection and the concomitant decline in immune function are associated with an increase in prevalence of HPV and progression of cervical lesions to malignancy.[118] In the next few years, an increase in incidence of cervical cancer can be expected as a consequence of the HIV pandemic.

Cervical Cancer: Program, Policy, and Research

It is possible that vaccines against HPV can be developed,[122] but the exact role of HPV as a factor in cervical cancer has to be better understood before that can happen. Cervical cancer therefore can be prevented only by decreasing risk factors in the community that lead to its development or by detecting the condition in an early stage through screening with a cervical smear (also called Pap smear). Reduction of risk factors requires changes in sexual behaviors that are difficult to achieve. Prevention programs in industrialized countries, based mainly on a cytology screening strategy have been highly successful in decreasing frequency and deaths from cervical cancer, but such programs are very rare in developing countries.[119]

Program Recommendations and Policy Implications

Prospects for primary prevention of cervical cancer are good, because epidemiological and experimental data have succeeded in identifying risk factors. Multiple sexual partners and early onset of sexual activity, by both males and females, are key behavioral risk factors. Therefore, information and education programs on the role of sexual behavior in cervical cancer and on the use of barrier contraceptives are strongly recommended, particularly for young people. The growing importance of incurable sexually transmitted infections, especially HIV infection, has greatly increased attention to health promotion and behavioral modification as methods for STD prevention.[120,121] The general principles for STD prevention, which also apply to HPV infection, are to promote safer sexual practices—namely, avoidance of multiple sex partners and casual sex; the use of barrier contraception, particularly condoms; and medical examination when lesions or other symptoms are noticed. At the same time, health education activities should strongly encourage people not to smoke.

The rationale for early detection (i.e., secondary prevention) is that the cure rate for cervical cancer is higher if the disease is detected during its preclinical phase than if it develops to an advanced stage. Invasive carcinoma evolves most often after a long period (10 years or more) of preinvasive disease. A Pap smear (exfoliative cytology) is a simple and sensitive method for detecting preinvasive cervical cancer. If adequately treated, preinvasive disease is virtually 100 percent curable through simple surgical procedures.[70] In industrialized countries, cytological screening has been implemented through nationwide programs.

The technology is relatively simple, and increased efforts for cervical cancer prevention can and should be implemented in developing countries. Operations research is urgently needed to determine how this can be most effectively done in a context of balanced health services development. A stepwise approach to screening implementation is recommended: (1) screen every woman between the ages of 35 and 40 years once in her lifetime; (2) if additional resources are available, screen women aged 35–55 every 10 years; (3) if greater resources are available, screen women aged 35–55 once every five years; (4) optimally, screen women aged 25–60 once every three years. A positive screening test or Pap smear has to be confirmed by a more elaborate test, most often a biopsy; if that test is positive, treatment should follow. Therefore, screening activities should be in tune with the development of diagnostic and treatment facilities for cervical cancer.

Research Needs

Important research issues related to the prevention of cervical cancer are as follows:

1. Applied and operations research are needed to develop appropriate and cost-effective screening strategies for developing countries, where the incidence of cancer of the cervix remains high and where resources for disease prevention and control are highly limited. The feasibility of downstage screening—i.e., visual inspection of the cervix by paramedical personnel in an attempt to find cases at an early stage—should be studied in those areas where cytological screening cannot yet be introduced. Studies should also determine why certain women do not seek screening and why resistance to screening exists in certain populations.

2. The exact role of HPV infections in cervical cancer, the natural history of these infections, and their interactions with host cells in the development of malignant tumors should be further studied, as should the contribution of other potentially carcinogenic factors (e.g., smoking, HSV-2 infections, exogenous hormones, mutagenic metabolites of bacteria, and protozoa in chronic inflammation) and their possible interaction with HPV.

3. The associations between sexual behavior and cervical cancer urgently need investigation in developing countries to ascertain whether multiple sexual partners and early onset of sexual intercourse are relevant risk factors in these settings, to increase understanding of why risky behaviors are undertaken, and to assess strategies to reduce these behaviors.

4. The protective value of existing barrier methods of contraception and of genital hygiene deserves further study, along with development of improved barrier methods, especially those that can be used by women without the knowledge or necessarily the cooperation of their partners.

5. The possible relationships between hormonal contraceptives and risk of cervical or other cancers should be further assessed.

6. The long-term effects of different methods of treatment of precancerous lesions and the optimal use of colposcopy and local ablation should be further investigated.

REFERENCES

1. Weström L, Mårdh P-A. Salpingitis. In: Holmes KK, Mårdh P-A, Sparling PF et al., eds. Sexually transmitted diseases, New York: McGraw-Hill, 1984:615–32.
2. Weström L. Incidence, prevalence and trends of acute pelvic inflammatory disease and its consequences in industrialized countries. Am J Obstet Gynecol 1980; 138:880–92.
3. Barbacci MB, Spence MR, Kappus EW, Burkman RC, Rao L, Quinn TC. Postabortal endometritis and isolation of Chlamydia trachomatis. Obstet Gynecol 1986; 68:686–90.
4. Osser S, Persson K. Postabortal pelvic infection associated with Chlamydia trachomatis and the influence of humoral immunity. Am J Obstet Gynecol 1984; 50:699–703.

5. Qvigstad E, Skang K, Jerve F, Fying P, Ulstrup JC. Pelvic inflammatory disease associated with Chlamydia trachomatis infection after therapeutic abortion. Br J Vener Dis 1983; 59:189–92.

6. Burkman RT, Tonascia JA, Atienza MF, King TM. Untreated endocervical gonorrhea and endometritis following elective abortion. Am J Obstet Gynecol 1976; 126:648–51.

7. Eschenbach DA, Buchanan TM, Pollock HM et al. Polymicrobial etiology of acute pelvic inflammatory disease. N Engl J Med 1975; 293:166–71.

8. Wasserheit JN, Bell TA, Kiviat NB et al. Microbial causes of proven pelvic inflammatory disease and efficacy of clindamycin and tobramycin. Ann Intern Med 1986; 104:187–93.

9. Weström L, Mårdh P-A. Acute pelvic inflammatory disease (PID). In: Holmes KK, Mårdh P-A, Sparling PF et al., eds. Sexually transmitted diseases, second edition, New York: McGraw-Hill, 1990:593–613.

10. Weström L. Effect of acute pelvic inflammatory disease on fertility. Am J Obstet Gynecol 1975; 121:707–13.

11. Wasserheit JN. The significance and scope of reproductive tract infections among third world women. Int J Gynaecol Obstet 1989; Suppl 3:145–68.

12. Carty MJ, Nzioki JM, Verhagen AR. The role of gonococcus in acute pelvic inflammatory disease in Nairobi. E Afr Med J 1972; 49:376–9.

13. Grech ES, Everett JV, Mukasa F. Epidemiological aspects of acute pelvic inflammatory disease in Uganda. Trop Doc 1973; 3:123–7.

14. Muir DG, Belsey MA. Pelvic inflammatory disease and its consequences in the developing world. Am J Obstet Gynecol 1980; 138:913–28.

15. Plummer FA, Laga M, Brunham RC et al. Postpartum upper genital tract infections in Nairobi, Kenya: epidemiology, etiology and risk factors. J Infect Dis 1987; 156:92–8.

16. Ratnam AV, Din SN, Chatterjee TK. Gonococcal infection in women with pelvic inflammatory disease in Lusaka, Zambia. Am J Obstet Gynecol 1980; 138:965–73.

17. Rosenberg MJ, Schulz KF, Burton N. Sexually transmitted diseases in sub-Saharan Africa. Lancet 1986; 2:152.

18. Meheus A, Reniers J, Coet M et al. Chlamydia trachomatis in women with acute salpingitis and infertility in Central Africa. In: Oriel D, Ridgway G, Schachter J, Taylor-Robinson D, Ward M, eds. Chlamydial infections. Proceedings of the sixth international symposium on human chlamydial infections, Cambridge University Press, 1986:241–4.

19. Mabey DCW, Ogbaselassie G, Robertson JN, Heckels JE, Ward ME. Tubal infertility in the Gambia: chlamydial and gonococcal serology in women with tubal occlusion compared with pregnant controls. Bull WHO 1985; 63:1107–13.

20. De Muylder X, Laga M, Tennstedt C, Van Dyck E, Aelbers GN, Piot P. The role of Neisseria gonorrhoeae and Chlamydia trachomatis in pelvic inflammatory disease and its sequelae in Zimbabwe. J Infect Dis 1990; 162:501–5.

21. Wertheim LJ, Abren A, Valdés-Vivo P. Problems and approaches in the surveillance and control of sexually transmitted diseases: the Cuban experience. Am J Obstet Gynecol 1980; 138:1082–7.

22. Eschenbach DA, Rosene K, Tompkins LS, Watkins H, Gravett MG. Endometrial cultures obtained by a triple-lumen method from afebrile and febrile postpartum women. J Infect Dis 1986; 153:1038–45.

23. World Health Organization. Maternal mortality: a global factbook, Geneva: World Health Organization 1991.

24. Mason PR, Katzenstein DA, Chimbira THK, Mtimavalye L, Puerperal Sepsis Study Group. Vaginal flora of women admitted to hospital with signs of sepsis following normal delivery, caesarian section or abortion. Cent Afr J Med 1989; 35:344–50.

25. Armon PJ. Maternal deaths in the Kilimanjaro region of Tanzania. Trans Roy Soc Med Hyg 1979; 73:284–8.

26. Caffrey KT. Maternal mortality: a continuing challenge in tropical practice. A report from Kaduna, northern Nigeria. East Afr Med J 1979; 56:274–7.

27. Mahokha AE. Maternal mortality: Kenyatta National Hospital 1972–1977. East Afr Med J 1980; 57:451–60.

28. Crowther CA. Maternal deaths at Harare Maternity Hospital during 1983. S Afr J Med 1986; 69:180–3.

29. Mason PR, Katzenstein DA, Chimbira THK, Mtimavalye L, Puerperal Sepsis Study Group. Microbial flora of the lower genital tract of women in labor at Harare Maternity Hospital. Cent Afr J Med 1989; 35:337–44.

30. Temmerman M, Laga M, Ndinya-Achola JO et al. Microbial aetiology and diagnostic criteria of postpartum endometritis in Nairobi, Kenya. Genitourin Med 1988; 64:172–5.

31. Perine PR, Duncan ME, Krause DW, Awoke S. Pelvic inflammatory disease and puerperal sepsis in Ethiopia. 1. Etiology. Am J Obstet Gynecol 1980; 138:969–73.

32. Cohen L, Veie JC, Calkins BM. Improved pregnancy outcome following successful treatment of chlamydial infection. JAMA 1990; 263:3160–3.

33. Venugopal MS, Bhaskaran CS. Puerperal and postabortal sepsis: a bacteriological study. J Obstet Gynecol India 1968; 18:70–8.

34. Lavaois P, Rioux JE, Côté L. Chlamydial infection among females attending an abortion clinic: prevalence and risk factors. Can Med Assoc J 1987; 137:33–7.

35. Nasah BT, Nguematcha R, Eyong M, Godwin S. Gonorrhoea, trichomonas and candida among gravid and nongravid women in Cameroun. Int J Gynaecol Obstet 1980; 18:48–52.

36. Chanduri P, Sng EH, Yuen WS. Chlamydia trachomatis infection in unmarried women seeking abortion. Genitourin Med 1986; 62:17–8.

37. Odujinrin OMT. Sexual activity, contraceptive practice and abortion among adolescents in Lagos. Int J Gynaecol Obstet 1991; 34:361–6.

38. Osinusi BO. The role of previous abortions on secondary infertility in Ibadan. J Obstet Gyn East Cent Afr 1986; 5:37–8.

39. Nichols D, Lapido OA, Paxman JM, Otolorin EO. Sexual behavior, contraceptive practice and reproductive health among Nigerian adolescents. Stud Fam Plann 1986; 17:100–6.

40. Nichols D, Woods ET, Gates DS, Sherman J. Sexual behavior, contraceptive practice, and reproductive health among Liberia adolescents. Stud Fam Plann 1987; 18:169–76.

41. Weström L. Pelvic inflammatory disease: bacteriology and sequelae. Contracept 1987; 36:111–28.

42. Cates W, Rolfs RT, Aral SO. Sexually transmitted diseases, pelvic inflammatory disease, and infertility: an epidemiologic update. Epidemiol Rev 1990; 12:199–220.

43. Frank O. Sterility in women in sub-Saharan Africa. IPPF Med Bull 1987; 21:6–8.

44. World Health Organization. Programme of research, development and research training in human reproduction, 1985, annual report, Geneva: World Health Organization, 1985.

45. Cates W, Farley TMM, Rowe PJ. Worldwide patterns of infertility: is Africa different? Lancet 1985; 2:596–8.

46. Marchbanks PA, Annegers JF, Coulam CB, Strathy JH, Kurland LT. Risk factors for ectopic pregnancy: a population-based study. JAMA 1988; 259:1823–7.

47. Thorburn J, Bernstsson C, Philipson M, Lindblom B. Background factors of ectopic pregnancy. I. Frequency distribution in a case-control study. Eur J Obstet Gynecol Reprod Biol 1986; 23:321–31.

48. Thorburn J, Philipson M, Lindblom B. Background factors of ectopic pregnancy. II. Risk estimation by means of a logistic model. Eur J Obstet Gynecol Reprod Biol 1986; 23:333–40.

49. Chow JM, Yonekura ML, Richwald GA, Greenland S, Sweet RL, Schachter J. The association between Chlamydia trachomatis and ectopic pregnancy. A matched-pair, case-control study. JAMA 1990; 263:3191–2.

50. Kihlstrom E, Lindgren R, Ryden G. Antibodies to Chlamydia trachomatis in women with infertility, pelvic inflammatory disease and ectopic pregnancy. Eur J Obstet Gynecol Reprod Biol 1990; 35:199–204.

51. Tuomivaara LM. Ectopic pregnancy and genital infections: a case-control study. Ann Med 1990; 22:21–4.

52. Miettinen A, Heinonen PK, Teisala K, Hakkarainen K, Punnonen R. Serologic evidence for the role of Chlamydia trachomatis, Neisseria gonorrhoeae, and Mycoplasma hominis in the etiology of tubal factor infertility and ectopic pregnancy. Sex Transm Dis 1990; 17:10–4.

53. Weström L, Bengtsson LPH, Mårdh P-A. Incidence, trends, and risks of ectopic pregnancy in a population of women. Br Med J 1981; 282:15–8.

54. Daisley H. Ectopic pregnancies in Trinidad. A clinico-pathological study of 154 consecutive surgically treated cases. West Indian Med J 1989; 38:222–7.

55. Picaud A, Nlome Nze AR, Ogowet Igumu N, Faye A, Loundou J. La grossesse extra-utérine. Etude de 509 cas traités chirurgicalement au CHU de Librevie. J Gynécol Obstét Biol Reprod (Paris) 1989; 18:714–20.

56. Lindow SW, Moore PJ. Ectopic pregnancy: analysis of 100 cases. Int J Gynaecol Obstet 1988; 27:371–5.

57. Oransaye U. Reproductive performance among patients with ectopic pregnancy. Nig Med J 1979; 9:247–51.

58. Centers for Disease Control. Ectopic pregnancies—United States 1987; MMWR 1990; 39 (24):401–4.

59. Johnsen HM, Becker-Christensen F. Ectopic pregnancy in Greenland. An epidemiological study. Arctic Med Res 1990; 49:43–7.

60. Olatunbosun OA, Okonufua FE. Ectopic pregnancy—the African experience. Postgrad Doct Afr 1986; 8:74–8.

61. World Health Organization. Maternal health and safe motherhood programme, 1990. Unpublished data, Geneva.

62. Makinen JI, Salmi TA, Nikkanen VP, Koskinen EY. Encouraging rates of fertility after ectopic pregnancy. Int J Fertil 1989; 34:46–51.

63. Ogunniyi SO, Faleyimu BL. Fertility after ectopic pregnancy in an African population. Int J Gynaecol Obstet 1989; 30:245–8.

64. Meheus A, Schulz KF, Cates W. Development of prevention and control programs for sexually transmitted diseases in developing countries. In: Holmes KK, Mårdh P-A, Sparling PF et al., eds. Sexually transmitted diseases, second edition, New York: McGraw-Hill, 1990:1041–6.

65. World Health Organization. Management of patients with sexually transmitted diseases, WHO, Technical Reports Series 810, Geneva: World Health Organization, 1991.

66. Expert Committee on Pelvic Inflammatory Disease. Pelvic inflammatory disease—research directions in the 1990s. Sex Transm Dis 1991; 18:46–64.

67. Stanley K, Stjernswärd J, Koroltchouk V. Women and cancer. World Health Stat Quart 1987; 40:267–78.

68. Standaert B, Meheus A. Le cancer du col utérin en Afrique. Méd Afr Noire 1985; 32:407–15.

69. Parkin DM, Läärä E, Muir CS. Estimates of the worldwide frequency of sixteen major cancers in 1980. Int J Cancer 1988; 32:407–15.

70. WHO Meeting. Control of cancer of the cervix uteri. Bull WHO 1986; 64:607–18.

71. Muir CS, Waterhouse J, Mack T, Powell J, Lohelan S. Cancer incidence in five continents. IARC Scientific Publications, No. 88, Lyon: IARC, 1988.

72. Briggs RM, Holmes KK, Kiviat N, Barker E, Eschenbach DA, DeJong R. High prevalence of cervical dysplasia in STD clinic patients warrants routine cytologic screening. Am J Public Health 1980; 70:1212–4.

73. Hill GB, Adelstein AM. Cohort mortality from carcinoma of the cervix. Lancet 1967; 2:606–7.

74. Johnson SR, Smith EM, Guenther SM. Comparison of gynecologic health care problems between lesbian and bisexual women. J Reprod Med 1987; 32:805–11.

75. Cross HE, Kennel EE, Lilienfeld AM. Cancer of the cervix in an Amish population. Cancer 1968; 21:102–8.

76. Larsson E, Webb AT. Cancer survey: experiences in mass screening of cervical smears. Obstet Gynecol 1963; 22:630–5.

77. Lyon JL, Klauber MR, Gardner JW, Smart CR. Cancer incidence in Mormons and non-Mormons in Utah, 1966–1970. N Engl J Med 1976; 294:129–33.

78. Boyd JT, Do R. A study of the aetiology of carcinoma of the cervix uteri. Br J Cancer 1964; 18:419–34.

79. Lancaster WD, Norrild B. Diagnosis of HPV by DNA hybridization techniques. In: Munoz N, Bosch FX, Jensen OM, eds. Human papilloma virus and cervical cancer. IARC Scientific Publications, No. 94, Lyon: IARC, 1989.

80. McCance DJ, Walker PG, Dyson J, Coleman DV, Singer A. Presence of human papilloma virus DNA sequences in cervical intraepithelial neoplasia. Br Med J 1983; 287:784–8.

81. Zur Hausen H. Papilloma viruses and human cancer. Cancer 1987; 59:1692–6.

82. McCance DJ, Kalache K, Ashdown K, Andrade-Menezes F, Smith P, Do R. Human papilloma virus type 18 in carcinoma of the penis in Brazil. Int J Cancer 1986; 37:55–60.

83. Crum CP, Ikenberg H, Richart RM, Gissmann L. Human papilloma virus type 16 and early cervical neoplasia. N Engl J Med 1984; 310:880–3.

84. Walker PG, Singer A, Dyson JL, Shah KV, To A, Coleman DV. The prevalence of human papilloma virus antigen in patients with cervical intraepithelial neoplasia. Br J Cancer 1983; 48:99–101.

85. Editorial. Human papilloma viruses and cervical cancer: a fresh look at the evidence. Lancet 1987; 1:725–6.
86. World Health Organization. Genital human papilloma virus infections and cancer: memorandum from a WHO meeting. WHO Bull 1987; 65:817–27.
87. zur Hausen H. Human genital cancers: synergism between two virus infections or synergism between a virus infection and initiating events? Lancet 1982; 2:1370–2.
88. Galloway DA, McDougall JK. The oncogenic potential of herpes simplex viruses: evidence for a "hit-and-run" mechanism. Nature 1983; 302:21–4.
89. Iwasaka T, Yokoyama M, Hayashi Y, Sugimori H. Combined herpes simplex virus type 2 and human papilloma virus type 16 or 18 deoxyribonucleic acid leads to oncogenic transformation. Am J Obstet Gynecol 1988; 159:1251–52.
90. Schachter J: Chlamydial infection. N Engl J Med 1978; 298:490–5.
91. Rotkin ID. A comparison review of key epidemiological studies in cervical cancer related to current searches for transmissible agents. Cancer Res 1973; 22:1353–67.
92. Harris RCW, Brinton LA, Cowde RH et al. Characteristics of women with dysplasia or carcinoma in situ of the cervix uteri. Br J Cancer 1980; 42:359–69.
93. Buckley JD, Harris RCW, Do R, Vessey MP, Williams PT. Case-control study of the husbands of women with dysplasia or carcinoma of the cervix uteri. Lancet 1981; 2:1010–5.
94. Cuzick J, De Stavola B, McCance D et al. A case-control study of cervix cancer in Singapore. Br J Cancer 1989; 60:238–43.
95. Reeves WC, Brinton LA, Brenes MM, Quiroz E, Rawls WE, De Britton RC. Case-control study of cervical cancer in Herrera Province, Republic of Panama. Int J Cancer 1985; 36:55–60.
96. Slattery ML, Robison LM, Schuman KL et al. Cigarette smoking and exposure to passive smoke as risk factors for cervical cancer. JAMA 1989; 261:1593–8.
97. Richardson AC, Lyon JB. The effect of condom use on squamous cell cervical intraepithelial neoplasia. Am J Obstet Gynecol 1981; 140:909–13.
98. Wright NH, Vessey MP, Kenward B, McPherson K, Do R. Neoplasia and dysplasia of the cervix uteri and contraception: a possible protective effect of the diaphragm. Br J Cancer 1978; 38:273–9.
99. Hendershot GE. Coitus-related cervical cancer risk factors: trends and differentials in racial and religious groups. Am J Public Health 1983; 73:299–301.
100. Hildesheim A, Brinton LA, Main K et al. Barrier and spermicial contraceptive methods and risk of invasive cervical cancer. Epidemiol 1990; 1:266–72.
101. Beral V, Hannaford P, Kay C. Oral contraceptive use and malignancies of the genital tract. Results from the Royal College of General Practitioners' Oral Contraception Study. Lancet 1988; 2:1331–5.
102. Brinton LA, Huggins GR, Lehman HF et al. Long-term use of oral contraceptives and risk of invasive cervical cancer. Int J Cancer 1986; 38:339–44.
103. Brinton LA. Oral contraceptives and cervical neoplasia. Contracept 1991; 43:581–95.
104. Skegg DCG, Corwin PA, Paul C, Do R. Importance of the male factor in cancer of the cervix. Lancet 1982; 2:581–3.
105. Kjaer SK, de Villiers EM, Dahl C et al. Case-control study of risk factors for cervical neoplasia in Denmark. I: Role of the "male factor" in women with one lifetime sexual partner. Int J Cancer 1991; 48:39–44.
106. Zunzunegui MV, King MC, Coria CF, Charlet J. Male influences on cervical cancer risk. Am J Epidemiol 1986; 123:302–307.

107. Kennaway EL. The racial and social incidence of cancer of the uterus. Br J Cancer 1948; 2:177–212.
108. Wynder EL. Environmental factors in cervical cancer: an approach to its prevention. Br Med J 1955; 1:743–7.
109. Megafu U. Cancer of the genital tract among Ibo women in Nigeria. Cancer 1979; 44:1875–8.
110. Dodge OG, Linse CA, Davies JNP. Circumcision and the incidence of carcinoma of the penis and the cervix. East Afr Med J 1963; 40:440–4.
111. Abou-Daoud. Epidemiology of carcinoma of the cervix uteri in Lebanese Christians and Moslems. Cancer 1967; 20:1706–14.
112. Boyd JT, Do R, Gurd CH. Cancer incidence in Fiji. Int J Epidemiol 1973; 2:177–8.
113. Winkelstein W Jr. Smoking and cervical cancer—current status: a review. Am J Epidemiol 1990; 131:945–57.
114. Schiffman MH, Haley NJ, Felton JS et al. Biochemical epidemiology of cervical neoplasia: measuring cigarette smoke constituents in the cervix. Cancer Res 1987; 47:3886–88.
115. Parizzini F, La Vecchia C, Negri E, Cecchetti G, Fedele L. Reproductive factors and the risk of invasive and intraepithelial cervical neoplasia. Br J Cancer 1989; 59:805–9.
116. Brinton LA, Reeves WC, Brenes MM et al. Parity as a risk factor for cervical cancer. Am J Epidemiol 1989; 130:486–96.
117. Schneider V, Kay S, Lee HM. Immunosuppression as a high risk factor in the development of condyloma acuminata and squamous neoplasia of the cervix. Acta Cytol 1983; 27:220–4.
118. Byrne MA, Taylor-Robinson D, Munday PE, Harris JRW. The common occurrence of human papilloma virus infection and intraepithelial neoplasia in women infected by HIV. AIDS 1989; 3:379–82.
119. Devesa SS, Young JL Jr, Brinton LA, Fraumeni JF Jr. Recent trends in cervix uteri cancer. Cancer 1989; 64:2184–90.
120. World Health Organization. Sixth report of the WHO Expert Committee on Venereal Diseases and Treponematoses, WHO Technical Reports, Series 736, Geneva: World Health Organization, 1986.
121. World Health Organization meeting. Prevention and control of sexually transmitted diseases/acquired immuno-deficiency syndrome in young people, Geneva: World Health Organization, 1987.
122. McCance DJ. A vaccine to genital papilloma viruses: is it feasible? In: Meheus A, Spier R, eds. Vaccines for sexually transmitted diseases, London: Butterworths, 1989; 147–65.

FAMILY PLANNING: THE RESPONSIBILITY TO PREVENT BOTH PREGNANCY AND REPRODUCTIVE TRACT INFECTIONS

Willard Cates, Jr., M.D., M.P.H.
Director, Division of Training
Epidemiology Program Office

Katherine M. Stone, M.D.
Clinical Research Investigator
Division of STD/HIV Prevention

Centers for Disease Control
1600 Clifton Road, Mailstop EO2
Atlanta, GA 30333

INTRODUCTION

Using contraception has two main benefits: prevention of unplanned pregnancy and protection against reproductive tract infections (RTIs).[1-4] But technology development, policy emphasis, and service delivery have focused almost solely on preventing pregnancy, with little attention paid to reducing RTIs. Abstinence from sexual intercourse provides nearly absolute protection against both outcomes. For those choosing to be sexually active, contraception reduces, but does not eliminate, the risk of either pregnancy or RTIs. Unfortunately, the contraceptives with the best record for pregnancy prevention provide minimal RTI protection. Some contraceptives may even raise the risk of certain infections. Thus, decisions about contraception by individuals, communities, and policymakers should involve balancing the relative need to prevent both RTIs and unplanned pregnancy.

At the personal level, contraceptive *use* by couples is affected by the perceived risks and costs of either RTIs or pregnancy.[5,6] These involve such complex individual factors as partner selection, coital frequency, timing of coitus within the menstrual cycle, safety of the contraceptive method, availability of the method, cost of the method, and acceptance of the method by the sex partner.[7,8,9]

At the community level, contraceptive *acceptance* is affected by the social norms of particular cultures. This involves such complex community factors as the relative value of fertility within specific societies,[10,11] local customs about sexual activities at early ages,

Reproductive Tract Infections, Edited by A. Germain *et al.*
Plenum Press, New York, 1992

community pressures on teenagers to bear children, societal norms about genital manipulation, and religious proscriptions against use of particular contraceptives.

At the policy level, contraceptive *emphasis* by policymakers is affected by the aggregate risk and costs of RTIs and unplanned pregnancy in that particular society.[8,9,12–14] These involve such complex public health factors as the local prevalence of RTIs and unplanned pregnancy, the level of unprotected sexual activity, the political acceptance of individual choice over sexual and reproductive decisions, and the economic capacity of the society to support the existing population growth rate. To date, most national and international contraceptive policies have tended to downplay the risks of RTIs relative to those of unplanned pregnancy.

The situation is further complicated when considering the longer-range reproductive implications of contraception. Contraceptive use has an influence not only on the acute risks of RTIs and unplanned pregnancy, but also on the eventual reproductive capacity of those making contraceptive decisions. Therefore, personal choices, community programs, or policy decisions made in the short run to prevent RTIs and unplanned pregnancy can simultaneously improve or harm chances of planned procreation in the long run.[15]

This background paper explores similarities and differences between the fields of RTIs and unplanned pregnancy, examines the scientific evidence of contraceptive influence on RTIs, presents estimates of the relative effectiveness of different contraceptive methods in preventing unplanned pregnancy and RTIs, and recommends areas where sexually transmitted disease (STD) control and family planning programs might build on each other's efforts.

RTIs AND UNPLANNED PREGNANCY—SIMILARITIES

The health conditions of RTIs and unplanned pregnancy resemble each other in a variety of ways. First, sexual contact, usually intercourse, is necessary for the transmission of both. Thus, behavioral lessons learned about how to modify unsafe sexual practices can be applied to reducing the risks of both RTIs and unplanned pregnancy. Recent worldwide attention paid to preventing human immunodeficiency virus (HIV) infection has led to behavioral research investments at both the community and the individual levels that provide spinoff opportunities for simultaneously preventing RTIs and unplanned pregnancy.[1,16]

Second, both RTIs and unplanned pregnancy discriminate biologically against women. Anatomic differences make RTIs more easily transmissible to, yet more difficult to diagnose in, women;[17] for example, the diagnosis of vaginal discharge is more difficult than that of urethral discharge.[18] STDs are more frequently asymptomatic in women than in men, and clinical symptoms are more subtle in women. Even worse, the long-term complications in women are far more common and serious.[17] Salpingitis is more frequent than its male counterparts, epididymitis and prostatitis.[19–21] This intrinsic gender breakdown also exists with unplanned pregnancy; women obviously bear the entire burden of the health risks associated with it.

Third, those concerned with both RTIs and unplanned pregnancy must contend with the power imbalance between genders that favors men. In some cultures, women frequently have little say about when, with whom, and under what conditions sexual relations occur.[17,22] This situation influences whether any preventive measures are used against RTIs, unplanned pregnancy, or both. Moreover, in many societies where the woman's status depends on her role as a wife and a mother, she is expected to bear children and is ostracized if she does not or cannot.[22] Where RTIs impair her ability to reproduce, a cruel paradox results.

Fourth, the groups most likely to be affected by RTIs and unplanned pregnancy are remarkably similar. Those younger than 25 have the highest levels of STDs and unintended pregnancies. For example, this age group accounts for two thirds of both the reported gonorrhea cases[23] and the legally induced abortions[24] in the developed countries. Also, those with lower incomes have higher rates of both STDs and unintended conceptions, even after one controls for the effects of age.[25] A similar socioeconomic profile exists in the developing world for these conditions. Thus, the poor represent those at greatest risk for both sexually transmitted infections and unplanned pregnancies around the globe.

RTIs AND UNPLANNED PREGNANCY—DIFFERENCES

While similarities might create a bond between those interested in STDs and those whose focus is unplanned pregnancy, important differences between these two conditions drive them apart (Table 1). First, compared with the proportion of individuals able to achieve pregnancy, a relatively small percentage of men and women in most communities are capable of transmitting STDs at any one time; depending on the STD battery of diagnostic tests, fewer than one in five members of the general population will be infected at any time, and thus be capable of bacterial STD transmission.[26] Only in selected communities, or with more prevalent viral STDs, do STDs exceed this level. However, a vastly different situation exists for unplanned pregnancy. In most areas of the world, over nine in 10 men and women under age 35 years are fertile, and thus capable of conception.[27]

Table 1. Differences between RTIs and Unplanned Pregnancy

Characteristic	RTIs	Unplanned pregnancy
Percentage susceptible	20%	90%
Transmission risk per coital event	Male, 60% Female, 30%	0–20%
Prevention focus	Partner selection	Coital frequency
Basic science focus	Microbiologic	Physiologic
Treatment	Antibiotics	Hormones, surgery
Approach to patient	Directive	Nondirective
Gender focus in clinics	Male	Female
Health care emphasis	Crisis (symptomatic)	Preventive (asymptomatic)
Type of contact for transmission	Genital contact, discharge	Spermatozoa

Second, for each coital episode, the risk of transmitting a bacterial lower genital tract infection is much higher than the chance of producing a pregnancy. If the man is infected, he transmits gonorrhea to a susceptible female approximately two thirds of the time;[28] if the woman is infected, she transmits the organism to a susceptible male approximately one third of the time.[29] Other sexually transmitted bacterial organisms probably have slightly lower risks of transmission per given sexual act.[30] However, the rate of "transmitting" pregnancy is markedly lower. Depending upon the timing of intercourse within the woman's cycle, the likelihood of pregnancy is 0–20 percent.[31] The probability of pregnancy is greatest if intercourse occurs the day before ovulation. Even then, the woman's risk of becoming *pregnant* from a coital act is approximately one quarter that of becoming *infected* if her partner has gonorrhea.

Third, the first two concepts combine to create different foci for prevention, depending on whether the major concern is reducing RTIs or unplanned pregnancies. Those interested in designing interventions to prevent RTIs care primarily about with *whom* the intercourse occurs; those concerned with unplanned pregnancy count *how many times* and *when* intercourse takes place. From the STDs standpoint, if an infected partner is chosen, the risk of transmission is relatively high. Thus, the number and choice of sexual partners are key behavioral parameters.[32] From the family planning standpoint, the number of *partners* is less important than the number of *times* unprotected intercourse occurs. Because such a high percentage of people are capable of "transmitting" pregnancy, the low risk of becoming pregnant per act of intercourse becomes cumulatively quite high if coitus is frequent throughout the menstrual cycle. This basic difference between STDs and family planning in their behavioral prevention focus creates a subtle philosophic hurdle that hinders communication.

Fourth, the primary researchers in both disciplines have different backgrounds. The basic science focus of those interested in RTIs is microbiology, whereas for those interested in family planning, it is physiology. Scientific advances on the STDs frontier have been made by developing new technologies for diagnosing infections, discovering new antimicrobials to more effectively treat infections, and introducing new vaccines for primary prevention. Advances on the family planning frontier have been largely endocrinologic: the amino acid sequencing of peptide hormones, the identification of opiate receptors in the brain, and the development of new antiprogestin analogues to control human reproductive function are all examples of contraceptive breakthroughs.[33] The major scientific meetings that the two groups attend are also vastly different. Thus, little scientific overlap or exchange exists between the two groups. Without a common scientific arena, it is not unusual that relatively few efforts have been made to promote a common discipline.

Fifth, as clinical entities, STDs and unplanned pregnancies have different treatment approaches. For bacterial STDs, antibiotic therapy is usually indicated. In situations such as pelvic inflammatory disease (PID), in which the long-term consequences are serious and the causative microorganisms are polymicrobial, broad-spectrum antibiotic coverage is recommended.[34] Unplanned pregnancies are treated either hormonally (postcoital estrogens, RU-486 in early pregnancy) or surgically (induced abortion) if women seek termination.

Sixth, those in the RTIs and family planning fields differ in their fundamental approach to patients in particular, and to public health in general. With couples desiring to prevent unplanned pregnancies, the family planning provider will ideally present the benefits and risks of the different contraceptives in a *nondirective* manner and counsel the couple to choose that method most in line with their values.[35] Family planning clients are usually assumed to be healthy and are being supported to take preventive action. With patients diagnosed as having an STD, the counseling is more directive, since the person is already infected. Not only are STD patients educated about the nature and prognosis of their infection, but they are also *directively* counseled[36] to take their medicines as prescribed, to abstain from sexual intercourse until therapy is completed, and to use condoms in any high-risk sexual settings. Simultaneously, STD patients are coached in methods of notifying their sex partners, and if they so desire, they are offered provider referral services to get their partners treated.[36] Thus, while the fundamental goal of *birth* control providers is to provide information that helps individuals or couples choose their method of contraception, the objective of *infection* control personnel is to prevent transmission of the organism within the community, as well as to cure the patient.

Seventh, those providing clinical care for persons seeking STD or family planning services differ in their gender focus. Nearly all types of clinical facilities providing contraception serve women as their primary constituency.[37] This occurs in both the developed and the developing worlds. By contrast, most persons seeking care for RTIs are men: in the developed world, approximately two thirds of the patients receiving care in STD clinics are male; in the developing world, over 90 percent of those receiving treatment for clinical RTIs are men.[38] These gender differences affect the attitude toward, and the staffing patterns of, the two types of facilities.

Eighth, the health care emphasis between the two fields is vastly different. Those providing family planning services deal with asymptomatic clients, who are seeking preventive services in a proactive manner. The family planning clients, realizing they are sexually active and at risk of unplanned pregnancy, have already made decisions to reduce their risks; thus, they are seeking contraceptive methods that best fit their personal circumstances. Moreover, because the emphasis is on prevention, clinic staffing patterns can be planned for, allowing the best use of personnel, space, and time. However, with care for STDs, the situation is much more crisis-oriented. Most patients seek medical services either because they are symptomatic or because they have been screened and found to be infected. Therefore, the urgency of diagnosis and treatment is important both to the individual and to the community. In addition, the demand for such services is unpredictable, being based on the level of infection within the community and the degree of screening emphasized by public health authorities. Thus, in the midst of this "crisis" mentality, clinicians serving in STD clinics are less likely to tolerate the time-consuming preventive counseling messages.

Ninth, the conditions of unplanned pregnancy and STDs are spread by slightly different methods of genital contact. Unplanned pregnancy requires that active spermatozoa be deposited in the vagina. However, depending on the particular organism, STDs can be transmitted by genital contact alone (e.g., genital ulcers) or by genital discharge (e.g., gonorrhea, chlamydia, trichomonas) devoid of any sperm. Thus, while pregnancy requires ejaculation to take place, mere genital contact, even without ejaculation, can transmit STDs.

EFFECTS OF RTIs ON CONTRACEPTIVE USE

At the individual level, the impact of RTIs on the family planning practitioner depends on whether the infection is symptomatic or asymptomatic, whether the infection is curable, and what STD services are available from the contraceptive provider. If the RTI is symptomatic, it should be diagnosed and treated during the same patient visit in which contraceptive services are requested.[35] If no symptoms are present, the visit by sexually

active women to family planning providers offers the opportunity to screen for asymptomatic infections that can be treated in the lower genital tract before they result in
complications. If the patient has a history of RTIs, this should trigger both screening for
current RTIs and counseling regarding safer sexual practices to reduce future risks of
becoming infected. Finally, additional contraceptive methods should be encouraged that
have the greatest influence on reducing future RTIs, even though these methods may be
less effective in preventing pregnancy (see next section).

At the community level, some hypothesize that RTIs may have a negative impact on
family planning programs.[39] High prevalence of RTIs can serve to decrease acceptance or
continuation of family planning methods in two ways: the first way is directly—an RTI, if
perceived as a "side effect" of contraceptive methods, may result in nonuse or discontinuation of the methods. For example, in Nigeria, trends in oral contraceptive use were directly
related to adverse publicity about its alleged risks, including infection. The second way is
indirectly—an RTI, by compromising healthy childbearing in a community, may hinder any
willingness to delay initial childbearing or to space live births.[39] These direct and indirect
perceptions of RTIs must be overcome by effective community health education programs
and by improvements in the quality of family planning services, so that provision and use
of health services to reduce RTIs will be regarded as essential for ensuring a healthy
reproductive future.

EFFECTS OF CONTRACEPTIVE USE ON RTIs

The recent scientific literature has been replete with reviews of the effects of different
contraceptives on the risk of RTIs.[1,2,40–46] In general, they all come to the same conclusion—condoms alone, spermicides alone, and combinations of mechanical and chemical
methods all provide good protection against most RTIs. The impact of hormonal
contraception on RTIs is still unsettled. The IUD appears harmful, especially during the
interval after its insertion.

Our summary of the contraceptive and RTI literature has revised and updated tables
available in previously published reviews. We have arranged the evidence in chronologic
order, by strength of study design,[47] from weakest to strongest. In general, descriptive or
cross-sectional designs are most vulnerable to methodologic problems, with case-control
studies, cohort investigations, and randomized clinical trials ascending in their scientific
strength. Nonetheless, no study is perfect; thus, we must examine the consistency of
evidence in toto to assess our current state of knowledge.

Condoms

Condom quality, use, and effectiveness have been recently reviewed.[48] If men are
willing to use them properly, condoms protect against transmission of STDs by preventing
direct contact with semen, genital discharge, some genital lesions, and infectious secretions.
To be effective, condoms must be applied prior to genital contact, must remain intact, and,
most important, must be used *consistently and correctly*.[49]

A growing number of laboratory studies confirm that condoms provide an impervious
barrier to most STD pathogens. In experimental transmission models, condoms have been
shown to be effective barriers against herpes simplex virus (HSV),[50,51] *Chlamydia
trachomatis*,[50] cytomegalovirus,[52] and HIV.[53]

"Natural membrane" condoms, made of sheep intestinal membrane, may not be as effective as synthetic condoms. Latex condoms have been reported to be impermeable to high concentrations of hepatitis B surface antigen (HBsAg) particles, while natural membrane condoms are not.[54] The larger intact virus particle (HBV) passed through natural membrane condoms as well.[55] This permeability may relate to the size of pores in the intestinal membranes. HIV and HSV may also pass through natural membrane condoms.[56,57] Thus, limited data suggest that natural membrane condoms may offer less protection than latex condoms, but no empirical evidence exists to evaluate natural membrane condoms in practice.

In human studies, condoms have been found to protect men against *Neisseria gonorrhoeae* and *Ureaplasma urealyticum* infection (Table 2). In an Irish cross-sectional study of men attending an STD clinic for the first time, condom users were less likely to be infected with gonorrhea than were nonusers.[58] Among asymptomatic college men in Boston, regular use of condoms afforded significant protection against colonization with *Ureaplasma urealyticum*; this effect persisted despite the number of sex partners.[59] A similar study from England[60] showed an even stronger protection against gonorrhea.

Three cohort studies have also reported that men receive a protective effect from using condoms (Table 2). Among Australian soldiers returning from Vietnam, those who had used condoms were significantly less likely to report having had an STD than were those who had not;[61] however, substantial methodologic flaws limit the utility of this study. In the Philippines,[29] no seamen who reported using condoms while in port acquired gonorrhea.

Table 2. Efficacy of Condom Use in Preventing STDs in Men

Study location and publication year	Study design	Study population	Outcome	Measure of effect	95% confidence interval
Belfast, 1972[58]	Cross-sectional	Males, STD clinic	Urethral gonorrhea	0.51	0.33–0.80
Massachusetts, 1973[59]	Cross-sectional	Male college volunteers	Urethral (U. urealyticum)	0.33	0.16–0.68
London, 1977[60]	Cross-sectional	Males, STD clinic	Urethral gonorrhea	0.25	0.11–0.59
Vietnam, 1974[61]	Cohort	Australian soldiers	Self-reported STD	0.00	
Philippines, 1978[29]	Cohort	Naval crewman	Urethral gonorrhea	0.00	
California, 1989[62]	Cohort	Males, STD clinic	Urethral gonorrhea	0.34	0.10 1.13

Source: updated from reference 1.

In Sacramento, California,[62] men attending an STD clinic were given free condoms, then examined three months later. Those who always used condoms had less risk of gonorrhea than did men who never used them. Although traditional statistical significance was not achieved, these data, taken together, are consistent with an increasing body of knowledge indicating that condoms are protective.

Women may be protected by condoms against some STDs as well, although the data are more equivocal (Table 3). In part, this may be due to the wider variety of organisms studied and the varying time frame for the partners' condom use. In Costa Rica, women whose partners used condoms had significantly lower risks of being infected with HSV-2 than those whose partners used other methods.[63] Among these women, duration of condom use was associated with a dose-response protective effect against HSV-2 infection. In an Alabama STD clinic, women whose partners had used condoms in the past three months had a lower risk of gonorrhea than women whose partners had not used condoms, although statistical significance was not achieved.[64] However, a Scandinavian study[65] found no protective effect of condoms against human papilloma virus (HPV) infections of the cervix.

Table 3. Efficacy of Condom Use in Preventing STDs in Women

Study location and publication year	Study design	Study population	Outcome	Measure of effect	95% confidence interval
Costa Rica, 1989[63]	Cross-sectional	Female controls from a case-control study of cervical cancer	HSV-2 sero-positivity	0.60	0.40–0.80
Alabama, 1984[64]	Case-control	Females, STD clinic	Cervical gonorrhea	0.87	0.64–1.19
Finland, 1984[65]	Case-control	Females, obstetrics and gynecology clinics	Cervical HPV infection	1.35	0.72–2.78
Colorado, 1989[66]	Case-control	Females, STD clinic	Cervical gonorrhea	0.66	0.52–0.84
			Cervical chlamydia	0.97	0.60–1.57
			Vaginal trichomoniasis	0.70	0.55–0.89
United States, 1982[67]	Case-control	Hospitalized women	PID	0.60	0.40–0.90
United States, 1987[68]	Case-control	Women seeking infertility services	Tubal infertility	0.70	0.50–1.10

Source: updated from reference 1.

In Finland, the histories of women with cytologic evidence of HPV infections were compared with histories of women with normal Pap smears; those whose partners used condoms had slightly higher HPV risks, though not significantly so. In Colorado, among women attending STD clinics, those whose partners had used condoms during the previous month were less likely to have gonorrhea or trichomoniasis, but just as likely to have chlamydia or bacterial vaginosis.[66] Thus, these observational studies of condoms and STDs in women provide less-convincing evidence of a protective effect than those investigations in men.

Condoms may have a greater aggregate protective impact on upper than lower genital tract infections, though this probably reflects protection against cervical gonorrhea or chlamydia (Table 3). In a large, multicenter, case-control study of PID in the United States,[67] women who relied on condoms for contraception had a significantly lower risk of being hospitalized for PID than did women who used no contraception. In a different multicenter, case-control study of tubal infertility in the United States,[68] condom use alone was associated with a 30 percent reduced risk of infertility. Moreover, when condoms plus vaginal spermicides had been used for contraception, the protection increased to 50 percent.

Table 4. Efficacy of Condom Use in Preventing HIV in Women, by Type of Use

Study location and publication year	Study design	Study population	Use	Outcome	Measure of effect
Zaire, 1987[69]	Cross-sectional	CSWs	≥50% vs. <50% ≥50% vs. none	HIV seropositivity	0.00 (p=0.046) 0.00 (p=0.090)
California, 1987[70]	Cross-sectional	Partners of HIV positive men	Not specified	HIV seropositivity	0.6 (0.3–1.3)
Maryland, 1988[71]	Cross-sectional	STD clinic patients	Always vs. never	HIV seropositivity	0.6 (0.00–4.1)
United States, 1988[72]	Cross-sectional	Partners of hemophiliacs	Routine vs. none	HIV seroconversion	0.5 (p=0.5)
Greece, 1988[73]	Cross-sectional	Partners of HIV positive men	Regular vs. none	HIV seropositivity	0.0 (p <0.00)
Florida, 1987[74]	Cohort	Spouses of AIDS patients	Regular	HIV seroconversion	0.1 (0.00–0.40)
Kenya, 1988[75]	Cohort	CSWs	Any vs. none	HIV seroconversion	0.3 (0.13–0.92)
France, 1989[76]	Cohort	Partners of hemophiliacs	Always vs. other	HIV seroconversion	0.0 (p=0.15)
Zaire, 1991[77]	Cohort	Partners of HIV positive men	Sporadic	HIV seroconversion	HIV incidence = 1.9 per female person-year
Rwanda, 1991[78]	Cohort	Women attending pediatric/ prenatal clinic	Sporadic	HIV seroconversion	HIV seroconversion lower after increased condom use than before (3.4% per year vs. 4.6% per year)

Much recent work has evaluated the condom's influence in protecting women against HIV (Table 4). In general, the initial low prevalence of infection in women has reduced the power of existing studies to demonstrate statistically significant associations. Nonetheless, in a study of commercial sex workers (CSWs) in Zaire, those who used condoms frequently appeared to have a significantly lower level of HIV infection than those who used condoms less frequently.[69] Three cross-sectional studies in the United States showed lower rates of HIV seropositivity in high-risk women whose partners regularly used condoms.[70,71,72]

The cohort studies of condoms and HIV, by concentrating on such high-risk populations as CSWs and spouses of AIDS patients, were more conclusive. In Florida, use of condoms by AIDS patients was related to a marked reduction in the risk of HIV seroconversion in their spouses.[74] In Kenya, regular use of condoms by the clients of CSWs led to lower HIV seroconversion rates in the CSWs.[75] In France, none of the female partners of HIV-seropositive men with hemophilia who always used condoms became infected with the virus.[76] In Zaire, only two seronegative female partners of 80 HIV-infected men who sporadically used condoms became seropositive during an average of 15 months of observation; the estimated HIV incidence was less than two per person-year.[77] In Rwanda, the rate of HIV seroconversion declined in a population of urban women who increasingly used condoms.[78]

Taken together, these clinical studies suggest that the protective effect of condoms against many STDs can be important, yet the variation in the data imply that other factors affect their impact. Future investigations will help clarify the behavioral and biologic determinants of more effective condom use.

Condom Failure

Condom failure may be due to nonuse, incorrect use, breakage, or leakage. In turn, breakage and leakage may be due to poor manufacture, improper storage, or incorrect use.[49] Some physicians and laymen question condom quality and effectiveness to prevent STDs, since the typical condom *contraceptive* failure rate is at least 12 percent.[79,80] However, most of this failure in both developed and developing countries is likely due to nonuse or incorrect use rather than poor condom quality. At the present time, quality control tests by the U.S. Food and Drug Administration show that defective condoms manufactured in the United States are uncommon.[81]

In developing countries and tropical climates, condom quality may be less reliable. Because of transportation difficulties, condom inventories may linger on shelves under less-than-ideal storage conditions. Temperature extremes, humidity, ultraviolet light, ozone, and other environmental factors are known to contribute to condom deterioration.[82] Moreover, the quality of locally produced condoms may not conform to the standards in developed countries. During the past 10 years, numerous examples of advanced condom deterioration have been found in condoms stored in developing countries.[82] To ensure high quality, a system for monitoring condom quality in the field is necessary. Condom quality management laboratories have been established in Bangladesh, Guatemala, Indonesia, Mexico, Pakistan, the Philippines, and Thailand; additional facilities have been planned in the People's Republic of China, Egypt, and 10 other African countries.

Condom effectiveness increases with duration of use,[79] and a contraceptive failure rate as low as 0.6 percent has been documented among experienced users, although this was in women aged 40–44 years.[83] Incorrect use (not placing the condom on the penis at the very start of sexual activity) was clearly documented in a prospective study[62] among men who acquired gonorrhea despite condom use.

Little is known about condom breakage. However, several published studies have found that condom breakage is uncommon in developed countries (Table 5). Self-reported breakage rates in a 6–12-month period ranged from 1 percent to 7 percent for anal intercourse;[84–87] in one survey, the 12-month condom breakage rate during vaginal intercourse was 0.6 percent.[84] A survey in an Atlanta family planning clinic[88] found that 36 percent of women reported condom breakage during their lifetime. On the basis of woman-years of condom use, this proportion translates into 12-month breakage rates of 0.8 percent. Breakage rates did not differ by age or number of sexual partners. Among women asked to recall circumstances of the most recent condom breakage, a majority reported short periods of foreplay (and likely inadequate lubrication); however, no comparison group was similarly questioned. Another study, conducted prospectively, found breakage rates in a four-month period for anal and vaginal intercourse of 0.5 percent and 0.8 percent,[89] respectively. In this study, all breaks occurred prior to ejaculation, and more than half were attributed to improper use (oil-based lubricants, fingernail tears). The proportion of breakages due to improper storage conditions (temperature extremes, exposure to light) is unknown,[82,90] but could play a larger role in developing world conditions.

Few published data on breakage rates in developing countries are available. One survey of condom users in Bangladesh[91] estimated that 0.7–1.1 condoms broke yearly per user. If the number of condoms used in a year is assumed to be 100, the 12-month breakage rate is 1 percent, which is similar to the 12-month rates reported in the United States (Table 5). Another survey, in Nigeria,[92] found that 12 percent of men in a family planning clinic reported condom breakage; however, no breakage *rates* were estimated. Two unpublished studies of condom use suggest somewhat higher breakage rates. One study,[93] conducted in Bangladesh, Honduras, Ghana, Mali, and Egypt, found that 6 percent of users of one brand and 11 percent of another brand reported condom breakage in a one-month period. Considering the number of condoms used, one-month breakage rates were 1.2 percent and 1.8 percent, respectively, for the two brands. Similar one-month breakage rates might be expected in developed countries as well. A large study in the eastern Caribbean[94] found a

Table 5. Condom Breakage Rates

Study location and publication year	Study design	Study population	Recall period	Breakage rate
United States, 1989[84]	Cross-sectional	Men and women	12 months	1% (anal) 0.6% (vaginal)
England, 1989[85]	Cross-sectional	Gay men	12 months	3–5% (anal)
Sydney, Australia, 1989[86]	Cross-sectional	Gay and bisexual men	6 months	5–7% (anal)
United States, 1991[88]	Cross-sectional	Women	Lifetime	1%
		Family planning clinic clients	12 months	0.8%
Sydney, Australia, 1988[89]	Cohort	Male CSWs	4 months	0.5% (anal) 0.8% (vaginal)

more alarming situation. Breakage rates reported by men in Barbados and St. Lucia over a three-month period were 13 percent and 10 percent, respectively. More than half of the breaks occurred near the closed end of the condom, the area most vulnerable to deterioration.[82] Breakage did not appear to be strongly related to improper home storage conditions or use of oil-based lubricants. When a sample of condoms from the same manufacturing lot as those used in that study were used by men in North Carolina, the breakage rate was only 7 percent.[95] This suggests that culture-specific sexual practices may affect condom breakage rates.

Female Condoms

Several "female condoms" (intravaginal pouches, vaginal condoms) have been developed and are being tested for permeability, safety, and acceptability in the United States and elsewhere.[48] Basically, these products are pouches made of polyurethane (under the brand name Reality [in Europe, Femshield and Femidom], manufactured by Wisconsin Pharmacal) or latex (brand names Women's Choice and Condomme, manufactured by M.D. Personal Products) that line the vagina. Another newly developed vaginal barrier is a latex panty (The Bikini Condom from International Pharmaceuticals) with a built-in pouch. As with condoms, protection against STDs is likely only if these products provide an intact barrier to bacteria and viruses that stays properly positioned during intercourse, and if they are used consistently. In vitro testing of one product (Reality) showed it to be an effective barrier to HIV and cytomegalovirus.[96] However, the high cost and low acceptability of female condoms, as compared with those of male condoms,[48] are likely to limit their usefulness, especially in developing countries.

Spermicides

In vitro studies have shown that contraceptive spermicides kill or inactivate most STD pathogens. The main spermicidal agent in the United States is nonoxynol-9, a nonionic surfactant that damages the cell walls of sperm—and STD pathogens. Laboratory tests have documented activity against *Neisseria gonorrhoeae*,[91-99] *Trichomonas vaginalis*,[98] HSV,[100,101] HIV,[102] and *Treponema pallidum*.[91] *Ureaplasma urealyticum*[103] also is inactivated by spermicides. Reports on the effect of spermicides on *Chlamydia trachomatis* are conflicting: some[104-106] found that nonoxynol-9 inactivated chlamydial organisms, while others[107] found no such effect.

Clinical studies provide further support for a protective effect of spermicides (Table 6). In two southern United States STD clinic populations, investigators[64,108] observed reductions in the risk of cervical gonorrhea, although the magnitude of reduced risk differed. One community-based trial[109] also noted significant protection against this infection. In two large case-control studies, protection was found against cervical gonorrhea[110] and PID.[67] In a large, multicenter, case-control study of tubal infertility,[68] spermicide used alone had no impact on this outcome. When combined with either condoms or diaphragms, a powerful protective effect resulted (50 percent reduction).

The best-designed investigation of spermicides to date[111] supported their clinical efficacy in protecting against gonorrhea and chlamydia. In Alabama, regular use of nonoxynol-9 gel by women attending an STD clinic reduced cervical gonorrhea by 24 percent and cervical chlamydial infections by 22 percent. Two other randomized trials,[112,113] albeit with greater methodologic problems, also found that spermicides protected against cervical gonorrhea.

Table 6. Efficacy of Spermicides in Preventing STDs in Women

Study location and publication year	Study design	Study site	Spermicide	Outcome measure	Measure of effect	95% confidence interval
Tennessee, 1985[108]	Cross-sectional	STD clinic	Not specified	Cervical gonorrhea	0.39	0.31–0.50
Florida, 1980[109]	Descriptive community trial	STD clinic	Phenylmercuric acetate	Cervical gonorrhea	0.51	0.32–0.80
Alabama, 1984[64]	Case-control	STD clinic	Not specified	Cervical gonorrhea	0.90	0.47–1.73
Seattle, 1982[110]	Case-control	Health maintenance organizaton	Octoxynol or nonoxynol-9	Cervical gonorrhea	0.13	0.04–0.40
United States, 1982[67]	Case-control	16 hospitals	Not specified	PID	0.7	0.4–1.4
United States, 1987[68]	Case-control	Infertility centers	Not specified	Tubal infertility	1.0	0.6–1.8
Alabama, 1988[111]	Randomized clinical trial	STD clinic	Nonoxynol-9	Cervical gonorrhea Cervical chlamydia	0.76 0.78	0.59–0.98* 0.64–0.96*
Pennsylvania, 1979[112]	Randomized clinical trial	STD clinic	Nonoxynol-9	Cervical gonorrhea	0.11	0.02–0.55
Mexico, 1980[113]	Randomized clinical trial	Outpatient clinic	Phenylmercuric acetate	Cervical gonorrhea	0.30	0.08–1.14

* 90% confidence interval.
Source: updated from reference 1.

Whether spermicides alone, without any mechanical barriers, protect against HIV has not been determined. Despite nonoxynol-9's in vitro activity against HIV,[102] preliminary results from an ongoing study in Rwanda suggested little impact in vivo.[78] During the first year and a half, HIV seroconversion rates among Rwandan women using only spermicidal suppositories for contraception implied that spermicides were not effective in preventing HIV infection. Such methodologic issues as the type of delivery system (e.g., suppository vs. cream) and the population studied (e.g., CSW vs. other) clearly play a crucial role in allowing correct interpretation of studies involving spermicides and barriers.

Combined Barrier Contraceptives

Several studies have described a protective effect for combined mechanical and chemical barrier contraceptives (Table 7). In some studies, however, the authors did not distinguish between condoms and diaphragms. The diaphragm is nearly always used with a spermicide, which has a protective effect itself, as described above. In three cross-sectional studies, one in a family planning clinic,[114] and two in STD clinics,[108,115] the risk of cervical gonorrhea was lower among combination barrier users. In three case-control studies, diaphragm use was associated with at least a 50 percent reduction in cervical gonorrhea,[64] hospitalization for PID,[67] and tubal infertility,[68] respectively.

Table 7. Efficacy of Contraceptive Barrier Use in Preventing STDs in Women

Study location and publication year	Study design	Study site/ population	Barrier	Outcome	Measure of effect	
Louisiana, 1975[114]	Cross-sectional	Family planning clinic	Condom/ diaphragm, foam	Cervical gonorrhea	0.53	(0.18–1.59)
Tennessee, 1985[108]	Cross-sectional	STD clinic	Diaphragm, condom	Cervical gonorrhea	0.11	(0.08–0.17)
Colorado, 1988[115]	Cross-sectional	STD clinic	Diaphragm	Cervical gonorrhea	"protective"	(p<0.001)
				Cervical chlamydia	0.00	(0.00–0.20)
Thailand, 1987[116]	Randomized clinical trial	CSWs	Nonoxynol-9 sponge	Cervical gonorrhea	0.67	(0.42–1.07)
				Cervical chlamydia	0.31	(0.16–0.60)
Greenland, Denmark, 1990[117]	Cross-sectional	Population-based	Condom/ diaphragm	Cervical HPV infection	1.0	(0.70–1.40)
Alabama, 1984[64]	Case-control	STD clinic	Diaphragm	Cervical gonorrhea	0.45	(0.12–1.67)
United States, 1984[67]	Case-control	16 hospitals	Diaphragm	PID	0.4	(0.2–0.7)
United States, 1987[68]	Case-control	Infertility centers	Diaphragm	Tubal infertility	0.5	(0.3–0.7)

Source: updated from references 1 and 34.

In Thailand, women at high risk of STDs who used the contraceptive sponge (with spermicide in it) were protected against cervical gonorrhea and, to a lesser extent, against cervical *Chlamydia trachomatis*. However, vaginal infection with *Candida albicans* was more likely in sponge users.[116] In a large population-based study, women in Greenland and Denmark who had ever used condoms or diaphragms were not protected from cervical HPV infection.[117]

Recent concerns have been raised about potential harmful effects of combined mechanical and chemical barrier methods. A cohort study of users of foam and condoms and users of a diaphragm and spermicide showed that both methods were associated with vaginal colonization and bacteriuria with *Escherichia coli*.[118] Because facultative anaerobic microbial domination of vaginal flora (e.g., bacterial vaginosis) has been associated with RTIs,[119] the implications of this finding are of concern. Potential mechanisms for the *Escherichia coli* colonization include alteration of the vaginal ecosystem by the spermicide and a mechanical effect of the diaphragm.

A greater potential problem involves the hypothetical effect of combined barrier methods on HIV transmission. Although in vitro studies show that barrier methods are impervious to HIV, and that chemical barriers are toxic to HIV, studies in humans suggest some adverse outcomes. Among CSWs in Nairobi, women who were randomly assigned to use the nonoxynol-9 contraceptive sponge had significantly higher acquisition of genital ulcers than a placebo group.[120] Similarly, HIV seroconversion was also higher, although the increase was not statistically significant. In Vancouver, Canada, among a small sample of CSWs, over one third of women who had used nonoxynol-9-lubricated condoms stated that they had experienced vaginal irritation after their use.[121] We feel these data are hypothesis-generating at best because the amount of spermicide in spermicidally lubricated condoms is so small,[122] the population studied was atypical, and no comparison group was used. Nonetheless, such hypothetical irritation could act as a pathway for HIV acquisition.

Therefore, carefully controlled studies need to assess the relative value of the different mechanical and chemical barrier methods used together in preventing transmission of all STDs, not only HIV. Moreover, the investigations need to compare these methods not only in the highest risk core groups, but also in women in the general population. The "real world" effectiveness of combination methods remains to be proven.

Oral Contraceptives

Oral contraceptives (OCs) have an array of noncontraceptive health benefits. But their influence on STDs, PID, and eventual reproductive sequelae remains unsettled. The majority of studies have found an increased risk of cervical infections with *Chlamydia trachomatis* among users of OCs as compared with nonusers.[123-126] The association between OC use and cervical infection with *Chlamydia trachomatis* may be mediated through the cervical ectropion commonly induced by OCs. In one study,[127] *Chlamydia trachomatis* was isolated more frequently among women with ectropion than among women without ectropion, regardless of the method of birth control used.

However, the influence of OCs on the upper genital tract may be different than that on the lower genital tract. Studies from Europe and the United States[128-131] have revealed that women using OCs are half as likely to be hospitalized for PID as women who are sexually active but who do not use contraception. In a multicenter, case-control study from the United States,[132] the protection was observed only among women who had been using OCs for more than 12 months. Past use of pills conferred no protection. In Lund, Sweden,[133] OC use was associated with a significant reduction in the risk of chlamydial PID, although the protective effect was not as strong as that for gonococcal PID. By contrast, in Seattle, women using OCs were apparently differentially protected against chlamydial, as compared with gonococcal, PID.[134] OC users tend to have milder infection with *Chlamydia trachomatis*, as manifested by antibody response.[135] Moreover, primary tubal infertility is not increased among former users of most current OCs, as might be expected if use led to an increased risk of either overt or silent chlamydial PID.[68] However, among users of OCs with estrogen levels higher than 50 mcg, an increased risk of tubal infertility occurred.

Possible mechanisms for the hypothetical protective effect remain speculative. The progestin component of combination OCs thickens the cervical mucus. Changes in mucus composition or immunologic properties might account for this protection. An alternative explanation relates to the decreased menstrual blood loss associated with pill use. About 90 percent of women with normal fallopian tubes experience retrograde menstruation; this flow of potentially contaminated material into the tubes may initiate PID. In pill users, the inoculum introduced into the tubes may be smaller because of reduced menstrual-blood loss.

Use of OCs also seems to modify the course of PID favorably. As judged by laparoscopic examination, women with PID who were using OCs had milder inflammation than women not using OCs.[136] Among women with chlamydial salpingitis, use of OCs protected against Fitz-Hugh-Curtis syndrome.[135] In addition, pill users had a significantly lower titer of antibodies against *Chlamydia trachomatis* than did nonusers.[135] While the mechanisms remain unknown, sex steroids do modify immunologic function.[137]

As with barrier methods, the effect of OCs on HIV transmission, acquisition, or disease progression remains unsettled.[138] Studies of CSWs in Nairobi, Kenya, have provided support for the hypothesis that OC use could facilitate HIV transmission.[139] Potential biologic mechanisms by which hormonal contraception might facilitate HIV transmission include increased cervical ectropion caused by OC use; increased cervical chlamydial infection (see above), possibly associated with the ectropion; systemic immunologic changes associated with some exogenous steroids;[137] and, if long-acting hormonal contraception is used, irregular uterine bleeding. In addition, the particular type of estrogens and progestins contained in the oral contraceptive (or in injectable hormonal preparations) may be important factors relating to any impact on HIV acquisition or transmission.

The range of investigations (most unpublished) examining the relationship of hormonal contraceptive use and HIV received an extensive review (Table 8) in a conference in October 1990.[138] In summary, the best study to date[139] showed OC use was independently associated with acquisition of HIV among a group of highly exposed CSWs. A variety of biases could have influenced these results, just as with any epidemiologic study. For example, the comparison group included women using barrier methods, which would protect against HIV transmission and thus tend to spuriously elevate the OC risk. However, a thorough analysis examining the measurable potential confounders was not able to adjust away the higher HIV seroconversion risk associated with OC use. All other studies,[140-148] except for one in Rwanda, found little association between OC use and HIV seropositivity. A more recent study in Rwanda found a history of OC use was not related to seroconversion.[78] While the issue remains unsettled, because of the crucial role OCs and other hormonal contraception play in international family planning programs, and because the HIV pandemic is the world's most important health problem, policymakers and scientists in these fields must assign the highest research priority to resolving this question.

IUDs

Few publications have objectively examined the effect of the IUD on lower genital tract infections. One review article concluded the IUD was unrelated to cervical chlamydial infection.[149] However, a recent analysis of cross-sectional data from a population-based sample of Seattle women found those who had ever used an IUD had a significantly higher percentage of chlamydial antibodies than those who had never used an IUD; the difference remained even after stratifying for number of sex partners.[150] In contrast, a prospective study in Antwerp found IUD users had ninefold lower rates of chlamydia than OC users;[126] however, the same study showed women using IUDs had nearly eight times higher rates of bacterial vaginosis.

The possible association between IUD use and the development of upper genital tract infection still remains a controversial topic in contemporary contraception.[151,152] The initial investigations in the 1970s[153] all found an increased risk of PID, ranging from twofold to ninefold, among IUD users. The consistency of these findings strongly suggested a causal association.

However, epidemiologic evidence derived in the 1980s showed the association between IUD use and PID to be overestimated. Three particular methodologic problems in the early studies contributed to their overly pessimistic assessment. First, women using barrier

Table 8. Studies of the Association between OC Use and HIV Infection

Study location and publication year	Study design	Study population	Comparison	Relative risk (95% confidence interval)	
Kenya, 1991[139]	Cohort	CSWs	Ever-use never-use	4.5	(1.4–13.8)
Zambia, 1990[140]	Cross-sectional	AIDS referral clinic clients	Current/ noncurrent	1.1	(0.9–1.3)
Kenya, 1990[141]	Cross-sectional	CSWs	Current/ noncurrent	2.0	(1.2–3.4)
United States, 1990[142]	Case-control	CSWs	Recent/not in last five years	1.0	(0.4–2.2)
Rwanda, 1988[143]	Case-control	Couples	OC in last two years/no use	4.3	(1.4–15.4)
Zimbabwe, 1989[144]	Case-control	Couples	Current/ noncurrent	1.1	(0.4–3.3)
Thailand, 1989[145]	Case-control	CSWs	OC use/ nonuse	0.7	(0.4–1.2)
Kenya, 1990[146]	Case-control	Family planning clients	Non-OC use	1.5	(0.7–3.0)
European Centers, 1989[147]	Discordant couples	Partners	OC use/no method	1.4	(0.4–5.9)
Italy, 1990[148]	Discordant couples	Partners	Current/ noncurrent	0.4	(0.3–1.8)
Rwanda, 1991[78]	Cohort	Women attending pediatric/prenatal clinic	Ever-use never-use	"Not associated"	

Source: updated from reference 138.

methods or OCs served as the comparison group in most studies.[153] Since these methods *reduce* the risk of PID, such comparisons artifactually elevated the apparent risk associated with IUD use. Second, the PID diagnosis often rests on highly subjective symptoms and signs that are difficult to assess.[154] Since the putative association between IUD use and PID has been recognized since the 1960s, PID "diagnostic bias" might occur among IUD users. Namely, an IUD user with a cluster of lower abdominal signs and symptoms would be more likely to receive a diagnosis of PID than would a woman with similar complaints but without an IUD. This relative overdiagnosis of PID among IUD users would serve to inflate the risk estimate. Third, the early analyses did not adjust for type of IUD and the timing of its insertion. If either of these factors creates a disproportionate degree of PID risk, the overall crude risk for IUDs as a group is also spuriously elevated.[155,156]

Since 1983, a number of more sophisticated studies[157-162] have revised our understanding of the IUD–PID association (Table 9). These studies appropriately adjusted the comparison groups to include only women using no method of contraception,[158] and found the risk of PID associated with IUD to be below 2.0. In fact, depending on the design and analytic assumptions used, the same data base that produced slightly elevated risks of PID for IUD users also could be analyzed to find virtually no risk.[151] In contrast, in those studies where the comparison groups included women using methods that protected against PID,[157,159-161] the risks were between 2.3 and 8.6.

Current evidence suggests that the smaller, but still measurable, increased risk of PID associated with IUD use occurs around the time of insertion. Thus, contamination of the endometrial cavity at insertion may be more responsible for IUD-related PID than the device itself. Numerous studies[162] have noted an inverse relationship between risk of PID and duration of IUD use. The most explicit estimate[158] excluded Dalkon Shield users and found the relative risk associated with other IUDs was highest in the first month after insertion (3.8), lower in months 2–4 (1.7), and not significantly elevated above baseline (1.1) at five months and beyond.

Because IUD-related PID may in part be related to the timing of insertion, short-term antibiotics might help reduce the risks. In Kenya,[163] a randomized clinical trial of prophylactic doxycycline at the time of IUD insertion found that the antibiotic protected against PID and other complications. This finding lends further support to the concept that bacterial contamination of the endometrium at insertion may induce most cases of IUD-related PID. In Nigeria, however, a second study of prophylactic antibiotics during IUD insertion failed to show any protective effect.[164] Both African investigations found much lower rates of IUD-associated PID than expected, even among the placebo group. Further studies will need to resolve this question.

The particular type of IUD, especially the Dalkon Shield, also seems to be important. Because of the infrequency of IUD-related PID, even in the developing world, and because of the limited size of many studies, most data are insufficient to distinguish statistically among different types of IUDs. The largest study in the United States,[158] as well as others in developing countries[159] and England,[161] found the risk of PID with the Dalkon Shield to be 2–5 times that of other devices. In addition, the risk of PID associated with the Shield remained elevated beyond four months of use. However, recent reanalysis of the same data base has challenged this interpretation.[151] Nevertheless, the use of the Dalkon Shield has also been related to an increased risk of PID sequelae—primarily tubal infertility. In a multicenter study conducted in Boston,[165] women who had previously used Shields had a twofold increased risk. In a companion study from Seattle,[166] the relative risk was 2.6. However, among women who had used copper IUDs and who had had only one sex partner, no increase occurred in the risk of tubal infertility.

Because newer IUDs apparently are associated with lower rates of PID, even in the developing world,[163,164] they may be appropriate in certain settings where the risk of STDs is low. Further research may help establish the best circumstances in which to recommend the IUD for women who have difficulty with hormonal or coitally dependent methods.

Tubal Sterilization

Tubal sterilization protects against PID, but this protection is not absolute. Most typical

Table 9. Recent Studies of the IUD and PID

Study location and publication year	Comparison group	Measure of effect (95% confidence interval)	
United States/Canada, 1983[157]	Women using contraception other than IUD	8.6	(5.3–13.8)
United States, 1983[158]	Women using no contraception	1.9	(1.5–2.4)
Developing countries (World Health Organization international study), 1984[159]	Parous women using no contraception	2.3	(1.4–3.9)
England, 1990[161]	Parous women using no contraception or vasectomy		
Nonmedicated		3.3	(2.3–5.0)
Medicated		1.8	(0.8–4.0)

Source: adapted from reference 1.

cases of PID are thought to arise from ascent of pathogens from the cervix via the endometrial cavity; hence, disrupting the continuity of this passage should prevent inoculation of the distal fallopian tubes. Even though endometritis and proximal salpingitis are potentially possible, PID is rarely observed[167–170] among women after tubal sterilization. Anecdotal cases of PID[171] and tubo-ovarian abscess[172] continue to be reported. A more likely mechanism for poststerilization PID is iatrogenic contamination of the tubes during the operative procedure. In developing world settings, where sterile conditions are more difficult to maintain, this risk may be further elevated.

Abortion

Women who have cervical infection with *Neisseria gonorrhoeae* or *Chlamydia trachomatis* have an increased risk of endometritis following induced abortion performed under proper hygienic conditions. The risk appears to be at least tripled with either organism.[173,174,175] A number of studies suggest that use of prophylactic antibiotics at the time of the abortion procedure reduces the risk of infection by one half to two thirds.[176–184] While preoperative screening for infection with these organisms is desirable, a brief perioperative course of an antibiotic such as doxycycline seems both safe and cost-effective.[176] Women later found to be infected by *Neisseria gonorrhoeae* or *Chlamydia trachomatis* can be followed up with a full course of recommended antibiotics.

The greatest risk of RTIs associated with induced abortion occurs in circumstances where sterile conditions are not maintained. In countries where abortion services are restricted by law or practice, and especially in the developing world—where, even if abortion is legal, access to sanitary procedures is limited—postabortion infection poses risks not only to future fertility, but also to the woman's life.[185,186,187] More than half of abortion-related deaths occur in Southeast Asia; the next-largest proportion is in Sub-Saharan Africa, then Latin America and the Caribbean.[188]

Contraceptive Trade-offs

Under ideal circumstances, couples will use two contraceptive methods—one to prevent pregnancy and the other to prevent RTIs. If this occurs, and if use of both methods is consistent, prevention of pregnancy will be enhanced; depending on the methods used, prevention of RTIs may also be potentiated. However, because the contraceptives with the best record for pregnancy prevention provide little STD protection, if couples use only one method, trade-off choices are necessary.

For purposes of crude comparison, we have placed quantitative estimates on the effectiveness of different contraceptive methods on both unplanned pregnancy and gonorrhea (Table 10). The data for pregnancy are based on comprehensive reviews of the literature, conducted primarily in the developed world,[80] and are generally accepted by clinicians and policymakers. In addition, demographic surveys in developing countries[189] have confirmed these approximate levels of contraceptive failure (i.e., unplanned pregnancy). The data for gonorrhea are rough at best, and are based on the following assumptions: first, a "baseline" of 90 percent of women using no contraception will become infected by having regular intercourse for one year with a partner infected with gonorrhea; 10 percent will be "immune" for unknown reasons. Second, using data on relative risks from the tables in this manuscript, we multiplied the *lowest* and the *typical* relative risk for each contraceptive method by the "baseline" level of gonococcal infection. We emphasize that these estimates are imprecise at best, and are offered solely to facilitate a qualitative comprehension of the trade-off concept.

The relative strengths of each contraceptive method become obvious (Table 10). For those whose families are not completed, yet who do not currently wish to become pregnant, hormonal contraceptives remain the most effective single reversible method available to prevent pregnancy. However, hormonal methods provide no STD protection, at least in the lower genital tract level. Hence, for persons who are not mutually monogamous, addition of a barrier method, such as a condom, will help reduce the risk of STDs as well as that of unplanned pregnancy. Barrier methods are, however, substantially less effective in preventing conception than are hormonal methods, yet they offer important protection against STDs. To maximize protection against both unwanted pregnancy and STDs, a barrier method should be used in conjunction with a hormonal method.[190]

Worldwide, for couples whose families are completed, male or female sterilization is an increasingly popular method of contraception.[191] While these operations protect against upper genital tract infections in sterilized persons, they confer no protection against lower genital tract infections. Alternatives to sterilization are hormonal implants and the IUD; both are effective methods of reversible contraception, but offer no protection against RTIs. Sterilized persons would still need to use barrier methods to protect against infection.

Because both mechanical and chemical barrier prophylaxes are coitally dependent, their efficacy in preventing either infection or unplanned pregnancy depends entirely on compliance by the couple. Some populations have demonstrated high levels of barrier

Table 10. Estimated Failure Rates of Contraceptive
Methods to Prevent Pregnancy or STD

Contraceptive method	Pregnancy*		STD (cervical gonorrhea)†	
	Lowest	Typical	Lowest	Typical
None	85	85	90	90
Hormonal				
Combined oral	0.1	3	90	90
Injectable	0.3	0.3	90	90
Implants	0.03	0.03	90	90
Condom	2	12	0	55
Cap	6	18	u	u
Diaphragm (sponge)	6	18	62	62
Spermicide	3	21	69	69
IUD	0.8	0.5	90	90
Periodic abstinence	2	20	90	90
Continuous abstinence	0	0	0	0

* Percentage of women experiencing an unplanned pregnancy in the first year of
contraceptive use.
† Percentage of women becoming infected with gonorrhea in the first year of contraceptive
use through regular intercourse with an infected partner.
Note: Lowest = consistent users; typical = inconsistent users; u = unavailable.
Source: adapted from reference 80.

method use. For example, behavioral changes in response to HIV prevention recommendations—among them increased condom use—by homosexual men in HIV pattern I countries
have been associated with decreases not only in HIV transmission, but also in other STDs,
including rectal gonorrhea, syphilis, hepatitis B, and enteric infections.[192–195] Unfortunately,
to date, most heterosexual populations worldwide have not reported the same magnitude
of condom use[196,197] and have not experienced decreases in the traditional STDs. In
developed and developing countries, high levels of syphilis and chlamydia continue,
especially in the most economically deprived populations.

The discrepancy in gender power relations makes it difficult in some settings for a
woman to choose a male-dependent method. Moreover, cultural taboos against discussing
sex limit the practical negotiations that can take place.[22] In some societies, use of condoms

is associated with commercial sex, which makes condoms unacceptable for use in any primary relationship. In others, men consider condom use to be a major inhibition to their sexual satisfaction. In societies where a woman's status within her family and in her community depends on her being a wife and a mother, the trade-off decisions between preventing RTIs and avoiding unplanned pregnancy become even more cruel. If she insists on condom use, the woman may be beaten, deserted, or accused of infidelity. If she does not, she may expose herself to a tragic cycle of becoming infected with STDs acquired by her partner in other sexual relationships. These STDs can result in upper genital tract infections and eventual tubal infertility.

Another, more important aspect to assessing trade-off concerns is whether conditions exist for safe, sterile childbirth or abortion. If pregnancy itself, regardless of whether it is terminated or continued, carries markedly high "iatrogenic" risks of RTIs, then the *pregnancy* prevention efficacy of the contraceptive choice takes on greater weight. By preventing undesired pregnancy, the contraceptive methods simultaneously protect against pregnancy-associated RTIs. In the developing world, postabortal and puerperal infections are important causes of tubal infertility. In Africa, where the infectious etiology of infertility was most evident,[198] RTIs occurring both before and after the first pregnancy were associated with tubal occlusion. In Asia, abortion appeared to play a larger role than childbirth in contributing to infectious infertility, whereas in Latin America, the reverse was found.[199]

MERGING RTI AND FAMILY PLANNING SERVICES

Most publicly supported family planning, maternal-child health, and STD clinics in the developed world function as independent entities rather than one coordinated reproductive health unit. In contrast, the women being served by these clinics frequently have health needs that overlap. For example, in family planning clinics in developed countries, risk assessment surveys have found that approximately one quarter of women report behaviors that put them at increased risk for HIV and the other STDs.[200] In STD clinics, up to half of reproductive-age, sexually active women report using no method of contraception,[201] although most have histories of both STDs and unintended pregnancies.

In developing countries, this need for integrated care is even more acute. Since so few facilities are available for health care, they should not be fragmented. Moreover, because access to health services is usually more cumbersome and time-consuming in developing world settings, when patients avail themselves of a particular "categorical" service, the full range of clinical preventive care should be offered.

These overlapping needs provide those interested in RTIs and family planning with a unique opportunity to deliver more broad-based reproductive health care.[4,202] In the United States, this collaboration was initiated in the early 1970s, when family planning clinics became crucial allies for the federal gonorrhea control program.[203] By 1982, half of all women receiving family planning services were simultaneously screened for STDs, primarily gonorrhea; this screening appropriately targeted those women who had the highest RTI risks.[204] Moreover, efforts to screen for chlamydia in family planning settings have also been productive, especially when selective criteria are applied—such as age younger than 24, more than one sex partner in the past two months, or signs of cervical infection.[125,205-209]

Likewise, STD clinics in the United States increasingly have been willing to provide rudimentary contraceptive services. The condom, if used correctly, had been advocated for primary prevention of bacterial STDs. However, because secondary prevention (e.g., diagnosis and treatment) was available to control bacterial STDs, primary prevention often played a smaller role. Recent concerns with incurable viral STDs, especially HIV, have provided the necessary social environment and financial resources both to emphasize condom use during patient counseling sessions and to increase advertising of condoms in the media. However, as we described earlier, condom failure is usually due to nonuse, which itself depends primarily on the male's behavior. Thus, use of female-controlled mechanical or chemical contraceptives may be of further value in reducing risks of RTIs.[210,211] For this reason, diaphragms (which protect only the cervical os), spermicides, and eventually female condoms may play a wider role in upcoming efforts to prevent STDs.

The urgency of the HIV pandemic has furthered the need to integrate RTI and family planning services.[212] In HIV pattern II countries in the developing world, where heterosexual transmission predominates, family planning agencies can serve essential health functions by both counseling women on how to reduce their risks and providing services to diagnose or treat those STDs that themselves may further facilitate acquisition or transmission of HIV.[213] If the client's HIV status is known, more specific counseling is warranted. For seronegative women, culturally sensitive messages regarding ways to protect themselves from STD and HIV exposure are essential. For seropositive women, family planning choices are even more complicated. Complex personal ethical and policy issues are involved in protecting the woman's right to determine her reproductive future, improving her quality and duration of life, decreasing the risk of perinatal HIV transmission, and decreasing the risk of further HIV transmission within the community.[214,215,216]

In developed countries, recent concern with the rising percentage of heterosexual spread of HIV[217] has led many family planning clinics to offer HIV education, risk assessment, infection control, and patient referral services.[218] As resources increase to allow for additional HIV prevention activities in family planning settings, spinoff educational efforts directed to the other STDs must be incorporated. For example, the symptoms and signs of genital infections can be explained to the client seeking contraceptive services. STD clinical management can be integrated with other reproductive health care. Thus, in both the developing and the developed worlds, attention focused on HIV could facilitate a closer merger of the professionals interested in reproductive health from both an RTI and a contraceptive standpoint.

RESEARCH IMPLICATIONS

The above discussion has revealed many unanswered questions affecting the fields of RTIs and family planning. These involve issues of safety, contraceptive use, and new contraceptive methods. Regarding safety, the question of greatest importance is whether a woman's choice of hormonal contraception will directly affect her risk of acquiring HIV. If so, in countries with a high prevalence of HIV, the role of hormonal contraceptive methods will need reevaluation. A second safety issue is whether combined barrier contraception causes either microtrauma to the vaginal epithelium or colonization by potentially harmful anaerobic organisms. Finally, we must determine whether prophylactic antibiotics administered at the time of IUD insertion reduce the short-term infection risks of this method; answers to this question are especially important in communities with high levels of STD prevalence.

Consistent use of coitally dependent, barrier contraceptive methods with the best record of protecting against RTIs appears to be the major limiting factor to their effectiveness. Thus, a variety of intervention studies are underway to assess whether different approaches to encouraging or providing barrier methods will increase their cumulative and consistent use. The behavioral concept of community "social marketing" of contraceptives to prevent both RTIs and unplanned pregnancy is appealing, but as yet not widespread. Studies among homosexual men have shown that changing social norms to make it unacceptable to practice unsafe sex can lead to an aggregate impact on individual behaviors. This approach is being examined within adolescent populations and other communities with especially high levels of STDs.

Finally, perhaps most important, we need new and improved female-controlled contraceptive methods that have greater than 95 percent efficacy in preventing both pregnancy and RTIs.[210] A recent report from the Institute of Medicine called for a sizable increase in contraceptive research,[33] yet the primary emphasis was on pregnancy prevention. Those interested in reproductive health can no longer afford to champion methods to prevent one or the other of the adverse sexual outcomes—unplanned pregnancy vs. infection. Rather, researchers must increasingly commit both their bench-science technologies and their clinical investigations to develop methods that will reduce the need for trade-off decisions. This commitment may also serve to increase collaboration between the family planning and RTI professional communities.

POLICY IMPLICATIONS

Policymakers are also beset by a myriad of decision points. Recommendations regarding the trade-off priorities between preventing RTIs and preventing unplanned pregnancy must be considered differently from the standpoint of the developed vs. the developing world, the individual woman involved, the type of service provider, the safety of abortion and childbirth practices, and the type of political system in which policy decisions occur. As described in the introduction, each of these levels requires a careful balancing of multiple factors.

For example, the traditional measures of contraceptive efficacy used by studies conducted in the developed world may be misleading when applied to the developing world. OCs are more effective than barrier methods only in settings where they are available and consistently taken, and continuation rates are high. If diaphragms, condoms, and spermicides can be made available and used just as consistently, they can provide effective protection against both pregnancy and RTIs. We may have been too quick to assume that barrier methods cannot be effectively used in developing countries. Recent experience in Kenya[75] and Zaire[77] with condom promotion in high-risk settings has been encouraging. Perhaps policymakers should be further sensitized to the effect of social norms on increasing the aggregate use of combined barrier methods.

While integration of RTI and family planning services seems natural, many practical and ethical hurdles need to be overcome. Staff familiar with each field need to be cross-trained so that they can be sufficiently sensitive to, and informed about, the key issues of the other. More specifically, staff require the medical knowledge and cultural sensitivity to help clients make the best decisions to simultaneously reduce unplanned pregnancy and RTIs. Adequate supervision is necessary to ensure both that STD clients are properly counseled to avoid a method of contraception that may raise risks of reinfection, and that family planning clients with high-risk sexual behaviors are screened for possible STDs. As discussed above, counseling to improve condom use is a crucial skill for all providers of reproductive health care. Finally, continued advocacy by both groups for safer abortion and childbearing services is another means to both reduce RTIs and ensure planned, healthy births.

Integration of these services will require reallocation of resources (e.g., service costs, personnel, and time). Thus, cooperation in allocating family planning resources to preventing STDs, as well as STD resources to providing contraception, is needed from both groups. When family planning donors invest in STD control, they express their concern with the woman's total reproductive health rather than with just controlling her fertility. For those concerned with RTIs, provision of contraceptive services will avoid unplanned pregnancies and the risk of unsafe abortions or childbearing, especially in the developing world.

To conclude, these differing policy positions between the two camps imply competition for finite resources. Thus, certain priorities must be established. We believe donors need to invest in two key areas: development of female-controlled contraceptive methods effective against both pregnancy and infection (the female condom is as close as we have come so far, but its usefulness is probably limited); and support of demonstration projects, in both the developing world and low-income areas of the developed world, to evaluate integration of RTI and family planning programs. Without such investment, the types of trade-off decisions made by individuals, communities, and policymakers will frequently keep these two fields apart, rather than evolving toward a cooperative liaison.

Acknowledgments

This manuscript represents the cumulative efforts of many persons, especially our coauthor on previous reviews—David Grimes—and our colleagues at the International Women's Health Coalition—Adrienne Germain and Maggie Bangser. Others who made special contributions to update the current manuscript include Laurie Liskin, James Trussell, Carol Hogue, Bert Peterson, Judy Wasserheit, and Sandi Bowden. Our thanks to all.

REFERENCES

1. Grimes DA, Cates W, Jr. Family planning and sexually transmitted diseases. In: Holmes KK, Mårdh P-A, Sparling PF et al., eds. Sexually transmitted diseases, second edition, New York: McGraw-Hill, 1990:1087–94.
2. Harlap S, Kost K, Forrest JD. Preventing pregnancy, protecting health: a new look at birth control choices in the United States, New York: The Alan Guttmacher Institute, 1991.
3. DaVanzo J, Parnell AM, Foege WH. Health consequences of contraceptive use and reproductive patterns. JAMA 1991; 265:2692–6.
4. Cates W Jr. Sexually transmitted diseases and family planning. Strange or natural bedfellows? J Reprod Med 1984; 29:317–22.
5. Luker K. Contraceptive risk taking and abortion. Stud Fam Plann 1977; 8:190–6.
6. Horowitz DR, Oechsli W. Contraceptive risk-taking in a population with limited access to abortion. J Biosoc Sci 1980; 12:373–82.

7. Hatcher RA, Stewart FA, Trussell TJ, et al., eds. Contraceptive Technology, 1990–1992, 15th edition, New York: Irvington Press, 1990.
8. Hearst N, Hulley SB. Preventing the heterosexual spread of AIDS: are we giving our patients the best advice? JAMA 1988; 259:2428–32.
9. May RM, Anderson RM. Transmission dynamics of HIV infection. Nature 1987; 326:137–42.
10. Caldwell JC, Caldwell P. The cultural context of high fertility in Sub-Saharan Africa. Popul Develop Rev 1987; 13:409–37.
11. Caldwell JC, Caldwell P, Quiggin P. The social context of AIDS in Sub-Saharan Africa. Popul Develop Rev 1989; 15:185–234.
12. Fineberg HB. Education to prevent AIDS: prospects and obstacles. Science 1988; 239:592–6.
13. Eisenberg B. The number of partners and the probability of HIV infection. Statistics Med 1989; 8:83–92.
14. Reiss IL, Leik RK. Evaluating strategies to avoid AIDS: number of partners versus use of condoms. J Sex Res 1989; 26:411–33.
15. Cates W Jr, Rolfs RT Jr, Aral SO. Sexually transmitted diseases, pelvic inflammatory disease and infertility: an epidemiologic update. Epidemiol Rev 1990; 12:199–220.
16. Widdus R, Meheus A, Short R. The management of risk in sexually transmitted diseases. Daedalus 1990; 119:177–91.
17. Aral SO, Guinan ME. Women and sexually transmitted diseases. In: Holmes KK, Mårdh P-A, Sparling PF, Wiesner PJ, eds. Sexually transmitted diseases, first edition, New York: McGraw-Hill, 1984:85–9.
18. Sobel JD. Vaginal infections in adult women. Med Clin N Amer 1990; 74:1573–1602.
19. Rolfs RT, Galaid EI, Zaidi AA. Pelvic inflammatory disease: trends in hospitalizations and office visits, 1979–1988. Submitted for publication, 1991.
20. Drotman DP. Epidemiology and treatment of epididymitis. Rev Infect Dis 1982; Suppl 4:S788–93.
21. Krieger JN. Prostatitis syndromes: pathophysiology, differential diagnosis, and treatment. Sex Transm Dis 1984; 11:100–12.
22. Larson A. Social context of human immunodeficiency virus transmission in Africa: historical and cultural bases of East and Central African sexual relations. Rev Infect Dis 1989; 11:716–24.
23. Cates W Jr. The epidemiology and control of sexually transmitted diseases in adolescents. In: Schydlower M, Shafer M-A, eds. AIDS and the other sexually transmitted diseases. Adolesc Med State Art Rev 1990; 3:409–27.
24. Henshaw SK, Van Vort J. Abortion services in the United States, 1987 and 1988. Fam Plann Perspect 1990; 22:102–9.
25. Aral SO, Holmes KK. Epidemiology of sexual behavior and sexually transmitted diseases. In: Holmes KK, Mårdh P-A, Sparling PF et al., eds. Sexually transmitted diseases, second edition, New York: McGraw-Hill, 1990:19–36.
26. Johnson RE, Nahmias AJ, Magder LS, Lee FK, Brooks CA, Snowden CB. A seroepidemiologic survey of the prevalence of herpes simplex virus type 2 infection in the United States. N Engl J Med 1989; 321:7–12.
27. Mosher WD. Fecundity and infertility in the United States. Am J Public Health 1988; 78:181–2.

28. Platt R, Rice PA, McCormack WM. Risk of acquiring gonorrhea and prevalence of abnormal adnexal findings among women recently exposed to gonorrhea. JAMA 1983; 250:3205–9.

29. Hooper RR, Reynolds GH, Jones OG et al. Cohort study of venereal disease. I. The risk of gonorrhea transmission from infected women to men. Am J Epidemiol 1978; 108:136–44.

30. Brunham RC, Plummer FA. A general model of sexually transmitted disease epidemiology and its implications for control. Med Clin N Amer 1990; 74:1339–52.

31. Trussell J, Kost K. Contraceptive failure in the United States: a critical review of the literature. Stud Fam Plann 1987; 18:237–83.

32. CDC. Number of sex partners and potential risk of sexual exposure to human immunodeficiency virus. MMWR 1988; 37:565–8.

33. Mastroianni L Jr, Donaldson PJ, Kane TT. Development of contraceptives— obstacles and opportunities. N Engl J Med 1990; 322:482–4.

34. Peterson HB, Galaid EI, Zenilman JM. Pelvic inflammatory disease: review of treatment options. Rev Infect Dis 1990; 12(Suppl 6):S656–64.

35. Department of Health and Human Services, Office of Population Affairs. Guidelines for clinical practice for facilities funded under Title X, Washington, DC, 1989.

36. Parra W, Drotman DP, Siegel K, Esteves K, Baker T. Patient counseling and behavior modification. In: Holmes KK, Mårdh P-A, Sparling PF et al., eds. Sexually transmitted diseases, second edition, New York: McGraw-Hill, 1990: 1057–68.

37. Forrest JD. The delivery of family planning services in the United States. Fam Plann Perspect 1988; 20:88–98.

38. Bennett FJ. Control of sexually transmitted diseases in the tropics and developing countries. In: Osaba AO, ed. Sexually transmitted diseases in the tropics, London: Baillière-Tyndal, 1987:223–44.

39. Wasserheit JN. Reproductive tract infections. Presented at 117th Annual Meeting of the American Public Health Association, Chicago, October 17, 1989.

40. Stone KM, Grimes DA, Magder LS. Personal protection against sexually transmitted diseases. Am J Obstet Gynecol 1986; 155:180–8.

41. Stone KM, Grimes DA, Magder LS. Primary prevention of sexually transmitted diseases: a primer for clinicians. JAMA 1986; 255:1763–6.

42. McGregor JA, French JI, Spencer NE. Prevention of sexually transmitted diseases in women. J Reprod Med 1988; 33:109–18.

43. Feldblum PJ, Fortney JA. Condoms, spermicides, and the transmission of human immunodeficiency virus: a review of the literature. Am J Public Health 1988; 78:52–4.

44. Cates W Jr. STDs and contraceptive choice. Outlook 1988; 6(2):2–6.

45. North BB. Effectiveness of vaginal contraceptives in prevention of sexually transmitted diseases. In: Alexander NJ, Gabelnick HL, Spieler JM, eds. Heterosexual transmission of AIDS, New York: Wiley-Liss, 1990: 273–88.

46. Stone KM. Avoiding sexually transmitted diseases. Obstet Gynecol Clin N America 1990; 17:789–99.

47. Hulley SB, Newman TB, Cummings SR. Getting started: the anatomy and physiology of research. In: Hulley SB, Cummings RB, eds. Designing clinical research, Baltimore: Williams and Wilkins, 1988: 1–11.

48. Liskin L, Wharton C, Blackburn R et al. Condoms: the challenge. Popul Rep 1990; H-8.

49. CDC. Condoms for prevention of sexually transmitted diseases. MMWR 1988; 37:133–7.

50. Judson FN, Ehret JM, Bodin GF, Levin MJ, Rietjmeijer CAM. In vitro evaluation of condoms with and without nonoxynol-9 as physical and chemical barriers against Chlamydia trachomatis, herpes simplex virus type 2 and human immunodeficiency virus. Sex Transm Dis 1989; 16:51–6.

51. Conant MA, Spicer DW, Smith CD. Herpes simplex virus transmission. Sex Transm Dis 1984; 11:94–5.

52. Katznelson S, Drew WL, Mintz L. Efficacy of the condom as a barrier to the transmission of cytomegalovirus. J Infect Dis 1984; 150:155–7.

53. Conant M, Hardy D, Sernatinger J, Spicer D, Levy JA. Condoms prevent transmission of AIDS-associated retrovirus. JAMA 1986; 255:1706.

54. Minuk GY, Bohme CE, Bowen TJ. Condoms and hepatitis B virus infection. Ann Intern Med 1986; 104:584.

55. Minuk GY, Bohme CE, Bowen TJ, Cassol S. Condoms and prevention of AIDS. JAMA 1986; 256:1443.

56. Van de Perre P, Jacobs D, Sprecher-Goldberger S. The latex condom, an efficient barrier against sexual transmission of AIDS-related viruses. AIDS 1987; 1:49–52.

57. Lytle CD, Carney PG, Vohra S et al. Virus leakage through natural membrane condoms. Fifth International Conference on AIDS, Abstract No. M.A.P. 114, Montreal, June 4–9, 1989.

58. Pemberton J, McCann JS, Mahony DH, MacKenzie G, Dougan I, Hay I. Socio-medical characteristics of patients attending a VD clinic and the circumstances of infection. Br J Vener Dis 1972; 48:391–6.

59. McCormack WM, Lee Y, Zinner SH. Sexual experience and urethral colonization with genital mycoplasmas: a study in normal men. Ann Intern Med 1973; 78:696–8.

60. Barlow D. The condom and gonorrhoea. Lancet 1977; 2:811–12.

61. Hart G. Factors influencing venereal infection in a war environment. Br J Vener Dis 1974; 50:68–72.

62. Darrow WW. Condom use and use-effectiveness in high-risk populations. Sex Transm Dis 1989; 16:157–60.

63. Oberle MW, Rosero-Bixby L, Lee FK, Sanchez-Braverman M, Nahmias AJ, Guinan ME. Herpes simplex virus type 2 antibodies: high prevalence in monogamous women in Costa Rica. Am J Trop Med Hygiene 1989; 41:224–9.

64. Austin H, Louv WC, Alexander WJ. A case-control study of spermicides and gonorrhea. JAMA 1984; 251:2822–4.

65. Syrjanen K, Vayrynen M, Catren O et al. Sexual behavior of women with human papilloma virus (HPV) lesions of the uterine cervix. Br J Vener Dis 1984; 60:243–8.

66. Rosenberg MJ, Davidson AJ, Chen J-H, Douglas JM, Judson FN. Comparative
    effects of barrier contraceptives on sexually transmitted diseases in women.
    Submitted for publication, 1991.
67. Kelaghan J, Rubin GL, Ory HW, Layde PM. Barrier-method contraceptives and
    pelvic inflammatory disease. JAMA 1982; 248:184–7.
68. Cramer DW, Goldman MB, Schiff I et al. The relationship of tubal infertility to
    barrier method and oral contraceptive use. JAMA 1987; 257:2446–50.
69. Mann J, Quinn TC, Piot P et al. Condom use and HIV infection among prostitutes
    in Zaire. N Engl J Med 1987; 316:345.
70. Padian N. Male-to-female transmission of human immunodeficiency virus. JAMA
    1987; 258:3386–7.
71. Quinn TC, Glasser D, Cannon RO et al. Human immunodeficiency virus infection
    among patients attending clinics for sexually transmitted diseases. N Engl J
    Med 1988; 318:197–203.
72. Smiley ML, White GC, Becherer P et al. Transmission of human immunodeficiency
    virus to sexual partners of hemophiliacs. Am J Hematol 1988; 28:27–32.
73. Roumelioutou-Karayannis A, Nestoridou K, Mandalaki T et al. Heterosexual
    transmission of HIV in Greece. AIDS Res Hum Retroviruses 1988; 4:233–6.
74. Fischl MA, Dickinson GM, Scott GB, Limas N, Fletcher MA, Parks W. Evaluation
    of heterosexual partners, children, and household contacts of adults with AIDS.
    JAMA 1987; 257:640–4.
75. Ngugi EN, Plummer FA, Simonsen JN et al. Prevention of transmission of human
    immunodeficiency virus in Africa: effectiveness of condom promotion and
    health education among prostitutes. Lancet 1988; 2:887–90.
76. Laurian Y, Peynet J, Verroust F. HIV infection in sexual partners of HIV
    seropositive patients with hemophilia. N Engl J Med 1989; 320:183.
77. Kamenga M, Ryder RW, Jingu M et al. Evidence of marked sexual behavior
    change associated with low HIV-1 seroconversion in 149 married couples with
    discordant HIV-1 serostatus: experience in an HIV counseling center in Zaire.
    AIDS 1991; 5:61–7.
78. Allen S, Lindan CP, Hulley S, Carael M, Black D, Coates T. Behavior change
    among HIV– and HIV+ urban Rwandan women. Presented at National
    Institute of Mental Health Workshop on HIV Prevention and Behavior
    Change, Washington, DC, April 4, 1991.
79. Trussell J, Menken J. Lifetable analysis of contraceptive failure. In: Hermalin AI,
    Entwisle B, eds. The role of surveys in the analysis of family planning programs,
    Liège: Ordina Editions, 1982: 537–71.
80. Trussell J. Hatcher RA, Cates W Jr, Stewart FH, Kost K. Contraceptive failure in
    the United States: an update. Stud Fam Plann 1990; 21:51–4.
81. Nakamura RM, Coulson AH, Voeller R et al. In vitro condom testing [Abstract
    6510]. In: Program and abstracts, IV international conference on AIDS,
    Stockholm: Stockholm International Fairs, 1988.
82. Free MJ, Hutchings J. Condom quality management. In: Alexander NJ, Gabelnick
    HL, Spieler JM, eds. Heterosexual transmission of AIDS, New York: Wiley-Liss,
    1990:370–97.
83. Vessey MP, Villard-Mackintosh L, McPherson K, Yeates D. Factors influencing
    use-effectiveness of the condom. Br J Fam Plann 1988; 14:40–3.

84. Consumers Union. Can you rely on condoms? Consumer Rep 1989; (March): 135–41.
85. Golombok S, Sketchly J, Rust J. Condom failure among homosexual men. J AIDS 1989; 2:404–9.
86. Tindall B, Swanson C, Donovan B, Cooper DA. Sexual practices and condom usage in a cohort of homosexual men in relation to human immmunodeficiency virus status. Med J Aust 1989; 151:318–22.
87. vanGriensven GJP, deVroome EMM, Tielman RAP, Coutinho RA. Failure rate of condoms during anogenital intercourse in homosexual men. Genitourin Med 1988; 64:344–6.
88. Albert AE, Hatcher RA, Graves W. Condom use and breakage among women in a municipal hospital family planning clinic. Contraception 1991; 43:167–76.
89. Richters J, Donovan B, Gerofi J, Watson L. Low condom breakage rate in commercial sex. Lancet 1988; 2:1489.
90. Program for Appropriate Technology in Health, Program for Introduction and Adaptation of Contraceptive Technology. Monitoring condom quality. Outlook 1987; 5:2–5.
91. Ahmed G, Liner EC, Williamson NE, Schellstede WP. Characteristics of condom use and associated problems: experience in Bangladesh. Contracept 1990; 42:523–33.
92. Wright EA, Kapu MM, Wada I. Use of condoms as contraceptive and disease preventive measures among residents of Jos, northern Nigeria. Contracept 1990; 42:621–7.
93. Potter LS, Clarke K. Multicountry study of acceptability of spermicidally lubricated condoms: summary report, volume 1. Research Triangle Park, NC: Family Health International, 1988. Unpublished.
94. Population Council. Study of the determinants and quality of condom use in two eastern Caribbean countries: Barbados and St. Lucia. Final technical report, New York, 1990.
95. Piedrahita C, Hinson K, Foldesy R, Steiner M, Joanis C. Latex condom breakage study, Barbados and St. Lucia condom lot. Research Triangle Park, NC: Family Health International, 1990. Unpublished.
96. Drew WL, Blair M, Miner RC, Conant M. Evaluation of the virus permeability of a new condom for women. Sex Transm Dis 1990; 17:110–2.
97. Singh B, Cutler JC, Utdjiam HMD. Studies on the development of a vaginal preparation providing both prophylaxis against venereal disease and other genital infections and contraception. Br J Vener Dis 1972; 48:57–64.
98. Bolch OH Jr, Warren JC. In vitro effects of Emko on Neisseria gonorrhoeae and Trichomonas vaginalis. Am J Obstet Gynecol 1973; 115:1145–8.
99. Cowan ME, Cree GE. A note on the susceptibility of N. gonorrhoeae to contraceptive agent Nonyl-P. Br J Vener Dis 1973; 49:65–6.
100. Singh B, Postic B, Cutler JC. Virucidal effect of certain chemical contraceptives on type 2 herpes virus. Am J Obstet Gynecol 1976; 126:422–5.
101. Asculai SS, Weis MT, Rancourt MW, Kupfenberg AB. Inactivation of herpes simplex viruses by nonionic surfactants. Antimicrob Agents Chemother 1978; 13:686–90.
102. Hicks DR, Martin LS, Getchell JP et al. Inactivation of HTLV-III/LAV-infected cultures of normal human lymphocytes in vitro. Lancet 1985; 2:1422–3.

103. Amortegui AJ, Melder RJ, Meyer MP, Singh B. The effect of chemical intravaginal contraceptives and betadine on Ureaplasma urealyticum. Contracept 1984; 30:135–41.
104. Benes S, McCormack WM. Inhibition of growth of Chlamydia trachomatis by nonoxynol-9 in vitro. Antimicrob Agents Chemother 1985; 27:724–6.
105. Kelly JP, Reynolds RB, Stagno S, Louv WC, Alexander WJ. In vitro activity of the spermicide nonoxynol-9 against Chlamydia trachomatis. Antimicrob Agents Chemother 1985; 27:60–2.
106. Amortegui AJ, Myer MP. The in vitro effect of chemical intravaginal contraceptives on Chlamydia trachomatis. Contracept 1987; 36:481–85.
107. Kappus EW, Quinn TC. The spermicide nonoxynol-9 does not inhibit Chlamydia trachomatis in vitro. Sex Transm Dis 1986; 13:134–7.
108. Quinn TW, O'Reilly KR. Contraceptive practices of women attending the sexually transmitted disease clinic in Nashville, Tennessee. Sex Transm Dis 1985; 12:99–102.
109. Cole CH, Lacher TG, Bailey JC, Fairclough DL. Vaginal chemoprophylaxis in the reduction of reinfection of women with gonorrhoeae. Br J Vener Dis 1980; 56:314–18.
110. Jick H, Hannan MR, Stergachis A, Heidrich F, Perera DR. Vaginal spermicides and gonorrhea. JAMA 1982; 248:1619–21.
111. Louv WC, Austin H, Alexander WJ, Stagno S, Cheeks J. A clinical trial of nonoxynol-9 as a prophylaxis for cervical Neisseria gonorrhoeae and Chlamydia trachomatis infections. J Infect Dis 1988; 158:518–23.
112. Cutler JC, Singh B, Carpenter U. Vaginal contraceptives as prophylaxis against gonorrhea and other sexually transmissible diseases. Adv Planned Parent 1977; 12:45–56.
113. Rendon AL, Covarrubias J, McCarney KE, Marion-Landais G, Luna del Villar J. A controlled, comparative study of phenylmercuric acetate, nonoxynol-9 and placebo vaginal suppositories as prophylactic agents against gonorrhea. Curr Ther Res 1980; 27:780–3.
114. Berger GS, Keith L, Moss W. Prevalence of gonorrhea among women using various methods of contraception. Br J Vener Dis 1975; 51:307–9.
115. Magder LS, Harrison HR, Ehret JM, Anderson TS, Judson FN. Factors related to genital Chlamydia trachomatis and its diagnosis by culture in a sexually transmitted disease clinic. Am J Epidemiol 1988; 28:298–308.
116. Rosenberg MJ, Rojanapithayakorn W, Feldblum PJ, Higgins JE. Effect of the contraceptive sponge on chlamydial infection, gonorrhea, and candidiasis. A comparative clinical trial. JAMA 1987; 257:2308–12.
117. Kjaer SK, Engholm G, Teisen C et al. Risk factors for cervical human papilloma virus and herpes simplex virus infections in Greenland and Denmark: a population-based study. Am J Epidemiol 1990; 131:669–82.
118. Hooton RM, Hillier S, Johnson C, Roberts PL, Stamm WE. Escherichia coli bacteriuria and contraceptive method. JAMA 1991; 265:64–9.
119. Eschenbach DA, Hillier S, Critchlow C et al. Diagnosis and clinical manifestations of bacterial vaginosis. Am J Obstet Gynecol 1988; 158:819–28.
120. Kreiss J, Ruminjo I, Ngugi E, Roberts P, Ndinya-Achola J, Plummer F. Efficacy of nonoxynol-9 in preventing HIV transmission. Fifth International Conference on AIDS, Abstract No. MAO 361, Montreal, June 5, 1989.

121. Reckart ML, Barnett JA, Manzon LM, Wittenberg L, McNabb A. Nonoxynol-9: its adverse effects. Sixth International Conference on AIDS, Abstract No. SC 36, San Francisco, June 23, 1990.

122. Trap R, Trap B, Peterson CS. Evaluation of the amount of nonoxynol-9 available in condoms for the inhibition of HIV using a method based on HPLC. Int J STD AIDS 1990; 1:346–8.

123. Washington AE, Gove S, Schachter J, Sweet RL. Oral contraceptives, Chlamydia trachomatis infection, and pelvic inflammatory disease. JAMA 1985; 253:2246–50.

124. McCormack WM, Rosner B, McComb DE et al. Infection with Chlamydia trachomatis in female college students. Am J Epidemiol 1985; 121:107–15.

125. Handsfield HH, Jasman LL, Robert PL et al. Criteria for selective screening for Chlamydial trachomatis infection in women attending family planning clinics. JAMA 1986; 255:1730–34.

126. Avonts D, Sercu M, Heyerick P, Vandermeeren I, Meheus A, Piot P. Incidence of uncomplicated genital infections in women using oral contraception or an intrauterine device: a prospective study. Sex Transm Dis 1990; 17:23–29.

127. Harrison HR, Costin M, Meder JB et al. Cervical Chlamydia trachomatis infection in university women: relationship to history, contraception, ectopy, and cervicitis. Am J Obstet Gynecol 1985; 153:244–51.

128. Weström L. Incidence, prevalence, and trends of acute pelvic inflammatory disease and its consequences in industrialized countries. Am J Obstet Gynecol 1980; 138:880–92.

129. Eschenbach DA, Harnish JP, Holmes KK. Pathogenesis of acute pelvic inflammatory disease: role of contraception and other risk factors. Am J Obstet Gynecol 1977; 128:838–50.

130. Royal College of General Practitioners Oral Contraception Study. Oral contraceptives and health, New York: Pitman, 1974.

131. Panser LA, Phipps WR. Type of oral contraceptive in relation to acute, initial episodes of pelvic inflammatory disease. Contraception 1991; 93:91–9.

132. Rubin GL, Ory HW, Layde PM. Oral contraceptives and pelvic inflammatory disease. Am J Obstet Gynecol 1982; 144:630–5.

133. Wølner-Hanssen P, Svensson L, Mårdh P-A, Weström L. Laparoscopic findings and contraceptive use in women with signs and symptoms suggestive of acute salpingitis. Obstet Gynecol 1985; 66:233–8.

134. Wølner-Hanssen P, Eschenbach DA, Paavonen J et al. Decreased risk of symptomatic chlamydial pelvic inflammatory disease associated with oral contraceptive use. JAMA 1990; 263:54–9.

135. Wølner-Hanssen P. Oral contraceptive use modifies the manifestations of pelvic inflammatory disease. Br J Obstet Gynaecol 1986; 93:619–24.

136. Svensson L, Weström L, Mårdh P-A. Contraceptives and acute salpingitis. JAMA 1984; 251:2553–5.

137. Grossman C. Possible underlying mechanisms of sexual dimorphism in the immune response, fact and hypothesis. J Steroid Biochem 1989; 34:241–51.

138. Hunter DJ, Mati JK. Contraception, family planning, and HIV. Presented at the International Workshop on AIDS and Reproductive Health, Bellagio, Italy, October 1990. To be published by Plenum Press in AIDS and Women's Health.

139. Plummer FA, Simonsen JN, Cameron DW et al. Cofactors in male-female sexual
     transmission of human immunodeficiency virus type 1. J Infect Dis 1991;
     163:233–39.
140. Hira SK, Kamanga J, Macuacua R, Feldblum PJ. Oral contraceptive use and HIV
     infection. Int J STD AIDS 1990; 1:447–8.
141. Simonsen JN, Plummer FA, Ngugi EN et al. HIV infection among lower
     socioeconomic strata prostitutes in Nairobi. AIDS 1990; 4:139–44.
142. Darrow WW, CDC Collaborative Group. Human immunodeficiency virus type 1
     and other sexually transmitted infections in American prostitutes. Am J
     Epidemiol, 1991 (in press).
143. Carael M, Van de Perre PH, Lepage PH et al. Human immunodeficiency virus
     transmission among heterosexual couples in Central Africa. AIDS 1988;
     2:201–5.
144. Latif AS, Katzenstein DA, Bassett MT, Houston S, Emmanuel JC, Marowa E.
     Genital ulcers and transmission of HIV among couples in Zimbabwe. AIDS
     1989; 3:519–23.
145. Siraprasiri T, Thanprasertsuk S, Rodklay A et al. Study of risk factors for HIV
     infection among prostitutes in Chiengmai, Thailand. Presented at Field
     Epidemiology Training Program Second International Conference, Puebla,
     Mexico, January 1990.
146. Mati J, Maggwa A, Chewe D et al. Contraceptive use and HIV infection among
     women attending family planning clinics in Nairobi. Sixth International
     Conference on AIDS, Abstract No. Th.C.99, San Francisco, June 24, 1990.
147. European Study Group. Risk factors for male to female transmission of HIV. Br
     Med J 1989; 298:411–15.
148. Musicco M, The Italian Partners' Study. Oral contraception, IUD, condom use and
     man to woman sexual transmission of HIV infection. Sixth International
     Conference on AIDS, Abstract No. Th.C. 584, San Francisco, June 24, 1990.
149. Edelman DA. The use of intrauterine contraceptive devices, pelvic inflammatory
     disease, and Chlamydia trachomatis infection. Am J Obstet Gynecol 1988;
     158:956–9.
150. Daling JR, Department of Epidemiology, University of Washington, School of
     Public Health. Personal communication, March 28, 1991.
151. Kronmal RA, Whitney CW, Mumford SD. The intrauterine device and pelvic
     inflammatory disease: the Women's Health Study reanalyzed. J Clin Epidemiol
     1991; 44:109–22.
152. Burkman RT, Lee NC, Ory HW, Rubin GL. Response to "The intrauterine device
     and pelvic inflammatory disease: the Women's Health Study reanalyzed." J Clin
     Epidemiol 1991; 44:123–5.
153. Senanayake P, Kramer DG. Contraception and the etiology of pelvic inflammatory
     disease: new perspectives. Am J Obstet Gynecol 1980; 138:852–60.
154. Kahn JG, Walker CK, Washington AE, Landers DV, Sweet RL. Diagnosing pelvic
     inflammatory disease: a comprehensive analysis and new algorithm. JAMA,
     1991 (in press).
155. Paavonen J, Vesterinen E. Intrauterine contraceptive device use in patients with
     acute salpingitis. Contraception 1980; 22:107–14.
156. Burkman RT, Women's Health Study. Association between intrauterine device and
     pelvic inflammatory disease. Obstet Gynecol 1981; 57:269–76.

157. Kaufman DW, Watson J, Rosenberg L et al. The effect of different types of intrauterine devices on the risk of pelvic inflammatory disease. JAMA 1983; 250:759–62.
158. Lee NC, Rubin GL, Ory HW, Burkman RT. Type of intrauterine device and the risk of pelvic inflammatory disease. Obstet Gynecol 1983; 62:1–6.
159. Witoonpanich P, Koetsawang A, Koetsawang S et al. PID associated with fertility regulating agents. Contraception 1984; 30:1–21.
160. Vessey MP, Yeates D, Flavel R, McPherson K. Pelvic inflammatory disease and the intrauterine device: findings in a large cohort study. Br Med J 1981; 282:855–7.
161. Buchan H, Villard-Mackintosh L, Vessey M, Yeates D, McPherson K. Epidemiology of pelvic inflammatory disease in parous women with special reference to intrauterine device use. Br J Obstet Gynaecol 1990; 97:780–88.
162. Grimes DA. Intrauterine devices and pelvic inflammatory disease: recent developments. Contracept 1987; 36:97–109.
163. Sinei SKA, Schulz KF, Lamptey PR et al. Preventing IUD-related pelvic infection: the efficacy of prophylactic doxycycline at insertion. Br J Obstet Gynaecol 1990; 97:412–9.
164. Ladipo OA, Farr G, Otolorin E et al. Prevention of IUD-related pelvic infection: the efficacy of prophylactic doxycycline at IUD insertion. Adv Contracept 1991; 7:43–54.
165. Cramer DW, Schiff I, Schoenbaum SC et al. Tubal infertility and the intrauterine device. N Engl J Med 1985; 312:941–7.
166. Daling JR, Weiss NS, Metch DJ et al. Primary tubal infertility in relation to the use of an intrauterine device. N Engl J Med 1985; 312:937–41.
167. Falk HC. Interpretation of the pathogenesis of pelvic infection as determined by cornual resection. Am J Obstet Gynecol 1946; 52:66–72.
168. Haji SN. Does sterilization prevent pelvic infection? J Reprod Med 1978; 20:289–90.
169. Vessey M, Huggins G, Lawless M, Yeates D, McPherson K. Tubal sterilization: findings in a large prospective study. Br J Obstet Gynaecol 1983; 90:203–9.
170. Huggins GR, Sondheimer SJ. Complications of female sterilization: immediate and delayed. Fertil Steril 1984; 41:337–55.
171. Vermesh M, Confino E, Boler LR, Friberg J, Gleicher N. Acute salpingitis in sterilized women. Obstet Gynecol 1987; 69:265–7.
172. Edelman DA, Berger GS. Contraceptive practice and tuboovarian abscess. Am J Obstet Gynecol 1980; 138:541–5.
173. Burkman RT, Tonascia JA, Atienza M, King TM. Untreated endocervical gonorrhea and endometritis following elective abortion. Am J Obstet Gynecol 1976; 126:648–51.
174. Osser S, Persson K. Postabortal pelvic infection associated with Chlamydia trachomatis and the influence of humoral immunity. Am J Obstet Gynecol 1984; 150:699–703.
175. Westergaard L, Philipsen T, Scheibel J. Significance of cervical Chlamydia trachomatis infection in postabortal pelvic inflammatory disease. Obstet Gynecol 1982; 60:322–5.
176. Grimes DA, Schulz KF, Cates W Jr. Prophylactic antibiotics for curettage abortions. Am J Obstet Gynecol 1984; 150:689–94.

177. Park TK, Flock M, Schulz KF, Grimes DA. Preventing febrile complications of suction curettage abortion. Am J Obstet Gynecol 1985; 152:252–5.
178. Darj E, Stralm E-B, Nilsson S. The prophylactic effect of doxycycline on postoperative infection rate after first-trimester abortion. Obstet Gynecol 1987; 70:755–8.
179. Qvigstad E, Skaug K, Jerve F, Vik ISS, Ulstrup JC. Therapeutic abortion and Chlamydia trachomatis infection. Br J Vener Dis 1982; 58:182–3.
180. Osser S, Persson K. Postabortal pelvic infection associated with Chlamydia trachomatis and the influence of humoral immunity. Am J Obstet Gynecol 1984; 150:699–703.
181. Barbacci MB, Spence MR, Kappus EW, Burkman RC, Rao L, Quinn TC. Post-abortal endometritis and isolation of Chlamydia trachomatis. Obstet Gynecol 1986; 68:686–90.
182. Heisterberg L, Möller BR, Manthorpe T, Sörensen S, Petersen K, Nielsen NC. Prophylaxis with lymecycline in induced first-trimester abortion: a clinical controlled trial assessing the role of Chlamydia trachomatis and Mycoplasma hominis. Sex Transm Dis 1985; 12:782–5.
183. Schioötz H, Csango PA. A prospective study of Chlamydia trachomatis in first trimester abortion. Ann Clin Res 1985; 17:60–3.
184. Giertz G, Kallings I, Nordenvall M, Fuchs T. A prospective study of Chlamydia trachomatis infection following legal abortion. Acta Obstet Gynecol Scand 1987; 66:107–9.
185. Liskin L. Complications of abortion in developing countries. Popul Rep 1980; F-7:1–32.
186. Coeytaux F. Induced abortion in Sub-Saharan Africa: what we do and do not know. Stud Fam Plann 1988; 19:186–90.
187. Sherris J. The impact of unsafe abortion in the developing world. Outlook 1989; 7(3):2–7.
188. Henshaw SK. Induced abortion: a world review, 1990. Fam Plann Perspect 1990; 22:76–89.
189. Moreno L, Goldman N. Contraceptive failure rates in developing countries: evidence from the Demographic and Health Surveys. Int Fam Plann Perspect 1991; 17:44–9.
190. Kestelman P, Trussell J. Efficacy of combined barrier contraceptives. Submitted to Fam Plann Perspect, 1991.
191. United Nations Family Planning Association. Levels and trends of contraceptive use as assessed in 1988, New York: United Nations, 1989.
192. Judson FN. Fear of AIDS and gonorrhea rates in homosexual men. Lancet 1983; 2:159.
193. Handsfield HH. Decreasing incidence of gonorrhea in homosexually active men—minimal effect on risk of AIDS. West J Med 1985; 143:469–72.
194. Alter MJ, Hadler SC, Margolis HS et al. The changing epidemiology of hepatitis B in the United States. JAMA 1990; 263:1218–22.
195. Sorvillo FJ, Lieb L, Mascola L, Waterman SH. Declining rates of amebiasis in Los Angeles County. Am J Public Health 1989; 79:1563–4.
196. Bertrand JR, Makani B, Hassig SE et al. AIDS-related knowledge, sexual behavior and condom use among men and women in Kinshasa, Zaire. Am J Public Health 1991; 81:53–8.

197. Goldberg HI, Lee NC, Oberle MW, Peterson HB. Knowledge about condoms and their use in less developed countries during a period of rising AIDS prevalence. Bull WHO 1989; 67:85–91.

198. Cates W Jr, Farley TMM, Rowe PJ, WHO Task Force on Infertility. Worldwide patterns of infertility: Is Africa different? Lancet 1985; 2:596–8.

199. WHO Task Force on Infertility (Cates W Jr, Farley TMM, Rowe PJ). Infections, pregnancies and infertility: perspectives on prevention. Fertil Steril 1987; 47:964–8.

200. Bowen GS, Aral SO, Magder LS, Reed DS, Dratman C, Wasser S. Risk behaviors for HIV infection in clients of Pennsylvania family planning clinics. Fam Plann Perspect 1990; 22:62–4.

201. Upchurch DM, Farmer MY, Glasser D, Hook EW III. Contraceptive needs and practices among women attending an inner city STD clinic. Am J Public Health 1987; 77:1427–30.

202. Bureau of Community Health Services. Guidelines for health promotion and disease prevention services in reproductive health care settings, Washington, DC, and Rockville, Maryland, 1981.

203. Brown ST, Wiesner PJ. Problems and approaches to the control and surveillance of sexually transmitted agents associated with pelvic inflammatory disease in the United States. Am J Obstet Gynecol 1980; 138:1096–1100.

204. Aral SO, Mosher WD, Horn MC, Cates W Jr. Screening for sexually transmitted diseases by family planning providers: is it adequate and appropriate? Fam Plann Perspect 1986; 18:255–8.

205. Schachter J, Stoner E, Moncada J. Screening for chlamydial infections in women attending family planning clinics—evaluation of presumptive indicators for therapy. West J Med 1983; 138:375–9.

206. Addiss DG, Vaughn ML, Holzhueter MA, Bakken LL, Davis JP. Selective screening for Chlamydia trachomatis infection in nonurban family planning clinics in Wisconsin. Fam Plann Perspect 1987; 19:252–6.

207. Bagshaw SN, Edwards D. Risk factors for Chlamydia trachomatis infection of the cervix: a prospective study of 2,000 patients at a family planning clinic. N Z Med J 1987; 100:401–3.

208. Binns B, Williams T, McDowell J, Brunham RC. Screening for Chlamydia trachomatis infection in a pregnancy counseling clinic. Am J Obstet Gynecol 1988; 159:1144–9.

209. Begley CE, McGill L, Smith PB. The incremental cost of screening, diagnosis, and treatment of gonorrhea and chlamydia in a family planning clinic. Sex Transm Dis 1989; 16:63–7.

210. Stein ZA. The need for methods women can use. Am J Public Health 1990; 80:460–2.

211. Aral SO, Cates W Jr, Beral V. Are sexually transmitted diseases (STD) inherently sexist? Gender as a risk factor in STD epidemiology. In: Blumenthal S, Eichler A, Weissman G, eds. Women and AIDS, Washington, DC: American Psychological Press (in press).

212. World Health Organization. AIDS prevention: guidelines for MCH/FP programme managers. I. AIDS and family planning. Geneva, 1990:29–38.

213. Wasserheit JN. Epidemiological synergy. Interrelationships between HIV infection and other STDs. Presented at the International Workshop on AIDS and Reproductive Health, Bellagio, Italy, October 29, 1990. To be published by Plenum Press in AIDS and Women's Health.
214. Bayer R. AIDS and the future of reproductive freedom. Milbank Quart 1990; 8(Suppl 2):179–204.
215. Levine C, Dubler NN. HIV and childbearing: 1) Uncertain risks and bitter realities: the reproductive choices of HIV-infected women. Milbank Quart 1990; 68:321–51.
216. Arras JD. HIV and childbearing: 2) AIDS and reproductive decisions: having children in fear and trembling. Milbank Quart 1990; 68:353–82.
217. Holmes KK, Karon JM, Kreiss J. The increasing frequency of heterosexually acquired AIDS in the United States, 1983–1988. Am J Public Health 1990; 80:858–62.
218. Donovan P. AIDS and family planning clinics: confronting the crisis. Fam Plann Perspect 1987; 19:111–38.

HUMAN IMMUNODEFICIENCY VIRUS INFECTION PREVENTION: THE NEED FOR COMPLEMENTARY STD CONTROL

Marie Laga, M.D., Ph.D.
Institute of Tropical Medicine
WHO Collaborating Centre on AIDS
Department of Microbiology
Nationalestraat 155
2000 Antwerp, Belgium

INTRODUCTION

The emergence of the AIDS epidemic in the 1980s has highlighted the importance of sexual transmission in the spread of infections, as well as the lack of control programs for sexually transmitted diseases (STDs) in many parts of the world.[1] Prior to AIDS, STDs were relatively neglected internationally. Since 1988, AIDS professionals have begun to think about possible connections between AIDS and other STDs, as they search for an explanation of the ravaging human immunodeficiency virus (HIV) epidemic in some parts of the world.

During the last decade, research on the relationship between HIV and other STDs has revealed interesting concepts. Sexual transmission of HIV may be facilitated by the presence of other STDs, which probably partly explains the differing rates of spread of HIV around the world.[1] On the other hand, the natural history, diagnosis, or response to treatment of STDs may be altered in HIV-infected people. Several modes of interaction between HIV and STDs have been postulated:

1. STDs may enhance sexual transmission of HIV by increasing susceptibility in HIV-negative persons or increasing infectivity in HIV-positive persons.
2. HIV infection and consequent immunodeficiency may alter the natural history, diagnosis, or response to treatment of other STDs.
3. STDs may influence the natural history of HIV—for example, by accelerating progression to clinical disease.
4. HIV infection may increase susceptibility to other STDs.

This paper examines the available data from around the world on the first two HIV-STD interactions, which are the best studied and most important from a public health

Reproductive Tract Infections, Edited by A. Germain *et al.*
Plenum Press, New York, 1992

point of view. Special emphasis will be given to implications for the Third World, as regards the future spread of HIV and STDs, and to program and policy implications for HIV and STD control.

Reproductive tract infections that are not sexually transmitted, such as iatrogenic infections (those acquired during medical procedures), or endogenous infections (those caused by overgrowth of organisms normally present in the genital tract), are not covered here, since published data on the interactions of these infections with HIV are not yet available.

HIV-STD INTERACTIONS

Problems Inherent in Studying HIV-STD Interactions

A critical analysis of studies of the relationship between HIV and STDs must consider several methodological problems.[2]

First, such studies are complicated by the fact that HIV itself is an STD. Because STDs and HIV are transmitted in the same way and share behavioral risk factors (e.g., multiple sexual partners, contact with commercial sex workers [CSWs]), infection with another STD may merely be a marker for a high-risk behavior rather than a causal link in HIV transmission. Accordingly, analyses that control for sexual behavior are essential in establishing whether STDs are independent risk factors for HIV transmission. Unfortunately, the reliability of sexual exposure data is often poor, especially in "one-time" cross-sectional studies when no relationship of confidence between the interviewer and the interviewed is established. Thus, in a cohort study among Kinshasa CSWs, women tended to give more reliable information on condom use and number of partners after they were familiar with the study and the interviewers, than they gave at the intake interview.

A second problem arises from the potential impact of HIV infection and related immunodeficiency on other STDs. For example, the frequency of genital herpes lesions in HIV-infected persons is increased (see below). Without prospective studies documenting the temporal sequence, it is impossible to determine if a higher rate of STDs such as genital ulcers among HIV-infected people indicates that STDs facilitate HIV transmission or whether the presence of an infection is a marker for HIV-related immunosuppression.

Measurement issues also arise in determining the presence or absence of STDs. This is mainly because laboratory identification of STDs is often not feasible or available, particularly in Third World settings. Though STDs can be defined on the basis of a clinical syndrome, the sensitivity and specificity of clinical signs and symptoms of nonulcerative STDs in women are poor. It is also important to distinguish between recent and old infections (when diagnosis is based on serology), and to differentiate between treated and untreated episodes of STDs. Furthermore, individuals can be coinfected with several STDs at once. Only comprehensive STD testing, based on laboratory confirmation, and analysis that adjusts for the presence of multiple STDs can prevent the detection of a false association between one STD and HIV.

It is clear from the methodological problems discussed above that cross-sectional studies are inadequate in addressing the problem of HIV-STD interaction, because of their inability to determine the sequence of events and the difficulty in adequately controlling for confounding factors. Only prospective studies (observational studies or intervention trials) in which confounding factors are adequately controlled for and comprehensive laboratory-based STD diagnosis is done can give convincing insights into HIV-STD interrelationships.

The Impact of STDs on the Sexual Transmission of HIV

Two questions arise when studying the impact of STDs on sexual transmission of HIV: First, are there STDs that increase susceptibility to HIV among individuals not infected with the virus? Second, are there STDs that enhance the infectivity of persons with HIV, increasing the probability of HIV transmission to sexual partners? At present, the biological variables that determine both infectivity of HIV and susceptibility to sexually transmitted HIV infection are poorly understood. This reflects in part the absence of simple, quantitative measures of levels of HIV in blood, semen, and cervical secretions.

However, the hypothesis that the presence of STDs enhances the sexual transmission of HIV is biologically plausible. First, STDs can cause disruption of the normal epithelial barrier (in case of genital ulceration) or microscopic discontinuity in cervical or vaginal mucosa (in case of gonococcal or chlamydial cervicitis or trichomonas vaginitis). Friability of genital mucosa (especially the cervix) is common in the presence of STDs. HIV has also been isolated directly from the ulcer base in both men and women.[3,4] All these factors could affect both susceptibility and infectiousness of HIV. Another mechanism by which STDs may facilitate HIV transmission is through the recruitment of HIV-target cells, such as lymphocytes and macrophages, in the genital tract. Although lymphocytes and macrophages are normally present in the male and female genital tract,[5,6] studies indicate that their numbers are strongly increased in case of genital tract inflammation.[7,8] Thus, STDs could potentially augment the susceptibility of HIV-negative partners by increasing HIV-susceptible cells and could augment the infectiousness of HIV-positive partners by increasing the number of HIV-infected cells.

The Role of Genital Ulcer Disease (GUD) in HIV Transmission. Numerous studies, mostly from Africa, have linked GUD—either as a nonspecific clinical syndrome or as an etiologic diagnosis, such as syphilis or genital herpes—with an increased risk of HIV infection.[9-28] However, the majority of the studies documenting a higher rate of HIV infection among persons with GUD, or a higher rate of genital ulcers among HIV-infected persons, used cross-sectional study designs. As discussed above, these studies cannot determine if GUD was a risk factor for HIV acquisition, a marker of HIV-related immunodeficiency, or simply a marker of high-risk behavior. This section will therefore focus on the results of the prospective studies on GUD and HIV transmission in which a multivariate analysis was performed (Table 1).

The most convincing evidence that GUD enhances HIV transmission comes from Cameron and colleagues.[9] They showed in a prospective study of male clients of female CSWs in Nairobi (with a known HIV infection rate of greater than 80 percent) that acquisition of a genital ulcer (usually chancroid) in these men was a highly significant independent risk factor for HIV seroconversion. The authors concluded that the presence of a genital ulcer in the women (adjusted odds ratio, 4.7) strongly increased the infectiousness to the male client. Additionally, their data showed that lack of male circumcision increased susceptibility for HIV among male partners.

Table 1. Selected Prospective Studies on
STDs as Risk Factors for HIV Transmission

Author and location	Population studied	STD (method of diagnosis)	Risk
Cameron, Kenya[9]	Heterosexual men (clients of CSWs)	GUD—mainly chancroid (culture)	4.7
Darrow, United States[10]	Homosexual men	Syphilis (serology)	1.5–2.2
Kingsley, United States[11]	Homosexual men	Herpes 2 (clinical syndrome–serology)	—
Holmberg, United States[12]	Homosexual men	Herpes 2 (serology)	3.5
Laga, Zaire[13]	Female CSWs	GUD—mainly chancroid (culture) Gonorrhea (culture) Chlamydial infection (antigen detection) Trichomoniasis (direct exam)	— 3.5 3.2 2.7
Plummer, Kenya[14]	Female CSWs	GUD (culture) Chlamydial infection (culture)	3.9 7.3

Another prospective study, among homosexual men in the United States, documented a strong association between herpes simplex virus type 2 (HSV-2) seroconversion and subsequent HIV seroconversion.[12] However, other investigators failed to demonstrate a significant association between history and serologic diagnosis of genital herpes and HIV seroconversion.[11] Darrow and coworkers found a significant association of HIV acquisition with both self-reported history of syphilis and serologic diagnosis of syphilis.[10]

Whereas in an early study of CSWs in Kenya, GUD was a strong independent risk factor for acquisition of HIV infection in women,[14] a prospective study of female CSWs in Kinshasa failed to demonstrate an association between GUD and HIV seroconversion.[22] However, the monthly incidence of GUD in the latter cohort was only 1 percent, which may have been too small to reveal such an association.

It seems plausible that GUD increases the susceptibility to HIV in an HIV-negative male partner or increases the infectivity of an HIV-positive man. However, the presence of ulcers may largely preclude sex because of the pain (though data confirming this hypothesis are not available). It is therefore more likely that the role of GUD in HIV transmission is mainly to increase susceptibility in HIV-negative females and to increase infectiousness in HIV-positive females.

Although data supporting GUD as a risk factor for HIV transmission are very convincing, more attention should be given to the population-attributable risk of this variable. What is the proportion of HIV infection that has occurred because of GUD in different populations? In other words, what proportion of HIV infections would be prevented if GUD could be completely eliminated? The prevalence and incidence of GUD are much lower than those of nonulcerative STDs, even in high-risk Third World populations.[29] For example, in a cohort study among female CSWs in Kinshasa, Zaire, the prevalence of GUD was 5 percent, and among 55 women who seroconverted during a two-year period, only four had an episode of GUD prior to seroconversion. Assuming that GUD was the responsible risk factor for HIV acquisition, prevention of GUD in this group would have prevented not more than 7 percent of the HIV seroconversion in this population. Similarly, in a survey of 7,068 male employees in Kinshasa, only 18 percent of the HIV-positive workers ever had experienced a genital ulcer during the last five years. The frequency of GUD is generally 2–5 times lower than that of nonulcerative STDs, even in countries with much higher prevalence and incidence rates of GUD than Zaire.[29] Thus, while the relative risk of HIV seroconversion in the presence of GUD is high, most seroconversions probably occur in its absence, even in Africa.

The Role of Nonulcerative STDs in HIV Transmission. Data obtained from prospective studies on the role of nonulcerative STDs and HIV infection are far more limited than those on the role of GUD. Two cohort studies from Africa have demonstrated that these syndromes may also facilitate HIV transmission. Plummer and coworkers found a significant association between chlamydial infection and HIV seroconversion in the Nairobi CSW cohort. Their data showed no association with gonorrhea and HIV, and trichomoniasis was not considered in this study.[14] In Kinshasa, 450 initially HIV-negative female CSWs were followed up for two years, with monthly STD checkups and HIV testing every three months. Women who seroconverted during the follow-up (55 cases, or 12 percent of the population) were compared with women who remained HIV-negative (controls). In the four-month period prior to seroconversion, the incidence of gonorrhea, chlamydial infection, and trichomoniasis was significantly higher in the cases than in the controls, after the investigators controlled for the number of clients and for condom use, with odds ratios of 3.5, 3.2, and 2.7, respectively.[13]

An association between genital warts and HIV infection is suggested from several studies, all cross-sectional, however.[30,31,32] Prospective studies on the role of genital warts and human papilloma virus (HPV) infection in HIV transmission are not yet available. Warts may enhance the efficiency of HIV transmission because they are not uncommonly traumatized during sexual activity, and secondary infection may occur in larger warts. However, in view of the pathogenesis of HPV infection, it seems more plausible that HPV infection and genital warts do not facilitate HIV transmission, but rather are themselves promoted by HIV-related immunosuppression.

If nonulcerative STDs in fact facilitate HIV transmission, the proportion of cases of HIV infection attributable to the nonulcerative STDs may far outweigh that due to GUD, because in most populations worldwide, such diseases as chlamydial infection, gonorrhea, and trichomoniasis are far more common than GUD. For example, in Africa, prevalence rates of gonorrhea may range from 1 percent to 15 percent in pregnant women, and from 20 percent to 60 percent in CSWs, while the prevalence of GUD ranges from 0.1 percent to 2 percent in pregnant women, and from 5 percent to 15 percent in CSWs.[29] The few available data on the incidence of STDs also indicate that incidence rates of GUD are much lower than those of the urethritis/cervicitis syndromes. Thus, the monthly incidence of GUD in Kinshasa CSWs was 1 percent, as compared with 12 percent for gonorrhea and 7 percent for chlamydial infection.

These results imply that STD control as part of HIV control programs should focus on all STDs, not merely on GUD, in order to have a considerable impact at the population level.

The Impact of HIV Infection on the Natural History, Diagnosis, and Response of Treatment of Other STDs

Because of its impact on the host immune response, HIV infection could theoretically affect other STDs in a number of ways (Table 2). HIV infection may, for example, alter the STD incidence or frequency of recurrence. HIV infection could conceivably give rise to atypical presentation of other STDs, including larger, more numerous, and more persistent lesions. HIV infection may also modify the natural history of other STDs, resulting in more frequent or more rapid development of complications, aberrant laboratory test results, or inadequate response to standard therapy.

Several methodological considerations discussed above also pertain to studies of these issues. Unfortunately, at the current time, few definite statements can be made about the impact of HIV infection on other STDs, because there are few well-controlled prospective studies with a suitable HIV-negative comparison group. Our overall understanding of the natural history of such STDs as syphilis, genital herpes, chancroid, and HPV infection in the absence of HIV infection is still relatively limited. In this context, case reports or even case series of HIV-infected persons without controls may be difficult to interpret and even misleading.

The Impact of HIV Infection on GUD. Evidence is now emerging that the frequency of GUD is higher among HIV-infected persons than among HIV-seronegative persons having the same sexual exposure. This finding may be attributable both to an increased number of clinical recurrences in persons with genital herpes and to an increased susceptibility to genital ulcers caused by *Haemophilus ducreyi* or other organisms. In a cohort study of 450 HIV-negative and 150 HIV-positive female CSWs in Zaire, the incidence of GUD was three times higher among those with HIV infection independently of sexual behavior.[33] This was largely explained by a higher rate of genital herpes recurrences, but chancroid (the most common etiology of GUD in most parts of Africa) was also more common in HIV-infected women.

Decreased responsiveness to single-dose therapy for chancroid was documented in Nairobi, where treatment failures were at least six times more common in HIV-positive than in HIV-negative patients.[34] In Zimbabwe, Latif found not only an increased risk of treatment failure for chancroid in HIV-positive people, but also more frequent atypical presentations, with larger lesions.[35]

Large chronic, persistent herpetic ulcerations are a frequent complication in HIV-infected persons with advanced immunodeficiency.[39,40] A number of reports also suggest an increased incidence of acyclovir-resistant infection with HSV-2 in HIV-infected patients.[36-38]

Table 2. Possible Impact of HIV Infection on the
Presentation, Natural History, Diagnosis, and Therapy of STDs

STD	Clinical presentation	Natural history	Performance of standard laboratory tests	Response to therapy
Syphilis		More persistent lesions More central neurological involvement	Lower sensitivity of serologic tests	Higher risk of treatment failure
Herpes	Larger lesions Atypical sites	Higher incidence		Higher incidence of acyclovir resistance
Chancroid	? Larger lesions	More persistent lesions		Higher failure with single dose regimens
Genital warts	Larger lesions	Higher incidence Higher progression to dysplasia or neoplasia	Higher viral load Higher HPV detection	Higher response to topical or laser therapy
Gonorrhea		? Higher incidence of gonococcal pelvic inflammatory disease		

Much attention has been focused on the impact of HIV infection on syphilis.[41–48] Numerous case reports suggest that the clinical presentation of syphilis may be atypical in the setting of HIV infection, progression to neurosyphilis more frequent, serologic tests more likely to give false negative or false positive results, and standard therapy for early infection inadequate. Most of these studies should be interpreted with caution, however, because they lack a comparison group of HIV-negative patients, and the numbers are often very small. It should also be stressed that the knowledge of the natural history, serologic diagnosis, and response to treatment of syphilis in the absence of HIV infection is still incomplete. In an elegant study, Lukehart and coworkers[41] compared 15 HIV-positive and 25 HIV-negative patients who had untreated primary or secondary syphilis: surprisingly,

Treponema pallidum was isolated by rabbit inoculation from cerebrospinal fluid (CSF) in similar proportions in both groups. However, the same study described three HIV-infected patients with early syphilis in whom routine therapy with benzathine penicillin failed to eradicate *Treponema pallidum* from CSF. In a study among Kinshasa CSWs, there was no significant difference between 40 HIV-positive and 50 HIV-negative women in the proportion with initial rapid plasma reagin (RPR) titers greater than or equal to 1–16, or in terms of the change in RPR titer one year following therapy.[48] Studies with larger numbers of syphilis cases in HIV-infected persons and a valid control group of syphilis cases among HIV-negative persons, and with facilities both for rabbit inoculation to isolate *Treponema pallidum* and for performing comprehensive clinical evaluations, will be needed to elucidate the very complex problem of syphilis in persons with HIV infection.

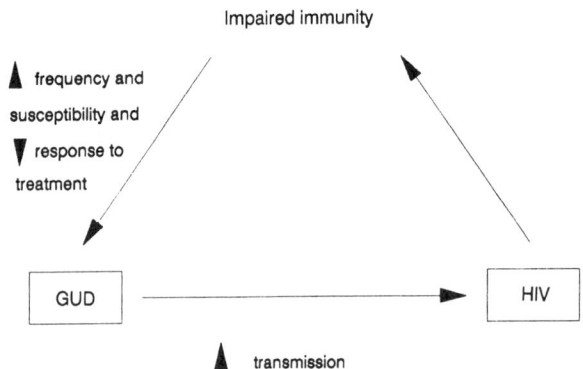

Figure 1. Interactions between GUD and HIV

The impact of HIV on the epidemiology of GUD is worrisome. If GUD facilitates transmission of HIV, and HIV-positive persons are more likely to have GUD (associated with more treatment failures), then these two infections are mutually reinforcing their spread, resulting in an increased prevalence of HIV and GUD in the community (Figure 1). This will have especially dramatic consequences in Sub-Saharan Africa (but also in Asia in the future), where both infections are already widespread. In addition, if GUD responds inadequately to standard antimicrobial therapy in HIV-infected patients, this interaction will become even stronger, and STD control programs in HIV-endemic countries will have to switch to more expensive alternative drugs for chancroid.

The Impact of HIV Infection on Nonulcerative STDs. The best-documented evidence of the effect of HIV infection on nonulcerative STDs is related to its impact on genital warts and HPV infection. HIV-infected people have higher rates of clinically manifested genital warts and high incidences of recurrence, and their response to standard therapy is probably altered.[30,31,32] For example, in 116 homosexual men treated with laser surgery for anal warts, the average number of recurrences was significantly greater among HIV-positive than among HIV-negative patients.[49]

One of the most worrisome impacts of HIV infection is its apparent ability to facilitate the development of anogenital dysplasia or neoplasia. Studies that incorporate HIV-negative comparison groups have consistently demonstrated that in both men and women, there is a significant association between HIV infection and cytological or histopathological evidence of neoplasia or preneoplastic abnormalities in cervical or anal specimens.[50-53] Longitudinal studies are now needed to confirm and clarify this issue. Even prior to the AIDS epidemic, East Africa had one of the world's highest cervical cancer rates, with an age-adjusted annual incidence of 23.3 per 100,000 women.[54] If both HPV infection and cervical cancer emerge as rapid opportunistic complications of HIV, mortality rates among young women may increase dramatically in Kenya and in other countries with no cervical cancer prevention programs.

There are currently no data to suggest that HIV infection alters the clinical presentation, diagnosis, or response to treatment of lower genital tract gonococcal, chlamydial, or trichomonal infections. However, the risk of complications of gonococcal disease may be increased. In a prospective study conducted among Nairobi CSWs, Plummer and coworkers[55] found that the incidence of gonococcal pelvic inflammatory disease among HIV-infected women was four times that among HIV-negative women. These findings need to be confirmed before any conclusions can be drawn.

STRATEGIC AND PROGRAMMATIC IMPLICATIONS OF HIV-STD INTERACTIONS

Besides the biological plausibility, several prospective studies, which controlled for behavioral risk factors, now support the hypothesis that the risk of HIV transmission is increased in the presence of GUD and nonulcerative STDs such as chlamydial infection, gonorrhea, and trichomoniasis. There is also increasing evidence that HIV infection may have an important impact on the clinical spectrum and management of other STDs. Therefore, the STD epidemic has severely aggravated the HIV epidemic in many parts of the world, while the HIV epidemic confronts us with additional obstacles in the fight against STDs (Figure 1). The program and policy implications of this interrelationship between HIV and other STDs are clear: since STDs are now recognized as readily modifiable risk factors for HIV transmission, STD prevention and control should become an integral part of HIV control programs. But there are many other reasons why close coordination between AIDS and STD programs is necessary:[56]

1 As the predominant modes of transmission of both HIV and other STDs are similar, primary prevention of either STDs or sexual transmission of HIV will help to reduce the other.
2. Many of the measures for preventing sexual transmission of HIV and STDs are the same, as are the target audiences for these interventions.

3. STD clinical services are an important access point for persons at high risk of both AIDS and STDs, not only for diagnosis and treatment, but also for education. For example, in the Kinshasa project, female CSWs started to change their behavior and use condoms once they gained confidence in health centers where they felt their STD problems were well taken care of.

4. Trends in STD incidence and prevalence can be useful early indicators of changes in sexual behavior and are easier to monitor than trends in HIV seroprevalence.

HIV-STD Program Coordination in Developing Countries

STD control has not been a political priority for most countries and development agencies, and very few countries have a functioning STD control program. Lack of awareness of the problem of STDs, competition with resources to control other important health problems, and, in some cases, reluctance to deal with diseases transmitted by sex have all played a role.[57] This situation seems now to be changing rapidly in many countries as a result of the launching of AIDS control programs, though the problem of resource allocation for HIV and STD control as compared with other health problems has not been resolved.

Coordination between AIDS and STD programs varies greatly from country to country. The extent of coordination is often related to the strength of the country's STD program at the time when AIDS first appeared. It is clear that in most developing countries, STD control programs were nonexistent or weak at the time the HIV epidemic emerged. Health planners were therefore badly prepared to develop strategies for HIV-STD coordination and integration activities. There is, however, growing interest in close coordination of AIDS and STD programs at the national and local levels. Coordination encompasses a spectrum of potential interactions, ranging from the peripheral level, where information can be shared through joint planning and implementation, to the central level, from which both programs can be run by a single manager.

Interventions to influence sexual behavior to prevent the transmission of STDs should be an integral part of any STD control program, though they have traditionally been neglected in favor of management of patients with STDs. These behaviors are receiving much attention now by AIDS prevention programs, which will undoubtedly also have an impact on the incidence of STDs. The AIDS pandemic further emphasizes the urgent need for increased support for broad programs of STD prevention, control, and research. At the national and international levels, STD and AIDS prevention and control programs should be combined or closely work together to develop strategies and effective means of program interaction and mutual support.

REFERENCES

1. Piot P, Laga M, Ryder R et al. The global epidemiology of HIV infection: continuity, heterogeneity and change. J AIDS 1990; 3:403–12.

2. Mertens TE, Hayes RJ, Smith PG. Epidemiological methods to study the interaction between HIV infection and other sexually transmitted diseases. AIDS 1990; 4:57–65.

3. Kreiss JK, Coombs R, Plummer FA et al. Isolation of human immunodeficiency virus from genital ulcers in Nairobi prostitutes. J Infect Dis 1989; 160:380–4.

4. Plummer FA, Wainberg MA, Plourde P et al. Detection of human immunodeficiency virus type 1 (HIV-1) in genital ulcer exudate of HIV-1-infected men by culture and gene amplification. J Infect Dis 1990; 161:810–1.

5. Krieger JN, Coombs R, Collier A et al. HIV recovery from semen: minimal impact of clinical stage of infection and minimal effect of semen analysis parameters. Sixth International Conference on AIDS, Abstract No. Th.C.102, San Francisco, June 20–24, 1990.

6. Van de Perre P, De Clercq A, Cogniaux-Leclerc J et al. Detection of IV p17 antigen in lymphocytes but not epithelial cells from cervicovaginal secretions of women seropositive for HIV: implications for heterosexual transmission of the virus. Genitourin Med 1988; 64:30–3.

7. Wolff H, Anderson DJ. Male genital tract inflammation associated with increased number of potential human immunodeficiency virus host cells in semen. Androl 1988; 20:404–10.

8. Mayer KH, Zierler S, Feingold L et al. Sexually transmitted diseases and genital tract inflammation among U.S. heterosexuals at increased risk for HIV infection. 30th ICAAC, Abstract No. 307, Atlanta, September 18–21, 1990.

9. Cameron DW, Lourdes JD, Gregory MM et al. Female to male transmission of human immunodeficiency virus type 1: risk factors for seroconversion in men. Lancet 1989; 2:403–7.

10. Darrow WW, Echenberg DF, Jaffe HW et al. Risk factors for human immunodeficiency virus (HIV) infections in homosexual men. Am J Public Health 1987; 77:479–83.

11. Kingsley LA, Armstrong J, Rahman A et al. No association between herpes simplex virus type-2 seropositivity or anogenital lesions and HIV seroconversion among homosexual men. J AIDS 1990; 3:773–9.

12. Holmberg SD, Stewart JA, Gerber AR et al. Prior herpes simplex virus type 2 infection as a risk factor for HIV infection. JAMA 1988; 259:1048–50.

13. Laga M, Nzila N, Manoka AT et al. Non ulcerative sexually transmitted diseases (STD) as risk factors for HIV infection. Sixth International Conference on AIDS, Abstract No. Th.C.97, San Francisco, June 20–24, 1990.

14. Plummer FA, Cameron DW, Simonsen N et al. Co-factors in male-female transmission of human immunodeficiency virus type 1. J Infect Dis 1991; 163:233–9.

15. Bulterys M, Chao A, Saah A et al. Risk factors for HIV-seropositive versus HIV-seronegative European expatriates in Africa. Sixth International Conference on AIDS, Abstract No. ThC.576, San Francisco, June 20–24, 1990.

16. Carael M, Van de Perre PH, Lepage PH et al. Human immunodeficiency virus transmission among heterosexual couples in Central Africa. AIDS 1988; 2:201–5.

17. De Vincenzi I, European Study Group. Risk factors for male to female transmission of HIV. Br Med J 1989; 298:411–5.

18. Greenblatt RM, Lukehart SA, Plummer FA et al. Genital ulceration as a risk factor for human immunodeficiency virus infection. AIDS 1988; 2:47–50.

19. Hira SK, Kamanga J, Macuacua R et al. Genital ulcers and male circumcision as risk factors for acquiring HIV-1 in Zambia. J Infect Dis 1990; 161:584–5.

20. Hudson CP, Hennis AJ, Kaaha P. Risk factors for the spread of AIDS in rural Africa: evidence from a comparative seroepidemiological survey of AIDS, hepatitis B and syphilis in southwestern Uganda. AIDS 1988; 2:255–60.
21. Latif AS, Katzenstein DA, Bassett MT. Genital ulcers and transmission of HIV among couples in Zimbabwe. AIDS 1989; 3:519–23.
22. Nzila N, Kivuvu M, Manoka AT et al. HIV risk factors in steady male partners of Kinshasa prostitutes. Sixth International Conference on AIDS, Abstract No. Th.C.579, San Francisco, June 20–24, 1990.
23. Piot P, Van Dyck E, Ryder RW et al. Serum antibody to Haemophilus ducreyi as a risk factor for HIV in Africa, but not in Europe. Fifth International Conference on AIDS, Abstract No. M.A.O.32, Montreal, June 4–9, 1989.
24. Ryder R, Ndilu M, Hassig S et al. Heterosexual transmission of HIV-1 among employees and their spouses at two large business in Zaire. AIDS 1990; 4:725–32.
25. Simonsen JN, Cameron DW, Gakinya MN et al. Human immunodeficiency virus infection among men with sexually transmitted diseases. N Engl J Med 1988; 319:274–8.
26. Simonsen JN, Plummer FA, Ngugi EN. HIV infection among lower socioeconomic strata prostitutes in Nairobi. AIDS 1990; 4:139–44.
27. Stamm WE, Handsfield HH, Rompalo AM et al. The association between genital ulcer disease and acquisition of HIV infection in homosexual men. JAMA 1988; 260:1429–33.
28. Van de Perre P, Clumeck N, Steens M et al. Seroepidemiological study on sexually transmitted diseases and hepatitis B in African promiscuous heterosexuals in relation to HTLV-III infection. Eur J Epidemiol 1987; 3:14–8.
29. Goeman J, Meheus A, Piot P. L'epidemiologie des maladies sexuellement transmissibles dans les pays en développement à l'époque du SIDA. Ann Soc Belge Méd Trop 1991 (in press).
30. Chiphangwi J, Dallabetta G, Saah A et al. Risk factors for HIV-1 infection in pregnant women in Malawi. Sixth International Conference on AIDS, Abstract No. M.B.P.57, San Francisco, June 20–24, 1990.
31. Kiviat N, Rompalo A, Bowden R et al. Anal human papilloma virus infection among human immunodeficiency virus-seropositive and -seronegative men. J Infect Dis 1990; 314:414–8.
32. Quinn TC, Glasser D, Cannon RO et al. Human immunodeficiency virus infection among patients attending clinics for sexually transmitted diseases. N Engl J Med 1988; 318:197–204.
33. Malele B, Kivuvu M, Nzila N et al. Genital ulcer disease (GUD) among HIV (+) and HIV (-) prostitutes in Kinshasa: prevalence, incidence and etiology. Fifth International Conference on AIDS in Africa, Abstract No. F.O.A.4., Kinshasa, Zaire, October 10–12, 1990.
34. MacDonald KS, Cameron W, D'Costa LJ et al. Evaluation of fleroxacin (RO 23-6240) as single-oral-dose therapy of culture-proven chancroid in Nairobi, Kenya. Antimicrob Agents Chemother 1989; 33:612–4.
35. Latif AS. Epidemiology and control of chancroid. Eighth ISSTDR, Abstract No. 66, Copenhagen, 1989.
36. Gold D, Corey L. Acyclovir prophylaxis for herpes simplex virus infection. Antimicrob Agents Chemother 1987; 31:361–7.

37. Thin RN. Management of genital herpes simplex infections. Am J Med 1988;
    85:3–6.
38. Conant MA. Prophylactic and suppressive treatment with acyclovir and the
    management of herpes in patients with acquired immunodeficiency syndrome. J
    Am Acad Dermatol 1988; 18:186–8.
39. Siegal FP, Lopez C, Hammer GS et al. Severe acquired immunodeficiency in male
    homosexuals, manifested by chronic perianal ulcerative herpes simplex lesions. N
    Engl J Med 1981; 305:1439–44.
40. Corey L, Genital herpes. In: Holmes KK, Mårdh P-A, Sparling PF et al. eds.
    Sexually transmitted diseases, second edition, New York: McGraw-Hill,
    1990:391–413.
41. Lukehart SA, Hook EW, Baker-Zander SA et al. Invasion of the central nervous
    system by Treponema pallidum: implications for diagnosis and treatment. Ann
    Intern Med 1988; 109:855–62.
42. Matlow AG, Rachlis AR. Syphilis serology in human immunodeficiency virus
    infected patients with symptomatic neurosyphilis: case report and review. Rev
    Infect Dis 1990; 12:703–7.
43. Terry PM, Page ML, Golmeier D. Are serological tests of value in diagnosing and
    monitoring response to treatment of syphilis in patients infected with human
    immunodeficiency virus? Genitourin Med 1988; 64:219–22.
44. Radolf JD, Kaplan RP. Unusual manifestations of secondary syphilis and abnormal
    humoral immune response to Treponema pallidum antigens in a homosexual
    man with asymptomatic human immunodeficiency virus infection. J Am Acad
    Derm 1988; 18:423–8.
45. Cusini M, Zerboni R, Muratori S et al. Atypical early syphilis in an HIV-infected
    homosexual male. Dermatologica 1988; 177:300–4.
46. Musher D, Hamille RJ, Baughn RE. Effect of human immunodeficiency virus
    infection on the course of syphilis and on the response to treatment. Ann Int
    Med 1990; 113:872–81.
47. Haas JS, Bolan G, Larsen S et al. Sensitivity of treponemal tests for detecting prior
    treated syphilis during human immunodeficiency virus infection. J Infect Dis
    1990; 162:862–6.
48. Manoka AT, Laga M, Kivuvu M et al. Syphilis among HIV-positive and HIV-
    negative prostitutes in Kinshasa: prevalence and serologic response to treatment.
    Sixth International Conference on AIDS, Abstract No. S.B.27, San Francisco,
    June 20–24, 1990.
49. Thomas G, Geraci A, Lavigne J et al. Recurrent anogenital warts and HIV status.
    Sixth International Conference on AIDS, Abstract No. Th.B.362,
    San Francisco, June 20–24, 1990.
50. Byrne MA, Taylor-Robinson D, Munday PE et al. The common occurrence of
    human papilloma virus infection and intraepithelial neoplasia in women infected
    by HIV. AIDS 1989; 3:379–82.
51. Milburn PB, Brandsma JL, Goldsman CI et al. Disseminated warts and evolving
    squamous cell carcinoma in a patient with acquired immunodeficiency
    syndrome. J Amer Acad Dermatol 1988; 19:401–5.
52. Palefsky J, Gonzales J, Greenblatt RM et al. Anal intraepithelial neoplasia and anal
    papilloma virus infection among homosexual males with group IV HIV disease.
    JAMA 1990; 263:2911–6.

53. Feingold AR, Vermund SH, Burk RD et al. Cervical cytologic abnormalities and papilloma virus in women infected with HIV. J AIDS 1990; 3:896–903.
54. Parkin DM, Loara E, Muir CS. Estimates of the world wide frequency of sixteen major cancers in 1980. Int J Cancer 1988; 41:184–97.
55. Plummer FA. Personnel communications.
56. WHO/GPA/INF/90.2 doc. Consensus statement from the consultation on global strategies for coordination of AIDS and STD control programs, Geneva, 1990.
57. Piot P, Laga M. Current approaches to STD control in developing countries. In: Wasserheit J, ed. Behavioral interventions for the control and prevention of sexually transmitted diseases, Washington, DC: American Society for Microbiology, 1991 (in press).

MATERNAL HEALTH AND CHILD SURVIVAL: OPPORTUNITIES TO PROTECT BOTH WOMEN AND CHILDREN FROM THE ADVERSE CONSEQUENCES OF REPRODUCTIVE TRACT INFECTIONS

Kenneth F. Schulz, M.B.A.
Associate Director, International Activities

Joann M. Schulte, D.O.
Medical Epidemiologist

Stuart M. Berman, M.D.
Special Assistant for Perinatal and Adolescent Studies

Division of STD/HIV Prevention
Centers for Disease Control
1600 Clifton Road (Mailstop E02)
Atlanta, GA 30333

INTRODUCTION

Although AIDS, human papilloma virus infection, and other newly identified sexually transmitted diseases (STDs) are attracting much attention, we must remain vigilant to the serious sequelae of conventional STDs, especially in areas where traditional "venereal diseases" have not been controlled. The problems currently associated with syphilis and gonorrhea during pregnancy in various parts of the world are strikingly reminiscent of those faced by the Western world in the early 1900s. Particularly compelling is the need to control fetal wastage, prematurity, and complications in neonates caused by reproductive tract infections (RTIs), especially in Third World countries.

We have compared the seriousness of the problems caused by RTIs in the Third World with that of the infectious diseases currently addressed by international donor agencies. RTIs appear to be at least as serious, if not more so. Syphilis during pregnancy, in aggregate, appears to cause infant death, adverse outcome, or syphilitic infant in over 5 percent of cases where the pregnancy survives beyond 12 weeks (Table 1). Gonococcal ophthalmia neonatorum (GON), potentially leading to blindness or even death, occurs in 2–6 percent of newborns. Most adverse outcomes occur before birth or during the first 30 days after birth.

Reproductive Tract Infections, Edited by A. Germain *et al.*
Plenum Press, New York, 1992

Table 1. RTIs: Manifestations, Prevalence, and Transmission Rate

RTIs	Prevalence of infections in pregnant women	Transmission rate	Without interventions, incidence of the manifestations	Severity of the manifestations
Adverse pregnancy outcomes caused by syphilis; Treponema pallidum	0.03–0.3% in industrialized countries; 3–22% in Sub-Saharan Africa, parts of South America, and Fiji	Almost 100% of early maternal syphilis; perhaps as low as 23% if late; overall, 40–70%	At a seroprevalence of 10%, over 5% of *all* pregnant women would have an adverse outcome: 2%, spontaneous abortions; 2.4%, perinatal deaths; and 1.4%, syphilitic infants	Spontaneous abortion, stillbirth, premature infant, or congenital syphilis
GON; Neisseria gonorrhoeae (GC)	Low: 1% or less, such as in Western Europe and some parts of North America High: 4–20%, such as in Sub-Saharan Africa and Thailand	47%; 68% when concomitantly infected with Chlamydia trachomatis	Published: 4–6% of births in Africa; 2–4% being common in much of Africa	Blindness can and does result; in the Third World, blindness is known to result, but the incidence is unknown, and, moreover, blind children have a high mortality rate.
Chlamydial ophthalmia neonatorum; Chlamydia trachomatis (CT)	Range: 2–37% Common: 4–12% Low: 0–5% Medium: 6–14% High: 15% and higher	Total: 60–70% Conjunctivitis: 15–50%; severe, 15–30%; coming to medical care, 25%	Assuming a 10% seroprevalence, 2.5% of pregnancies would result in infants with conjunctivitis who seek medical care.	Conjunctivitis: asymptomatic to moderately severe with no resultant blindness and no hospitalization required; morbidity can last for weeks.
Chlamydial pneumonia; Chlamydia trachomatis	Range: 2–37% Common: 4–12% Low: 0–5% Medium: 6–14% High: 15% or higher	Pneumonia: 5–15%; coming to medical care, 5%	Assuming a 10% seroprevalence, 0.5% of pregnancies would result in infants with pneumonia.	Pneumonia: most illnesses are prolonged but do not require hospitalization; severe cases require hospitalization; no fatalities in developed countries, but could occur in Third World.
Neonatal herpes; genital herpes simplex virus (HSV)	20–50% in the U.S. have developed antibodies to HSV; viral excretion at delivery is approximately 0.01–0.39%; prevalence appears lower in other parts of the world.	Primary infection: 50% Recurrent infection: 0.4–8%	Incidence is 0.2–0.33 per 1,000 live births in the U.S., with overall mortality being 0.14–0.23 per 1,000 live births.	80–85% of children with neonatal HSV infection have widespread organ involvement; 70% of children with infection die.
GC, CT, Mycoplasma hominis, Ureaplasma urealyticum, and bacterial vaginosis	GC and CT from above; Mycoplasma hominis, 7–70%, with an average of about 40%; Ureaplasma urealyticum, 60–90%; bacterial vaginosis, 10–19%	Most large prospective studies have provided inconclusive evidence that these organisms alone are causative agents for preterm delivery or low birth weight. The role of gonococcal infection as a cause of prematurity appears to be strongest, though it should be confirmed in large intervention studies. Bacterial vaginosis may also be associated with adverse outcome. Premature birth and low birth weight.		

By comparison, neonatal tetanus has been estimated to cause between 8 percent and 67 percent of all neonatal deaths; neonatal tetanus death rates are generally between 0.5 percent and 2.0 percent.[1,2] In the absence of any interventions, estimated death rates associated with specific perinatal, infant, or childhood infectious diseases are measles, 2 percent; polio, 0.5 percent; pertussis, 2 percent; and tetanus, 1 percent.[2,3] These death rates are measured over periods of approximately 2–4 years of life, except for tetanus, which is measured over the first month. Thus, the adverse outcomes and deaths caused by RTIs are at least of the same magnitude as those caused by the infectious diseases currently addressed, but their incidence density is greater; that is, they occur over a shorter time frame.

Not only are the problems caused by RTIs at least as serious as those caused by the immunizable diseases currently addressed, but their associated interventions appear to be more cost-effective. The cost per child for full immunizations in developing countries has been estimated to vary between US$5 and $15.[4] A recent cost estimate done in Gambia showed the per-childhood-death-prevented costs of immunization to be measles, $40.83; pertussis, $99.85; and neonatal tetanus, $152.53.[5] By comparison, in many locations in the Third World, $1.40 would avert one case of GON and $12 would avert an adverse outcome associated with syphilis during pregnancy (Table 2).

Although the problems caused by RTIs may be more serious and their related interventions more cost-effective, international donor agencies have allocated hundreds of millions of dollars to other infectious diseases, and virtually nothing to RTIs. This disproportionate allocation of resources should obviously be corrected.

In this paper, we describe the seriousness and extent of the consequences of selected STDs for pregnancy outcomes and child survival. For each disease, we examine available data on the prevalence in pregnant women, the transmission rate to fetus or infant, and the incidence of manifestations in the fetus and child. We suggest interventions to prevent the adverse outcomes and assess the likely cost-effectiveness of each, where possible. Lastly, we make summary recommendations for prevention and control initiatives and further research.

ADVERSE PREGNANCY OUTCOMES CAUSED BY SYPHILIS

Prevalence of Syphilis in Pregnant Women

Reported prevalences of syphilis seroreactivity in pregnant women attending antenatal clinics in African and Latin American countries range from 3 percent to 16 percent (Table 3). Not only are these findings consistently high across the Third World, but they may even be underestimates. In Zambia, researchers analyzed the rapid plasma reagin (RPR) test for syphilis and found a false positive rate of 5 percent and a false negative rate of 11–14 percent, which led them to conclude that the actual prevalence of syphilis may be slightly higher.[16] These serological findings likely reflect sexually acquired syphilis rather than nonvenereal treponemal infections.[11,17,18]

Transmission Rate

The best estimates of the outcome of pregnancies that continue to the third trimester among women with syphilis come from earlier Western data, which current Third World conditions appear to simulate. One study was published in 1917, in the era before effective

Table 2. Cost-effectiveness, Ease of Implementation, and Likelihood of Success for Suggested Interventions

Focus of intervention	Intervention	Cost per adverse outcome averted	Cost-effectiveness assumptions	Ease of implementation	Likelihood of success
Adverse outcomes caused by syphilis during pregnancy	Early antenatal care attendance, serologic screening of all attendees, and treatment of reactive women and their sexual partners	At a prevalence of 1%, $70.00; at 10%, $12.00; at 15%, $9.30	$0.10 for each rapid plasma reagin, $1.00 for treatment with benzathine penicillin; 20% of women retreated; 67% of spouses treated; amortized equipment costs	The test is simple, with results within five minutes, and treatment is a simple single injection; early antenatal visits and treating partners are problematic.	Very likely that demonstrable improvement can be achieved even under difficult circumstances
GON	Ocular prophylaxis at birth with tetracycline 1% eye ointment; silver nitrate 1% eye drops may be effective	At a prevalence of 10% and 1%, respectively, $2.90 and $22.00 with silver nitrate, $1.40 and $11.00 with tetracycline	Transmission rate of 47%; 85% efficacy, $0.10 per dose for silver nitrate; 94% efficacy, $0.05 per dose for tetracycline; $5.00 per dose for ceftriaxone	Very easy, no testing, all newborns would receive eye prophylaxis; instillation very simple	Easy and effective intervention, so it has a high likelihood of success
Chlamydial ophthalmia neonatorum	Ocular prophylaxis with 1% tetracycline, 1% silver nitrate, or 0.5% erythromycin within one hour of delivery	At a prevalence of 5%, $4.24; at 10%, $2.24; at 20%, $1.24	Transmission rate of 25%; tetracycline used at $0.05 per dose; 7.2% failure rate	Very easy, no testing; GON prophylaxis would normally cover	High likelihood
Chlamydial pneumonia	Maternal screening for cervical infection and treatment of positives with seven days of oral erythromycin	At a prevalence of 5%, $281; at 10%, $145; at 20%, $77	Transmission rate of 5%; cost for maternal screening of $4.00 per test; sensitivity of a single test of 80%; cost of maternal erythromycin treatment of $3.36, with 90% efficacy	Moderately difficult; poses some problems in locating women for treatment and then obtaining compliance; may not be logistically feasible in many settings	Low to moderate likelihood
Neonatal herpes	If herpes lesions are present, cesarean delivery. However, in many Third World settings, cesarean section should be reserved for patients who have typical herpetic lesions and in clinical settings where the morbidity of cesarean section is low.	In industrialized countries, $23,000; in Third World countries, $2,300	Of pregnant women with clinical herpes simplex virus infection at delivery, 7.5% would have a primary infection; cost for a cesarean delivery: industrialized, $3,000; Third World, $300	Straightforward but expensive; difficult to differentiate herpes from other genital ulcer diseases in many Third World settings	Moderately high in industrialized countries; low in Third World settings
Premature birth and low birth weight	Evidence of etiologic role for RTIs requires further definition; therefore, proposing public health interventions is premature. Further research is needed. Nevertheless, because several of these microbial agents cause considerable maternal and infant morbidity and mortality, interventions may currently be justified on other grounds.				

syphilis treatment was available (Table 4),[19] and the other was published in 1951, in the era before modern syphilis control programs were operational (Table 5).[20] These two prominent studies both reported that about one third of pregnancies yielded a noninfected infant, for a transmission rate of approximately 60–70 percent. The agreement between the two studies is remarkable, given both the disparity in time and the differences in study populations.

Table 3. Positive Reactions to Venereal Disease
Research Laboratory and RPR Tests in Pregnant Women

Country and year	% positive
Brazil, 1979[6]	16
Central African Republic, 1980[7]	10
Chile, 1977[8]	3
Ethiopia, 1977[9]	13
Ethiopia, 1970[10]	15
Mozambique, 1985[11]	5–15
Rwanda, 1982[12]	4
Swaziland, 1980[13]	14
Zambia, 1980[14]	15
Zambia, 1982[15]	14
Zambia, 1984[16]	13
Zambia, 1984[17]	15

When untreated, both early and late syphilis apparently produce widely disparate outcomes of pregnancy (Table 5). Although infectivity to sexual partners ceases after four years, infectivity to the fetus lasts longer, since syphilis is a blood-borne transplacental infection. A fetus is almost always infected in utero in early maternal syphilis. On the other hand, a mother with late syphilis has a 23 percent chance of having an adverse outcome (Table 5). Assumptions regarding the early or late status of syphilis are therefore essential

Table 4. Effect of Untreated Syphilis on Pregnancy Outcome, England, 1917

Outcome of pregnancy	%
Stillbirth or late miscarriage	17
Infant death	23
Infected infant	21
Noninfected infant	39
Total	100

Source: reference 19.

Table 5. Effect of Untreated Syphilis on Pregnancy Outcome,
Philadelphia General Hospital, 1951

Outcome of pregnancy	Early syphilis (%)	Late syphilis (%)	Early and late combined (%)
Stillbirth	25	12	22
Neonatal death	14	9	12
Infected infant	41	2	33
Noninfected infant	20	77	33
Total	100	100	100

Source: reference 20.

to the accurate estimation of outcome of pregnancy for women with syphilis. In the 1951 study, 73 percent of patients were classified as having early syphilis.[20] In a report from Zambia, RPR card test results for seroreactive women were analyzed: 70 percent of women had a titer of 1:8 or more, which corresponds to that found in early untreated syphilis.[17] The outcomes from the 1951 study seem to be roughly applicable to Zambia. Therefore, the overall transmission rate from women with syphilis to the fetus or infant in the Third World is approximately 40–70 percent, with 20–100 percent possible, depending on the mix of early and late maternal syphilis.

Incidence of Manifestations

Congenital Syphilis. Congenital syphilis in a live-born infant is an extremely serious condition that is often disfiguring and debilitating, if not fatal. Moreover, its manifestations appear to be much worse in the Third World than in the United States. Data on congenital syphilis are not as abundant as on syphilis in adults during pregnancy, but the data that are available are comprehensive. A study in Zambia established that nearly 1 percent of babies delivered at the University Teaching Hospital in Lusaka had signs of congenital infection at birth, and close to 7 percent were seroreactive at birth. These figures are consistent with prior reports, in that most congenital syphilis is not diagnosed until weeks or months after birth.[21] In another study from Zambia, seroreactivity in infants under six months old was 3 percent.[16] Half the seroreactive infants had two or more clinical features suggestive of early congenital syphilis; of these, 60 percent required hospitalization.

These data are consistent with what is known about the transmission of syphilis from mother to infant. A pregnant woman with untreated syphilis apparently has an approximately 33 percent chance of giving birth to a live infant with syphilis (Table 5). The prevalence of seroreactivity in the pregnant women in the studies from Zambia was 13–15 percent. Consequently, if syphilis in those women was not treated, we would expect that 33 percent of the pregnancies in infected women would produce live infants with syphilis —that is, 4–5 percent of babies born. The congenital syphilis seroreactivity rates of 3 percent and 7 percent are within the expected range, and the higher rate could, moreover, have been caused by passive antibody transfer at birth.

Further confirmation of the incidence and problems associated with early congenital syphilis in Zambia comes from two treatment studies. Early congenital syphilis was diagnosed in 9 percent of admissions in one of the nursery wards[22] and 8 percent of admissions to the intensive care unit.[23] Although perhaps an underestimate, a Zambia study found that 25 percent of pregnant women with syphilis bore infants with congenital syphilis.[24]

Perinatal, Neonatal, and Infant Deaths. The relation between syphilis during pregnancy and stillbirths is well established. A case-control study of the relation between stillbirths and high titer RPR card test seroreactivity in Zambia yielded a relative risk of 28 (95 percent confidence interval of 12–63).[17] This result is consistent with the 1951 study from the United States, which showed that the relative risk of stillbirths for a mother with untreated early syphilis was 32 times greater than that for a noninfected mother.[20] In pregnant women with untreated early syphilis, nearly 40 percent of pregnancies resulted in perinatal death (i.e., stillbirth or neonatal death); in pregnant women with untreated late syphilis, over 20 percent resulted in perinatal death (Table 5).

In the University Teaching Hospital in Lusaka, Zambia, 42 percent of stillbirths were attributed to syphilis during pregnancy.[15] In Zambia, congenital syphilis was implicated in 30 percent of the total perinatal infant mortality, which was 50 per 1,000 births.[15,16] In other words, 1.5 percent of all Zambian pregnancies that extend beyond 20–27 weeks end in deaths caused by syphilis. This is an underestimate, moreover, because it does not include postneonatal infants and because many stillborn infants do not have clinical evidence of congenital syphilis.

In Ethiopia, studies conducted on perinatal mortality identified syphilis as the fourth most common cause of perinatal death, accounting for 10 percent of about 70 perinatal deaths per 1,000 births.[25] Studies also found that syphilis causes nearly 5 percent of all postneonatal infant deaths.[25] Thus, at least 1 percent of Ethiopian pregnancies extending beyond 20–27 weeks end in perinatal or postneonatal infant deaths caused by syphilis. In absolute numbers, 15,000 fetal and infant deaths each year in Ethiopia are directly attributable to syphilis.[26]

Spontaneous Abortion. The largest absolute effect of syphilis during pregnancy could be spontaneous abortion during the second trimester and early in the third trimester. Researchers estimate that 5 percent of all pregnancies in Ethiopia are lost because of syphilis, a total of 75,000 pregnancy losses each year,[26] whereas in Zambia, 19 percent of miscarriages are attributable to syphilis.[15] Pregnant women in Ethiopia who were found to be seropositive to syphilis tests were five times more likely to have a spontaneous abortion or stillbirth than women who were seronegative.[10] These data strongly point to spontaneous abortion as a major adverse outcome of syphilis during pregnancy. The precise magnitude of the problem, however, is difficult to measure anywhere in the world, but especially in Africa, where women usually do not seek prenatal care until late in the third trimester.

The estimate from Ethiopia that many pregnancies are lost to spontaneous abortion due to syphilis during pregnancy appears to be plausible. Between 15–43 percent of postimplantation pregnancies in the Western world end in spontaneous abortion.[27,28] Given the nutritional and health status of most African women, we estimate that 45 percent of their pregnancies spontaneously abort.

Many spontaneous abortions would not be affected by syphilis, however, as first-trimester abortions are usually associated with phenotypic or chromosomal fetal abnormalities.[29] All available data suggest that syphilis is likely to cause a few spontaneous abortions in the first trimester, but has a very pronounced effect in the middle trimester and early in the third trimester.[30] Most miscarriages occur in the first trimester, so we estimate that two thirds could not be caused by syphilis, which leaves a baseline spontaneous abortion rate of 15 percent after the first trimester. The best available data indicate that a woman with untreated early syphilis is 3.3 times more likely to have a miscarriage or premature stillbirth than a noninfected woman.[20] This would appear to be a conservative estimate, as stillbirth at full-term is associated with a relative risk of about 30, as noted earlier. In fact, if an infection is acquired from an expectant mother with early syphilis in the second trimester, spontaneous abortion is the most probable outcome.[18] Thus, we would expect the spontaneous abortion rate in pregnant women with untreated syphilis to be 3.3 times 15 percent, or at least about 50 percent.

In conclusion, we estimate that of pregnancies that extend beyond 12 weeks' gestation, 15 percent in noninfected women and 50 percent in women with syphilis would spontaneously abort. These estimates are consistent with what we know about spontaneous abortion and the pathogenesis of syphilis during pregnancy. Nevertheless, for purposes of estimation, we will use the approximately 20 percent rate from the Zambian study as a conservative estimate for our calculations of cost-effectiveness.

Suggested Intervention

The suggested intervention is encouragement of early antenatal care, serologic screening by RPR test immediately during the first visit and again during the early third trimester, and treatment of all reactive women and their sexual partners with 2.4 million units of benzathine penicillin. The key to the success of this intervention in most Third World settings is the immediate RPR test by the staff at the antenatal clinic at the time of the woman's visit. By contrast, if blood is drawn and sent to a laboratory, precious time is lost, and the most likely outcome is that the laboratory results and the woman will never meet again.

Antenatal syphilis screening is not merely a theoretical intervention. It was implemented as a pilot project in Zambia with demonstrable success.[31] Postintervention adverse outcomes due to maternal syphilis were reduced by 61 percent.

Cost-effectiveness of the Intervention[32]

The cost-effectiveness of this intervention was calculated at prevalence levels of 1 percent, 10 percent, and 15 percent. Underlying assumptions were that an RPR test would cost $0.10, and benzathine penicillin would cost $1.00; 20 percent of initial reactors would be re-treated at a second visit; 67 percent of all spouses of reactors at the first and second visit would be treated; and fixed initial costs for material and equipment would be amortized over the 1,000 antenatal clinic attenders. The total cost and the cost per adverse outcome averted are displayed at the different prevalence levels in a cost-effectiveness model (Table 6).

This program is relatively inexpensive, considering that the cost of intervention for 1,000 pregnant women at 10 percent seroprevalence would be $600.00. If the intervention is perfectly effective, it could prevent 17 spontaneous abortions, 19 perinatal deaths, and 14 syphilitic infants for every 1,000 pregnant women (Table 7). The cost for 1,000 pregnant women at 1 percent seroprevalence would be $420.00; in this case, the intervention would prevent two spontaneous abortions, two perinatal deaths, and two syphilitic infants.

Such a program, however, could not be expected to be perfectly effective. First, women may attend the prenatal clinics late, sporadically, or never. Second, some women and spouses may not be treated. Third, the screening test is not 100 percent sensitive and specific. Nonetheless, this intervention reduced adverse outcomes by 61 percent in Lusaka.[31]

Ease of Implementation and Likelihood of Success

The RPR test is relatively simple, and results can usually be obtained in less than five minutes. Testing while the woman is still in the clinic is the key to success, as well as being much easier logistically. Moreover, the treatment is a simple, single injection. The major hurdles to overcome will be persuading women to make antenatal visits early enough to prevent spontaneous abortions, and persuading male partners to be treated. Nevertheless, because of the relative simplicity of this intervention, demonstrable improvement is likely to be achieved even under difficult circumstances, such as in Zambia. Achieving full effects will be difficult and take longer.

Table 6. Cost-effectiveness of the Syphilis Intervention
(Cost per 1,000 Attenders)

Measure	1% prevalence	10% prevalence	15% prevalence
Two tests per attender, at $0.10	$200.00	$200.00	$200.00
Treatment of all reactors at first visit, at $1.00 per treatment	$10.00	$100.00	$150.00
Treatment at subsequent visit, at $1.00 per treatment, assuming 20% will be re-treated	$2.00	$20.00	$30.00
Treatment of spouses, at $1.00 per treatment, assuming that 67% of spouses of reactors at first and second visits will be treated	$8.00	$80.00	$120.00
Amortized cost for development and behavioral and educational material	$100.00	$100.00	$100.00
Amortized cost for micro-centrifuges and lamps	$100.00	$100.00	$100.00
Total	$420.00	$600.00	$700.00
Adverse outcomes averted	6	50	75
Cost per averted adverse outcome	$70.00	$12.00	$9.28

ADVERSE PREGNANCY OUTCOMES CAUSED BY GON

Prevalence of Gonorrhea in Pregnant Women

The prevalence of *Neisseria gonorrhoeae* (GC) in pregnant women in the Third World is reported to be between 0.5 percent and 22 percent (Table 8). Many countries, including Cameroun, Kenya, Senegal, and Uganda, have documented rates of 18 percent or higher. Most of the studies that yielded these prevalence rates were undertaken in urban settings, and many researchers believe that gonorrhea is more prevalent in towns than in rural settings. Gonococcal infection, however, may be more common in some populations of rural women. For example, a study done at Yaoundé Central Hospital, an urban setting, in

Table 7. Reproductive Outcome Model, Assuming 10%
Seroreactivity in 1,000 Pregnant Women

Pregnancies and outcomes	Seroreactive pregnant women	Nonseroreactive pregnant women
Pregnancies	100	900
Spontaneous abortions in 2nd or early 3rd trimester	20 (20%)	27 (3%)
Excess spontaneous abortions due to syphilis	17	—
Pregnancies extending beyond 20–27 weeks	80	873
Perinatal deaths	24 (30%)	52 (6%)
Excess perinatal deaths due to syphilis	19	—
Syphilitic infants	14 (25%)	—

Source: reference 32.

the United Republic of Cameroun, yielded a gonorrhea infection rate of 14 percent.[33] The same authors found that 22 percent of rural women had gonorrhea. GON can be a more serious complication in a rural setting because of less-adequate medical care. Obviously, however, more data are needed from the rural areas of the Third World, as well as regions other than Africa.

Transmission Rate

The neonate acquires GON at delivery during passage through the infected birth canal. At least 30 percent of infants exposed to GC during birth will develop gonococcal eye infections if prophylaxis is not given.[43] In perhaps the best study to date, a transmission rate of 47 percent has been found in Kenya.[39,44] This same study demonstrated that the transmission rates of penicillinase producing GC (PPNG) and non-PPNG were similar. When the mother is concurrently infected with GC and Chlamydia trachomatis, the gonococcal transmission rate to the newborn is significantly higher—68 percent vs. 31 percent.[44]

Incidence of GON

The best estimates of the incidence of GON in the Third World place the rates between 0.5 percent and 5 percent.[43] These estimates look reasonable and are corroborated by available data from both East and West Africa. In Cameroun, 4 percent of neonates had GON;[33] a corresponding rate from a large hospital in Kenya was 3.6 percent, and in

Ethiopia, 6 percent.[44,45] These incidence rates were over 50 times higher than the rates from the Western world, which average 0.06 percent.[46]

Not only are the GON rates high in Africa and perhaps other parts of the Third World, but many cases may not be diagnosed because of inaccessibility to the health care system or lack of symptoms of disease. Moreover, only limited treatment is usually available for GON in general, with no treatment or only inadequate treatment possible for GON caused by PPNG infections. Many children are thus exposed to the risk of blindness and potentially, as a consequence, death.

Table 8. Prevalence of Neisseria Gonorrhoeae in Pregnant Women

Country	% positive
Cameroun (urban), 1984[33]	14
Cameroun (rural), 1984[33]	22
Cameroun, 1980[34]	15
Central African Republic, 1984[7]	15
Gabon (Franceville), 1984[35]	10
Gambia, 1982[36]	7
Ghana, 1983[37]	3
Ghana, 1985[38]	3
Kenya, 1988[39]	7
Kenya, 1983[37]	18
Malaysia, 1981[40]	1
Nigeria, 1983[37]	4
Senegal, 1983[37]	19
South Africa, 1983[37]	10
South Africa, 1986[41]	12
Swaziland, 1980[13]	4
Tanzania, 1983[37]	8
Thailand, 1981[40]	12
Uganda, 1983[37]	18
Zambia, 1986[42]	11

Severity of GON

GON, if untreated, often leads to blindness. In developing countries, blindness in children is not reported as being highly prevalent. The World Health Organization (WHO) concludes, however, that blind children in developing countries have a high mortality rate, so the true problem would not be apparent in prevalence surveys.[43,47] The incidence of blindness from GON in the Third World is unknown,[47] but historical data from industrialized countries on childhood blindness can provide some insight. At the turn of the last century, when prophylaxis and treatment for GON did not exist, and levels of gonococcal infection in pregnant women were similar to those now present in Third World countries, an estimated 20–40 percent of children in European homes for the blind were there as a result of GON.[43] Some estimates were even higher.

GON is no longer a cause of blindness in industrialized countries because of effective diagnosis and treatment of women during pregnancy or effective prophylaxis of neonates, or both (Table 9). In many parts of the Third World, ocular prophylaxis is not available, is incompletely applied, or has been discontinued.

Suggested Intervention[28]

Only limited treatment is available for GON in general; furthermore, an increasing number of gonococcal infections (10–80 percent) are caused by PPNG, for which frequently no or only inadequate treatment is available. Hence, we recommend priority attention to prophylaxis for GON rather than treatment of the woman. The transmission of GC from the maternal cervix to the newborn's eyes can be interrupted by instilling ocular prophylaxis immediately after birth. Ocular prophylaxis is undoubtedly the most feasible operational strategy, and the most cost-effective approach to GON prevention. Three

Table 9. Percentage of U.S. Children Blind because of GON,
and Number of States Requiring Prophylaxis

Period covered	% of blindness caused by GON	No. of states requiring prophylaxis
1906–11	24	1
1916–21	18	23
1926–31	9	39
1936–41	7	46
1946–51	2	47
1951–56	0.5	48
1958–59	0.3	50

Source: reference 48.

Table 10. Rates of GON among Exposed Newborns Receiving
Silver Nitrate, Tetracycline, and No Prophylaxis

Measure	Silver nitrate (%)	Tetracycline (%)	No prophylaxis* (%)
% of newborns exposed to GC[†] with GON	7	3	47
Efficacy of prophylaxis compared with no prophylaxis	85	94	na

* Infants from a historical cohort.
† The difference between the silver nitrate and tetracycline groups was 4 percent
  (95 percent confidence interval, −3.4 to 11.4).
Note: na=not applicable.
Sources: references 32 and 39.

regimens have been recommended: silver nitrate 1 percent eye drops; tetracycline 1 percent eye ointment; and erythromycin 0.5 percent eye ointment. Only the first two regimens have been evaluated prospectively in areas with a high proportion of PPNG.[32,39] Both silver nitrate and tetracycline were highly effective in the prevention of GON; tetracycline ointment was slightly more effective, albeit not statistically significantly so (Table 10). All other studies on the efficacy of the three regimens in preventing GON were retrospective, the prevalence of gonococcal infections in the mothers was often unknown, or the expected rate of GON was too low to discern any protective effect.[32]

Many potential explanations exist for the failure of ocular prophylaxis to prevent neonatal ophthalmia. The most prominent are acquisition of infection in utero following prolonged rupture of membranes, failure to instill the agent correctly into the conjunctival sac, flushing of the eye after administration of silver nitrate (to prevent chemical conjunctivitis), postpartum acquisition of GON either by autoinoculation or from other infected persons, and failure to differentiate chlamydial conjunctivitis from GON.

Silver nitrate is inexpensive, but is toxic if overconcentrated, primarily through evaporation. Single-dose ampules are much more expensive and less available than multidose containers. Tetracycline ointment is nontoxic and may remain longer in the eye because it is an ointment. It may be more effective, and multidose preparations are inexpensive and widely available in developing countries. Erythromycin ointment is expensive and not available in many Third World countries.

Delay in prophylaxis of more than four hours after birth is associated with a 4–5-fold increase in the risk of GON.[45] Prophylaxis should therefore be given as soon after birth as practical, preferably within one hour, for both hospital and home births. Traditional birth attendants' kits should include a single-dose dispensing system for eye prophylaxis.

Cost-effectiveness of the Intervention[32]

The cost-effectiveness of silver nitrate and tetracycline for ocular prophylaxis is compared with that of early diagnosis and treatment of GON in a group of 1,000 women with a 10 percent prevalence of gonococcal infection (Table 11). The cost for 1,000 prophylactic regimens is US$100 for silver nitrate and $50 for tetracycline. The Kenya study shows that 7 percent and 3 percent of the babies in the silver nitrate and tetracycline groups, respectively, will develop GON, compared with 47 percent of those who receive no prophylaxis. The price of one treatment regimen for GON varies from $5 (Ceftriaxone 125 mg IM single-dose) to $2 (Kanamycin 75 mg plus topical tetracycline). Optimum conditions are assumed in these examples, in that each case of GON would receive appropriate treatment in health care facilities.

The total costs of silver nitrate, tetracycline, and no prophylaxis per 1,000 women with a GC prevalence of 10 percent are $135, $65, and $235, respectively; the corresponding costs per adverse outcome averted are $2.87, $1.38, and $5.00 (Table 11). Indirect costs of visual impairment due to late or no adequate treatment are not taken into account.

Clearly, the strategy of ocular prophylaxis is more cost-effective than early diagnosis and treatment of GON. Furthermore, it is more convincing on humanitarian grounds, especially in areas where availability of efficacious drugs is low. In areas where prevalence of maternal gonococcal infection is low (e.g., less than 1 percent), the cost of ocular prophylaxis may be higher than the cost of treating GON (Table 12). Yet, the potential risk of blindness (if GON is not adequately treated) warrants use of ocular prophylaxis in all countries where the coverage of health care is not optimal.

Table 11. Cost-effectiveness of GON Control among 1,000 Pregnant
Women with a Prevalence of Gonococcal Infection of 10 Percent

Measure	Silver nitrate	Tetracycline	No prophylaxis
Price per dose	$0.10 (single-dose ampule)	$0.05 (multidose tubes)	na
Cost for 1,000 neonates	$100	$50	na
% of exposed newborns with GON*	7	3	47
Cost for treatment of GON (Ceftriaxone 125 mg IM; single dose, US$5)	$35	$15	$235
Total cost	$135	$65	$235
Cost per adverse outcome averted	$2.87	$1.38	$5.00

* Incidence rates based on Nairobi clinical trial.[39]
Note: na=not applicable.
Source: reference 32.

Table 12. Cost-effectiveness of GON Control among 1,000 Pregnant
Women with a Prevalence of Gonococcal Infection of 1 percent

Measure	Silver nitrate	Tetracycline	No prophylaxis
Price per dose	$0.10 (single-dose ampule)	$0.5 (multidose tubes)	na
Cost for 1,000 neonates	$100	$50	na
% of exposed newborns with GON*	0.7	0.3	4.7
Cost for treatment of GON (Ceftriaxone 125 mg IM; single-dose, US$5)	$3.5	$1.5	$23.5
Total cost	$103.5	$51.5	$23.5
Cost per adverse outcome averted	$22	$11	$5

* Incidence rates based on Nairobi clinical trial.[39]
Note: na=not applicable.
Source: reference 32.

Ease of Implementation and Likelihood of Success

The suggested intervention of ocular prophylaxis is very easy—all newborns would receive ocular prophylaxis, so it would require no testing. The instillation procedure is simple and takes a very short time. This intervention also has synergistic benefits in that it is also a prophylaxis for chlamydial ophthalmia neonatorum. Where deliveries are assisted by trained persons, this intervention would have a high likelihood of success.

ADVERSE PREGNANCY OUTCOMES CAUSED BY CHLAMYDIA

Prevalence of Chlamydia in Pregnant Women

Infection with *Chlamydia trachomatis* is the most common bacterial STD in the United States.[49] An estimated 4.65 million infections occur annually, and prevalence rates vary between 2 percent and 37 percent.[50,51] Studies published in the last two years have also found high prevalence in the developing world (Table 13). Reported African rates range from 4 percent to 20 percent. These findings mirror those in published studies of U.S. adolescents, in whom chlamydial infection rates of 8–37 percent have been reported.[50,58,62–64] An 8 percent rate of chlamydial infection was noted among 514 pregnant women screened during their first prenatal visit at a Taiwan (Taipei) clinic.[52] Chlamydial infections among

Table 13. Prevalence of Chlamydia Trachomatis in Pregnant Women

Country and year	% positive
Baltimore, USA, 1984[50]	37
Formosa, 1988[52]	8
Gabon, 1988[53]	18
Ghana, 1988[54]	4
Kenya, 1988[39]	9
Kenya, 1988[55]	20
Kenya, 1990[56]	8
New Mexico, USA, 1987[57]	22
Saudi Arabia, 1989[58]	9
Somalia, 1990[59]	18
South Africa, 1989[60]	11
Zimbabwe, 1989[61]	13

pregnant women are common even in socially restrictive countries, such as Saudi Arabia, where 9 percent of 106 asymptomatic pregnant women were infected, compared with 17 percent of 18 symptomatic women.[58]

Transmission Rate

Epidemiological evidence suggests infants become infected via delivery through an infected cervix.[65] Infection after cesarean section is rare.[66] Conjunctivitis can obviously develop after inoculation of an infant's eyes; it is unclear whether chlamydial pneumonia is acquired via direct aspiration of cervical or nasopharyngeal secretions or spread of infection from infected conjunctiva.[67] Risk of any chlamydial infection for infants born to infected mothers is estimated at 50–75 percent; chlamydial conjunctivitis that requires medical treatment is most common, developing in 25–50 percent of neonates born to infected mothers.[32,68] Chlamydial pneumonia develops in 5–10 percent of infants born to infected mothers.[32,56,68,69] The nasopharynx is thought to be the most common site of infection, but only 30 percent of infants so infected subsequently develop pneumonia.[68] Some infants may not have a clinically apparent infection, but may demonstrate poor weight gain and a concurrent rise in chlamydial antibody titers.[70] Possible associations between Chlamydia trachomatis and low birth weight, prematurity, fetal demise, and intrauterine growth retardation are discussed in a later section of this paper.

Incidence of Manifestations

The well-documented consequences of neonatal chlamydial infection are ophthalmia neonatorum and pneumonia. Ophthalmia neonatorum has declined in industrialized nations, but remains a problem in the developing world.[71] Chlamydial ophthalmia neonatorum was detected in 3 percent of 750 infants in a recent Gabon study,[72] 2 percent in Cameroun,[73] and a higher rate, of 8 percent, was noted in Kenya.[44] In contrast, the U.S. incidence is estimated at 0.4 percent.[74] Chlamydial pneumonia infects many infants in developing countries. In Costa Rica, 33 percent of 39 infants aged two weeks to six months had chlamydial Immunoglobin M (IgM) antibody identified by enzyme immunoassay (EIA) and microimmunofluorescent (MIF).[75] A prospective study of 112 consecutive infants less than six months of age in Bangkok, Thailand, found that 27 percent of pneumonia was caused by *Chlamydia trachomatis*.[76]

Severity of Manifestations

Typically, infected infants develop an inclusion conjunctivitis in the second or third week of life.[65] Chlamydial ophthalmia neonatorum differs from the gonorrhea version in that blindness does not develop, but corneal scarring and vascularization may occur.[68] Conjunctival infection may persist for months or years. On the other hand, untreated conjunctivitis may be self-limited, and conjunctival infection may be asymptomatic.

Pneumonia is the other major illness associated with maternal infection with *Chlamydia trachomatis*. Usually, infants present in the first three months of life with a prolonged history of cough that can be followed by cyanosis, a bluish discoloration indicating poor oxygenation.[77] The pneumonia has a slow onset, and the infant is typically afebrile. Three studies[78,79,80] have suggested persistently diminished respiratory function in children who had chlamydial pneumonia during infancy, but no specific pulmonary conditions, such as asthma, have been documented.

The severity of chlamydial pneumonia is quite variable. It is generally mild, but if untreated, it will result in morbidity that may last for weeks. Most illnesses do not require hospitalization, even without treatment. With treatment, the disease will still last at least 2–3 weeks. Some cases have to be hospitalized, usually because of cyanosis, initiated by paroxysms of coughing. Rarely, the intensity and persistence of cyanosis may require administration of oxygen and monitoring in an intensive care unit. No fatalities have been attributed to *Chlamydia trachomatis* pneumonia in the developed world. In the Third World, fatalities could be occurring but remain undetected.

Suggested Intervention

Erythromycin is currently the only drug available to treat cervical chlamydial infections in pregnant women, but it must be used in multiple-dose regimens, unlike the single dose that can eradicate gonorrhea.[66,74] Erythromycin's efficacy may be as high as 90 percent, but patient compliance may be reduced by the required number of doses and by side effects such as gastrointestinal disturbances.[81] Furthermore, where per capita health budgets are very limited, such expensive treatments are beyond reach.[82]

As with GON, we recommend ocular prophylaxis rather than treatment of the woman. Alternative approaches are silver nitrate, erythromycin, and tetracycline. A recent New

York study concluded that compared with silver nitrate, tetracycline or erythromycin did not significantly reduce the incidence of chlamydial conjunctivitis among infants born to infected women.[83] A prospective trial of ocular prophylaxis done among neonates in Kenya found tetracycline prophylaxis more effective than silver nitrate, although not statistically significantly so. Laga and colleagues recommended the use of tetracycline ointment for ocular prophylaxis.[39]

Cost-effectiveness of the Intervention[32]

The assumptions for the cost-effectiveness analysis include chlamydial prevalences of 5 percent, 10 percent, and 20 percent; a 25 percent transmission rate for chlamydial conjunctivitis; and a 5 percent transmission rate for pneumonia. Relative to ocular prophylaxis, we assumed a failure rate of 7.2 percent.[39] The cost of prophylaxis with tetracycline was assumed to be US$0.05 per dose. The cost of 14 days of treatment for an infant with oral erythromycin was $3.34. For maternal treatment, the additional assumptions include a diagnostic test cost of $4.00, which is reasonable for antigen detection tests, but perhaps could be lowered for mass applications. We assumed that the sensitivity of the tests to detect maternal infection is 80 percent, with a specificity of 98 percent. The cost of maternal erythromycin treatment is $3.36, based on a seven-day course of 2 grams per day. An efficacy of 90 percent is assumed for erythromycin.

The easiest intervention would be ocular prophylaxis of neonates within one hour of birth. The cost-effectiveness of tetracycline ocular prophylaxis contrasted with no ocular prophylaxis is calculated per 1,000 women (Table 14). At a 5 percent prevalence rate, the cost per adverse outcome averted is $4.24. At a prevalence of 10 percent, the cost per adverse outcome prevented is $2.24; at 20 percent, $1.24. Unfortunately, however, this treatment leaves the infant at risk for chlamydial respiratory infection.

The calculations are somewhat more complex regarding maternal treatment (Table 15). The universal cost of a screening test is included for the total example, although in these calculations, no charge has been assigned for the personnel cost in administering the test or personnel costs in the laboratory. Obviously, the cost of maternal screening and treatment is far greater than that of prophylaxis, but it may be more effective than indicated. The failure rates are based on cervical infection, as there are too few observations on prevention of neonatal disease. Again, as in the prophylaxis estimates, no medical care costs have been inserted.

Maternal treatment is more costly, but still may be cost-effective in developed countries. Some pneumonia cases will be hospitalized, often with periods in intensive care. Only one of these cases in a sample of 1,000 pregnant women could tip the scales in favor of maternal screening and treatment. Nevertheless, the strategy does not appear to be cost-effective for Third World countries. Obviously, ocular prophylaxis is the most cost-effective approach. Moreover, if ocular prophylaxis is directed against gonococcal conjunctivitis, chlamydial conjunctivitis generally will be covered as well.

Ease of Implementation and Likelihood of Success

Ocular prophylaxis with tetracycline ointment is the most easily implemented approach, the most affordable, and the most likely to succeed. While detection and treatment of all infected mothers could potentially prevent both conjunctivitis and pneumonia, important barriers could block its implementation. The laboratory testing and multiple antibiotic doses required to treat mothers decrease the likelihood of success. In addition, limited health budgets make it unlikely that many developing countries can afford such programs. In comparison, ocular prophylaxis is inexpensive, needs no laboratory

Table 14. Cost-effectiveness Estimates for Ocular Prophylaxis of Neonates to Prevent Chlamydia Trachomatis Neonatal Conjunctivitis among 1,000 Pregnant Women with Chlamydia Prevalences of 5%, 10%, and 20%

Measure	Tetracycline			No prophylaxis		
Prevalence in mother	5%	10%	20%	5%	10%	20%
Cost per dose	$ 0.05	$ 0.05	$ 0.05	NA	NA	NA
Cost per 1,000 infants	$50.00	$50.00	$50.00	NA	NA	NA
No. of infants with conjunctivitis	0.9	1.8	3.6	12.5	25	50
Treatment costs	$ 3.00	$ 6.01	$12.02	$41.75	$83.50	$167.00
Total cost	$53.00	$56.01	$62.02	$41.75	$83.50	$167.00
Cases averted or treated	12.5	25	50	12.5	25	50
Cost per adverse outcome averted	$4.24	$2.24	$1.24	$3.34	$3.34	$3.34

Note: NA=not applicable.
Source: reference 32.

testing, and requires one treatment at a point when infants are easily accessible. Gonococcal ocular prophylaxis should take priority over chlamydial prophylaxis because the former's consequences—blindness and possible death—exceed those of chlamydial infections. Yet, gonococcal prophylaxis will generally cover chlamydial ophthalmia neonatorum as well.

Table 15. Cost-effectiveness Estimates for Maternal Screening and Treatment to Prevent Chlamydia Trachomatis Neonatal Conjunctivitis and Pneumonia among 1,000 Pregnant Women with Chlamydia Prevalences of 5%, 10%, and 20%

Measure	5% prevalence	10% prevalence	20% prevalence
Diagnostic test (1,000 x $4.00)	$4,000.00	$4,000.00	$4,000.00
80% test sensitivity; cases identified	40	80	160
98% test specificity; false positives	19	18	16
Cost of maternal treatment ($3.34 per case)	$197.06	$328.92	$591.04
Failure of maternal therapy (10% of cases)	4	8	16
Maternal cases missed for diagnosis	10	20	40
Total maternal cases	14	28	56
Resultant infant diseases Conjunctivitis (25%) Pneumonia (5%)	3.5 0.7	7 1.4	14 2.8
Total requiring treatment	4.2	8.4	16.8
Total cost of treatment ($3.34 per case)	$14.03	$28.06	$56.11
Total cost of strategy	$4,211.89	$4,356.98	$4,647.15
No Maternal Screening			
Total infants exposed	50	100	200
Resultant infant diseases Conjunctivitis (25%) Pneumonia (5%)	12.5 2.5	25 5	50 10
Cost-Effectiveness			
Adverse outcomes averted	15	30	60
Cost per adverse outcome averted	$280.79	$145.23	$77.45

Source: reference 32.

GENITAL HERPES INFECTIONS OF THE NEWBORN

Prevalence of Herpes in Pregnant Women

Genital herpes simplex virus (HSV) infections are among the most common STDs in the United States. HSV-2, typically acquired via sexual contact, has an estimated prevalence of 50–60 percent in lower-income persons and 10–35 percent among higher-income strata.[84-87] No studies have specifically addressed the prevalence of HSV-2 antibodies in pregnant women. However, the prevalence of genital infection in pregnant women at delivery is considered to be less than 1 percent.[88] The actual incidence of women excreting the herpes virus at delivery time has been estimated at 0.01–0.39 percent, irrespective of herpes history.[88-91] Cervical virus shedding has been noted to be 0.56 percent in symptomatic women and 0.66 percent in asymptomatic women.[90-93]

Transmission Rate

According to current estimates, more than half the infants delivered vaginally become infected[94] when primary maternal infection is present at delivery; transmission rates of 0.4–8 percent have been estimated for a vaginally delivered infant with recurrent maternal infection.[92] Primary herpes infections are most likely to affect an infant because such infections are associated with the highest levels of viral particles, cervical infection, low levels of maternal antibody, and prolonged shedding.[92] However, many infants who develop neonatal disease have mothers who are completely asymptomatic at delivery.[87,92]

The vaginal route of infection, one of three possible mechanisms, accounts for 70–80 percent of the infections. In utero, infants may become infected via transplacental or ascending infections, no matter whether maternal infection is primary or recurrent.[95] Postnatal infection, usually with type 1 herpes virus, has been increasingly recognized and may account for 30 percent of all such infections.[96,97,98] Sources of the type 1 virus have included fathers, breast-feeding mothers, visitors, and hospital personnel.[99-102]

Incidence of Manifestations

Neonatal herpes has been estimated to develop in one of every 2,000–5,000 infants in the United States, but increasing trends have been noted.[88,92] One recent study found one HSV-infected infant in every 1,500 deliveries.[103] Developing countries, particularly Central African countries, have prevalences of HSV-2 antibodies at least as high as the U.S. rate, but only a few deliveries of infected infants have been reported.[104,105]

Severity of Manifestations

Primary herpes infections are the most damaging in terms of morbidity and mortality among both infected adults and neonates delivered by infected women. Outside the neonatal period, primary HSV infections often present with crops of painful vesicular lesions that ulcerate and heal over a 1–2-week period. Systemic symptoms, such as headache, fever, muscle aches, burning during urination, and malaise, may accompany the genital ulcers.[106] In contrast, the severity of neonatal infection depends upon which body sites are infected and how extensive viral replication is. The spectrum of HSV disease includes intrauterine infection; disseminated infection (involving multiple organs); encephalitis; and infections limited to the eyes, skin, or mouth.[92,107,108]

Typically, up to 85 percent of HSV-infected neonates have disseminated or central nervous system (CNS) manifestations.[92] Such infants have a 70 percent mortality rate if untreated; the rate decreases to 40 percent if acyclovir or vidarabine therapy is instituted.[109,110] Herpes infections localized to the skin, eyes, or mouth are associated with lower mortality, but up to 30 percent of children thus affected may have some neurological impairment or ophthalmological problems, including cataracts.[92,109,111–113]

The HSV mortality and morbidity patterns among neonates may be changing, according to recent studies. A 1988 study in the United States showed that localized HSV infection, restricted to eyes, skin, or mouth, occurs in 44 percent of cases, and that 56 percent of infected infants manifest disseminated or CNS infection.[88,112] In 1988, overall mortality following therapy was approximately 20 percent, and more than one half of infected children reportedly had normal development at their first birthdays.[112]

Suggested Intervention[32]

Weekly screening for herpes virus during the last 4–8 weeks prior to delivery of all pregnant women with a history of genital herpes is *not* recommended. In areas where genital herpes is the predominant cause of genital ulcer disease (GUD), cesarean delivery is recommended in women who have herpetic lesions in the genital tract at the time of rupture of membranes or during labor. This recommendation is suggested only if the patient presents within 4–6 hours.[32,114]

In areas where genital herpes is a relatively minor contributor to GUD (in areas with large case numbers of chancroid and syphilis), the predictive value of genital ulcers for genital herpes is low. Further, the morbidity of cesarean section may be much higher in such areas. In such situations, the risk of morbidity associated with the cesarean section may be greater than the risk of neonatal herpes.[32] Therefore, cesarean section should be reserved for patients who have typical herpetic lesions, especially women with typical primary genital herpes, and for clinical settings where the morbidity and mortality associated with cesarean section is low.

The two therapeutic choices for treatment of neonatal herpes infections are vidarabine and acyclovir;[109,112,115] increasing numbers of U.S. hospitals are switching to the latter.[110]

Cost-effectiveness of the Intervention[32]

Assuming that 8 percent of pregnant women with clinical herpetic infection at delivery would have a primary infection, and the cost of cesarean section is US$3,000 in industrialized countries and $300 in the Third World, the cost per case prevented has been estimated as $23,000 in developed countries and $2,300 in the Third World.

Ease of Implementation and Likelihood of Success

The implementation of this intervention in developed countries is relatively easy and straightforward but expensive. It would be problematic, however, in Third World settings, because the predictive value of genital ulcers for genital herpes is low and because the morbidity of cesarean section is generally much higher in such areas. Moreover, it is a prohibitively expensive intervention for developing countries and is not likely to succeed, because health budgets are limited and other neonatal infections are likely to merit higher priority. While the success rate would be moderately high in developed countries, it would be low in Third World settings. Thus, in Third World settings, this intervention is not cost-effective, is difficult to implement, and has a very low likelihood of success.

PREMATURE BIRTH AND LOW BIRTH WEIGHT

STDs can have other severe consequences for infants born to infected mothers, including prematurity, low birth weight, sepsis, and intrauterine growth retardation. RTIs can also cause spontaneous abortions or stillbirths. Such outcomes have been reported in infants whose mothers had gonorrhea, chlamydia, or bacterial vaginosis. More recently, the possibility of similar associations has been considered with ureaplasma and mycoplasma infections.

"Premature birth" refers to any infant born at less than 37 weeks' gestation (but more than 26 weeks' gestation). Such births generally result in low birth weight (less than 2,500 g). Other infants who are not premature can also be low birth weight because of in utero influences, such as infection or hypertension, that can cause intrauterine growth retardation.

New emphasis is being placed on links between RTIs and prematurity because the premature-birth rate has remained constant during the last three decades at 6–8 percent in the United States.[116] Premature infants account for 70–80 percent of all perinatal deaths in the United States after newborns with congenital malformations are excluded.[117]

Some 2–10 percent of all infants are low birth weight in developed countries, but the condition may occur in up to 30 percent of births in developing countries.[118] A recent Nairobi study found an 8 percent incidence of low birth weight.[119] The causes of low birth weight may be different in industrialized countries and the developing world. In the former, about two thirds of low birth weight infants are premature, while low birth weight infants in developing countries may more often be the product of intrauterine growth retardation.[120]

RTIs as a Possible Cause of Adverse Outcomes

STDs have been associated with both prematurity and low birth weight, and affect the fetus in varying ways. Usually, medical curricula about gonorrhea, for example, emphasize its association with ophthalmia neonatorum.[44] But gonorrhea has also been associated with chorioamnionitis, prematurity, and premature rupture of membranes.[121] A recent study in Nairobi found a maternal gonorrhea infection to be independently associated with preterm birth, an association that was independent of age, rupture of membranes, and hypertension.[122] Gonococcal infections were present in 4 percent of 175 controls and 11 percent of 166 cases; other STDs were not associated with preterm births. The authors suggest that successful treatment might reduce the prematurity rate by 14 percent. This new study confirms earlier studies that suggested a link between preterm birth and maternal gonorrhea, but were flawed by small sample sizes and the possible selection biases inherent in retrospective study designs.[123,124,125]

Maternal gonococcal infections and their relationship to prematurity have important implications for both the United States, where prevalence rates among pregnant women as high as 7 percent have been reported,[126] and the developing nations, where prevalence rates have been estimated as high as 22 percent.[33]

Between 25 percent and 40 percent of women infected with gonorrhea have a concurrent chlamydial infection,[127] which accounts for an estimated 4.65 million infections annually in the United States.[49] Depending on the population studied, chlamydial prevalence rates of 2–37 percent have been reported among U.S. women.[50] Reported prevalence rates among pregnant women in the developing countries have ranged from 4 percent to 20 percent.[54,60]

The association between *Chlamydia trachomatis* and prematurity and its related conditions is less clear than with gonorrhea, and more controversial. Some studies have suggested such associations, but these findings have not been replicated consistently in later studies. The earliest studies, in which most chlamydial infections were identified during the last trimester of pregnancy, did not reveal any statistically significant differences in regard to birth weight, prematurity, premature rupture of membranes, or stillbirth.[128,129,130] However, a prospective study of maternal chlamydial infection before 20 weeks' gestation found a 10-fold and fivefold increased risk of perinatal mortality and prematurity,[131] but was hampered by a small sample size. A more recent study found that women who were both culture-positive for chlamydia and seropositive for IgM antibodies against chlamydia had increased risk of delivering low birth weight infants and sustaining premature rupture of membranes.[132] Whether the IgM finding indicates a new chlamydial cervical infection or a more invasive one is uncertain.

A 1986 study of 47 women that used a multiple logistic analysis found an association between cervical chlamydial infection and preterm labor, premature rupture of membranes and low birth weight.[133] A much larger study of Native American women found that women with chlamydial infections had only a 1.5 relative risk of delivering a low birth weight infant, but a subset of women with an IgM seroconversion had a higher risk.[57] Another case-control study, involving 540 women, found only a subset of women with IgM antibodies were at higher risk of preterm delivery.[134] The usefulness of identifying pregnant women with chlamydial IgM antibodies merits further examination in both industrialized and developing nations.

Research examining any links between bacterial vaginosis and prematurity is limited, as are any studies of the syndrome based in the developing world. Such links are considered speculative; current thought is that increased intravaginal bacterial concentrations and a shift to potentially virulent flora may predispose a woman to premature delivery and its complications.[135] Organisms linked to bacterial vaginosis have been significantly associated with premature rupture of membranes, preterm labor, and amniotic fluid infection.[133,136] A diagnosis of bacterial vaginosis based on a gram stain has also been associated with preterm delivery.[137]

Fewer than 20 percent of women seen in a family practice clinic or a student health clinic were diagnosed with bacterial vaginosis,[138,139] but the condition has been diagnosed in 24–37 percent of women attending STD clinics.[140,141,142] The prevalence of bacterial vaginosis has been reported as 16–29 percent in pregnant U.S. women.[143,144,145] Two recent studies done in Zimbabwe are among the first to profile bacterial vaginosis in developing countries. One case-control study of maternity patients found clue cells in 20 percent of women who developed sepsis within 48 hours of a vaginal delivery, compared with 6 percent of controls.[61] Such clue cells are considered diagnostic of bacterial vaginosis. A second study found the vaginal flora to contain lactobacilli in 20 percent of prepartum women and a significant decrease postpartum.[146] Other studies have found 75 percent of women colonized vaginally with lactobacilli.

Initial results of the Vaginal Infection and Prematurity (VIP) Study, sponsored by the National Institutes of Health, are providing increased understanding of the possible role of bacterial vaginosis in prematurity and low birth weight. The study, involving 6,716 women, showed that pregnant women with bacterial vaginosis had a 40 percent increased risk of amniotic fluid infection;[147] mycoplasma and gardnerella organisms were weakly associated with such infections. Other researchers involved in the VIP study found carriage of *Trichomonas vaginalis* at midgestation weakly associated with premature rupture of membranes and low birth weight.[148]

Two other organisms, *Ureaplasma urealyticum* and *Mycoplasma hominis*, have gained increasing attention as possible causes of habitual abortion and stillbirth, chorioamnionitis, and low birth weight. Genital tract colonization of 40–80 percent has been reported for the former and 5–50 percent for the latter in U.S. studies.[149] *Ureaplasma urealyticum* has been cultured from amniotic fluid from 60 percent of patients with chorioamnionitis, and mycoplasma from 10 percent of such patients.[145] Other recent studies have suggested mycoplasma may be linked to CNS infection in preterm infants and chronic lung diseases. Studies have shown transient colonization with ureaplasma and mycoplasma in 15–59 percent of neonates.[150,151,152] Recolonization occurs with sexual contact;[153] Boston researchers have reported carriage rates as high as 54 percent for *Mycoplasma hominis* and 76 percent for *Ureaplasma urealyticum*.[154]

Women with a history of recurrent spontaneous abortion have had ureaplasma isolated more frequently than a control group,[155] but a majority of investigators have found no relationship between genital colonization with *Ureaplasma urealyticum* and fetal wastage.[156,157,158] However, *Ureaplasma urealyticum* is more frequently isolated from premature infants, spontaneously aborted fetuses, and stillborns than from full-term infants.[159,160] Some success in preventing such loss has been reported when such women are treated with antibiotics,[161,162] but the trials have been uncontrolled or had limited numbers.

Mycoplasma hominis and *Ureaplasma urealyticum* have also been associated with complications of chorioamnionitis later during pregnancy and low birth weight. *Ureaplasma urealyticum* have been isolated twice as frequently from neonates when chorioamnionitis was documented histologically.[163] Other studies, which specifically considered the length of rupture of membranes, have also found a significant association between mycoplasma infection and chiorioamnionitis.[164,165] Others have suggested that mycoplasma infection might result after membranes are ruptured, rather than being the causative agent.[166]

Mixed results have also come from studies examining the relationship between low birth weight and mycoplasma or ureaplasma infections. A prospective study of 484 prenatal patients, who were cultured at the time of the first visit, showed that both mycoplasma and ureaplasma cultures were associated with low birth weight.[153] Other studies have not found such an association.[158] Ureaplasma may cause infection after birth; a 1988 study of 100 neonates, mostly preterm, suggested ureaplasma may be associated with intraventricular hemorrhage and hydrocephalus.[167] Other reviews have suggested it may be related to chronic lung disease, especially in low birth weight neonates.[168,169] A recent review of nine cohort studies, two case-control studies, and one randomized clinical treatment trial found that the weight of the evidence did not support an association between mycoplasma species and prematurity or low birth weight.[170]

Suggested Intervention[32]

Currently available studies have provided inconclusive evidence that the organisms discussed in this section are causative agents for premature birth and low birth weight. The strongest case for an etiologic role in prematurity seems to exist for gonorrhea. Its role should be confirmed in large epidemiological studies. In Third World countries, where gonococcal infections are still highly prevalent in pregnant women, control of gonorrhea during pregnancy may have a substantial impact on prematurity and perinatal mortality. After gonorrhea, bacterial vaginosis is perhaps most likely to cause adverse outcomes.

Evidence of an etiologic role for the other organisms discussed above in prematurity and low birth weight is unclear. Part of the reason for these nebulous results may be methodologic. Suppose one of these organisms is truly causally related to adverse outcomes. It is also most likely correlated with many of the other organisms. If all of them are inserted into a multivariate analysis, multicollinearity could cause an analyst to conclude that none of the organisms are related to adverse outcomes even though at least one is. Yet, given the conflicting and unconvincing data that now exist, public health interventions specifically aimed at preventing premature birth and low birth weight caused by these agents are premature. Thus, cost-effectiveness analyses are not feasible.

SUMMARY

We have compared the seriousness of the problems caused by RTIs in the Third World with that of the infectious diseases currently addressed by international donor agencies. The problems caused by RTIs appear to be at least as serious as those infectious diseases, if not more so. Those associated with syphilis and gonorrhea during pregnancy are particularly well documented.

Not only are the problems caused by RTIs at least as serious as those caused by the immunizable diseases currently addressed in many locations in the Third World, but their associated interventions appear to be more cost-effective. For example, to avert one case of GON would cost about $1.40, and to avert one adverse outcome associated with syphilis during pregnancy, about $12.00. Comparative cost-effectiveness estimates for the immunizable diseases range from approximately $40 to $150 per adverse outcome averted.

Women's health benefits, furthermore, are not computed in our cost-effectiveness analyses. Synergistic effects to the woman in many instances would enhance the attractiveness of the interventions proposed. Of particular note are those interventions that we have deemed premature relative to pregnancy outcome and child survival, but that may be cost-effective and justifiable solely on maternal grounds.

A relatively minor amount of funds spent on interventions for syphilis during pregnancy and GON would yield large benefits. Consider a hypothetical country in East Africa, that has a population of 20 million, a crude birth rate of 50 per 100,000 (population), 1 million births per year, and approximately 1.5 million pregnancies per year. An intervention for GON would cost about $65,000 for 1 million births and would avert an estimated 47,000 cases of GON. An intervention to test and treat for syphilis during pregnancy would cost about $900,000 for 1.5 million pregnancies and would avert an estimated 75,000 adverse outcomes.

While the problems caused by RTIs may be more serious and their related interventions more cost-effective, international donor agencies have allocated hundreds of millions of dollars to other infectious diseases and virtually nothing to RTIs. This disproportionate allocation of resources should obviously be corrected.

SUMMARY RECOMMENDATIONS

- RTI interventions to prevent and control GON and the adverse outcomes caused by syphilis during pregnancy are the most important to reduce adverse outcomes of pregnancy and improve morbidity and mortality. They are the most cost-effective, and the most likely to succeed (Tables 1 and 2). Thus, funds must be committed by international donor agencies for programs to implement these interventions.

- Research must be done on the most cost-effective approaches for GON prophylaxis; on the most effective GON prophylaxis in various Third World settings, especially those with high PPNG prevalence; and on the prevalence of gonorrhea during pregnancy and of GON, especially in rural areas and in countries where prevalence studies have not been undertaken.

- Research must be conducted into the most cost-effective approaches to prevent and control the serious sequelae of syphilis during pregnancy; these approaches include contact tracing or partner notification and treatment procedures in Third World settings. Further research on the prevalence of syphilis during pregnancy should be initiated, especially in rural areas and in countries where prevalence studies have not been undertaken.

- For *Chlamydia trachomatis*, it is important to seek alternatives to erythromycin with increased efficacy and acceptability for treatment of pregnant women, and to seek less-expensive and simpler methods for culture or antigen detection.

- Intervention research aimed at one specific organism or at several organisms should be performed to assess the efficacy of antibiotic treatment and the role of genital infections in ascending intrapartum infection and prematurity.

- A simulation model should be developed that could be used to estimate the effects of different prevention strategies on pregnancy outcome and child survival.

ACKNOWLEDGMENTS

Many of the cost-effectiveness analyses and recommended interventions emanate from the proceedings of the World Health Organization (WHO) Consultation on Maternal and Perinatal Infections, held in Geneva, Switzerland, November 28–December 2, 1988. The primary organizers of the consultation were Dr. R. J. Guidotti, Scientist, Dr. M. A. Belsey,

Chief, Maternal and Child Health, Division of Family Health, and Dr. A. Meheus, the WHO Chief, Programme of Sexually Transmitted Diseases, Division of Communicable Diseases. The WHO Secretariat consists of Dr. Belsey, A. DeSchryver, Dr. Guidotti, A. Galazka, F. Gasse, D. Heymann, Dr. Meheus, A. Petros-Barvazian, K. F. Schulz (Temporary Advisor), and M. Thieren. The participants, and thereby contributors to this work, were the following: E. R. Alexander, Atlanta, Georgia; S. K. Hira, Lusaka, Zambia; K. Holmes (Consultation Chairperson), Seattle, Washington; S. Kietinun, Phathumtani, Thailand; M. Laga, Antwerp, Belgium; P. Piot, Antwerp, Belgium; R. Ryder, Kinshasa, Zaire; R. Stekettee, Atlanta, Georgia; E. Washington, Stanford, California; R. Whitley, Birmingham, Alabama; Z. Xu, Shanghai, People's Republic of China. Thanks!

REFERENCES

1. Hayden GF, Sato PKA, Wright PF et al. Progress in worldwide control and elimination of disease through immunization. J Pediatr 1989; 114:520–7.
2. Hinman AR, Foster SO, Wassilak SGF. Neonatal tetanus: Potential for elimination in the world. Pediatr Infect Dis 1987; 6:813–7.
3. Bart KF, Lin KFYC. Vaccine-preventable disease and immunization in the developing world. Pediatr Clin North Am 1990; 37:735–56.
4. Expanded program on immunization: economic appraisal, Sri Lanka. Weekly Epidemiol Record 1985; 50:191–4.
5. Robertson RL, Foster SO, Hull HF et al. Cost-effectiveness of immunization in the Gambia; J Trop Med Hyg 1985; 88:343–51.
6. Azulay RD, Ricart JC, Monteiro CA et al. Sifilis: inquerito sorologica em diferentes gupos socio-economicos na cidade de Niteroi. AMB Rev Assoc Med Bras 1979; 25(3):85–86.
7. Widy-Wirski R, D'Costa J. Maladies transmises par voie sexuelle dans une population rurale en Centrafrique. In: Rapport final, 13e conference technique, Yaoundé, Cameroun: OCEAC, 1980:651–4.
8. Grinspun M, Goldenberg R. Epidemiologia y control de al sifilis en el area sur, Santiago, Chile. Bol Ofic San Panamer 1977; 83:48–55.
9. Friedman PS, Wright DJM. Observations on syphilis in Addis Ababa. 2. Prevalence and natural history. Br J Vener Dis 1977; 53:276–80.
10. Larsson Y, Larsson V. Congenital syphilis in Addis Ababa. Ethiop Med J 1970; 8:163–72.
11. Liljestrant J, Bergstrom S, Nieuwenhuis F et al. Syphilis in pregnant women in Mozambique. Genitourin Med 1985; 61:355–8.
12. De Clercq A. Problèmes en obstetrique et gynecologie. In: Meheus A, Butera S, Eylenbosch W et al., eds. Santé et maladies au Rwanda, Brussels: Administration Générale de la Cooperation au Développement, 1982:627–56.
13. Meheus A, Friedman F, Van Dyck F et al. Genital infections in prenatal and family planning attendants in Swaziland. East Afr Med J 1980; 57:212–7.
14 Ratnam AV, Din SN, Chatterjee TK. Sexually transmitted diseases in pregnant women. Med J Zambia 1980; 14:75–8.
15. Ratnam AV, Din SN, Hira SK et al. Syphilis in pregnant women in Zambia. British J Vener Dis 1982; 58:355–8.

16. Hira SK. Epidemiology of maternal and congenital syphilis in Lusaka and Copperbelt Provinces of Zambia, Lusaka: Republic of Zambia, 1984:1–40.
17. Watts TE, Larsen SA, Brown ST. A case-control study of stillbirths at a teaching hospital in Zambia, 1979–80: serological investigations for selected infectious agents. Bull WHO 1984; 62:803–8.
18. World Health Organization Scientific Group. Treponemal infections. WHO Technical Report, 1982; 674:14–8.
19. Harman N. Staying the plague. London: Methuen, 1917. Cited in Murphy FK, Patamasucon P. Congenital syphilis. In: Holmes KK, Mårdh P-A, Sparling PF, Wiesner PJ, eds. Sexually transmitted diseases, New York: McGraw-Hill 1988: 821–42.
20. Ingraham NR. The value of penicillin alone in the prevention and treatment of congenital syphilis. Acta Dermatol Venereol 1951; 31(S24):60–88.
21. Hira SK, Bhat GJ, Ratnam AV et al. Congenital syphilis in Lusaka. II. Incidence at birth and potential risk among hospital delivered infants. East Afr Med J 1982; 59:306–10.
22. Hira SK, Ratnam AV, Sehgal DB et al. Congenital syphilis in Lusaka. I. Incidence in a general nursery ward. East Afr Med J 1982; 59:241–6.
23. Bhat GJ, Hira SK, Ratnam AV et al. Congenital syphilis in Lusaka. III. Incidence in neonatal intensive care unit. East Afr Med J 1982; 59:273–8.
24. Hira SK. Maternal and congenital syphilis in Zambia—some epidemiologic aspects. Afr J Sexual Transm Dis 1987; 3:3–6.
25. Naeye RL, Tafari N, Marboe CC et al. Causes of perinatal mortality in an African City. Bull WHO 1977; 55:63–5.
26. Bishaw T, Tafari N, Zewdie M et al. Prevention of congenital syphilis. In: Nsanze H, Widy-Wirski RH, Ellison RH, eds. Proceedings of the third African regional conference on sexually transmitted diseases, Basel: Ciba Geigy, 1983:148–53.
27. Biggers JD. In vitro fertilization and embryo transfer in human beings. N Engl J Med 1981; 304:336–42.
28. Miller JF, Williamson E, Glue J et al. Fetal loss following implantation: a prospective study. Lancet 1980; 1:554–6.
29. Poland BJ, Carr DH. Abortion: pathogenesis, cytogenetics. In: Chance GW, ed. Perinatal medicine: the basic science underlying clinical practice, Baltimore: Williams and Wilkins, 1976:48–56.
30. Brunham RC, Holmes KK, Eschenbach D. Sexually transmitted diseases in pregnancy. In: Holmes KK, Mardh P-A, Sparling PF, Wiesner PJ et al., eds. Sexually transmitted diseases, New York: McGraw-Hill, 1984:782–816.
31. Hira SK, Bhat GJ, Chikamata DM et al. Syphilis intervention in pregnancy: Zambian demonstration project. Genitourin Med 1990; 66:159–64.
32. World Health Organization. Consultation on maternal and newborn infections (meeting report). Geneva, 28 Nov–2 December 1988, Geneva (in press).
33. Galega FP, Heymann DL, Nasah BT. Gonococcal ophthalmia neonatorum: the case for prophylaxis in tropical Africa. Bull WHO 1984; 62:95–8.
34. Nasah BT, Nguematcha R, Eyong M et al. Trichomonas and candida among gravid and nongravid women in Cameroun. Int J Gynaecol Obstet 1980; 18:48–52.

35. Yvert, F, Riou JY, Frost E et al. Les infections gonococciques au Gabon, Haut Ogue. Pathol Biol 1984; 32:80–1.
36. Mabey DCW, Whittle HC. Genital and neonatal chlamydial infection in a trachoma-endemic area. Lancet 1982; 2:301–2.
37. Quarcoopome CO. Ophthalmia neonatorum: Problems of prophylaxis and treatment in Africa, Geneva: World Health Organization, 1983 (WHO publication no. PBL/ON/83–1, 1–4).
38. Bentsi C, Klufio, CA, Perine PL et al. Genital infections with Chlamydia trachomatis and Neisseria gonorrhoeae in Ghanaian women. Genitourin Med 1985; 61:48–50.
39. Laga M, Plummer FA, Piot P et al. Prophylaxis of gonococcal and chlamydial ophthalmia neonatorum. A comparison of silver nitrate and tetracycline. N Engl J Med 1988; 318:653–7.
40. Goh T, Ngeow YF, Teoh SK. Screening for gonorrhea in a prenatal clinic in Southeast Asia. Sex Transm Dis 1981; 8:67–9.
41. Welgemoed NC, Mahaffey A, Van den Ende J. Prevalence of Neisseria gonorrhoeae infection in patients attending an antenatal clinic. S Afr Med J 1986; 69:32–4.
42. Hira, S. Sexually transmitted diseases—a menace to mother and children. World Health Forum 1986; 7:243–7.
43. World Health Organization. Prevention and treatment of conjunctivitis in the newborn at the primary level, Geneva: 1984 (WHO publication no. PBL/84–4; 1–23).
44. Laga M, Plummer FA, Nzanze H et al. Epidemiology of ophthalmia neonatorum in Kenya. Lancet 1986; 2:1145–9.
45. Muhe L, Tafari N. Is there a critical time for prophylaxis against neonatal gonococcal ophthalmia? Genitourin Med 1986; 62:356–7.
46. Rothenberg R. Ophthalmia neonatorum due to Neisseria gonorrhoeae: prevention and treatment. Sex Transm Dis 1979; 6:187–91.
47. Fransen L, Nsanze H, Klauss V et al. Ophthalmia neonatorum in Nairobi, Kenya: the role of Neisseria gonorrhoeae and Chlamydia trachomatis. J Infect Dis 1986; 153:862–9.
48. Barsam PC. Specific prophylaxis of gonococcal ophthalmia neonatorum: a review. N Engl J Med 1966; 274:731–4.
49. Washington AE, Johnson RE, Sanders LL et al. Incidence of Chlamydia trachomatis infection in the United States: using reported Neisseria gonorrhoeae as a surrogate. In: Oriel D, Ridgeway G, Schachter J, Taylor-Robinson D, Ward M, eds. Chlamydial infections, Cambridge University Press, 1986: 487–90.
50. Hardy PH, Nell EE, Spence RS et al. Prevalence of sexually transmitted disease agents among pregnant inner-city adolescents and pregnancy outcome. Lancet 1984; 2:333–7.
51. Rettig PJ. Perinatal infections with Chlamydia trachomatis. Clin Perinatol 1988; 15:321–50.
52. Yang YS, Lee TY, Chang FM et al. Chlamydia trachomatis infection in pregnant women. J Formosan Med Assoc 1988; 87:1177–81.
53. Leclerc A, Frost E, Collett M et al. Urogenital Chlamydia trachomatis in Gabon: an unrecognized epidemic. Genitourin Med 1988; 64:308–11.

54. Drescher C, Elkins TE, Adkeo O et al. The incidence of urogenital Chlamydia trachomatis infections among patients in Kumasi, Ghana. Int J Gynecol Obstet 1988; 27:381–3.

55. Temmerman M, Laga M, Ndinya-Achola JO et al. Microbial aetiology and diagnostic criteria of postpartum endometritis in Nairobi, Kenya. Genitourin Med 1988; 64:172–5.

56. Braddick MR, Ndinya-Achola JO, Mirza NB et al. Toward developing a diagnostic algorithm for Chlamydia trachomatis and Neisseria gonorrhoeae cervicitis in pregnancy. Genitourin Med 1990; 66:62–5.

57. Berman SM, Harrison RH, Boyce WT et al. Low birth weight, prematurity and postpartum endometritis: association with prenatal cervical Mycoplasma hominis and Chlamydia trachomatis infections. JAMA 1987; 257:1189–94.

58. Bakir TMF, Hossain A, DeSilva S et al. Enzyme immunoassay in the diagnosis of Chlamydia trachomatis infection in diverse patient groups. J Hyg Epidemiol Microbiol Immunol 1989; 33:189–97.

59. Ismail SO, Ahmed HJ, Jama MA. Syphilis, gonorrhoeae and genital chlamydia infection in a Somali village. Genitourin Med 1990; 66:70–5.

60. O'Farrell N, Hoosen AA, Kharsany ABM et al. Sexually transmitted pathogens in pregnant women in a rural South African community. Genitourin Med 1989; 65:276–80.

61. Mason PR, Katzenstein DA, Chimbira THK et al. Microbial flora of the lower genital tract of women in labour at Harare maternity hospital. Cent Afr J Med 1989; 35:337–43.

62. Frazer JJ, Rettig PJ, Kaplan DW. Prevalence of Chlamydia trachomatis and Neisseria gonorrhoeae in female adolescents. Pediatr 1983; 71:333–6.

63. Golden N, Hammerschlag M, Neufhoff S et al. Prevalence of Chlamydia trachomatis cervical infection in female adolescents. Am J Dis Child 1984; 138:562–4.

64. Fisher M, Swenson PD, Risucci D et al. Chlamydia trachomatis in suburban adolescents. J Pediatr 1987; 111:617–20.

65. Alexander ER, Harrison HR. Role of Chlamydia trachomatis in perinatal infection. Rev Inf Dis 1983; 5:713–9.

66. Hammerschlag MR. Chlamydial infections. J Pediatr 1989; 114:727–34.

67. Harrison HR, Alexander ER. Chlamydial infections in infants and children. In: Holmes KK, Mårdh P-A, Sparling PF et al., eds. Sexually transmitted diseases, New York: McGraw-Hill, 1990:812.

68. Hammerschlag MR, Chandler JW, Alexander ER et al. Longitudinal studies of chlamydia infections in the first year of life. Pediatr Infect Dis 1982; 1:395–401.

69. Beem MO, Saxon EM. Respiratory-tract colonization and a distinctive pneumonia syndrome in infants infected with Chlamydia trachomatis. N Engl J Med 1977; 296:306–10.

70. Schachter J, Grossman M, Holt J et al. Prospective study of chlamydial infection in neonates. Lancet 1979; 2:377–80.

71. Fransen L, Klauss V. Neonatal ophthalmia in the developing world: epidemiology, etiology, management and control. Int Ophthalmol 1988; 11:189–96.

72. Frost E, Yvert F, Ndong JZ et al. Ophthalmia neonatorum in a semi-rural African community. Tran R Soc Trop Med Hyg 1987; 81:378–80.

73. Buisman NJF, Abong-Mwemba T, Garrigue G et al. Chlamydia ophthalmia neonatorum in Cameroun. Doc Ophthalmol 1988; 70:257–64.

74. CDC. Chlamydia trachomatis infections: Policy guidelines for prevention and control. MMWR 1985; 34:S53.

75. Farrow JM, Mahony JB. Chlamydial pneumonia in Costa Rica: results of a case control study. Bull WHO 1988; 66:365–8.

76. Limudonporn, Prapphal N, Pongpun N et al. Afebrile pneumonia associated with chlamydial infection in infants less than 6 months of age: initial results of a three year prospective study. Southeast Asian J Trop Med Public Health, 1989; 20:286–90.

77. Harrison HR, English MG, Lee CK et al. Chlamydia trachomatis infant pneumonitis: comparison with matched controls and other infant pneumonitis. N Engl J Med 1978; 298:702–8.

78. Harrison HR, Taussig LM, Fulginiti VA. Chlamydia trachomatis and chronic respiratory disease in childhood. Pediatr Infect Dis 1982; 1:129–33.

79. Weiss SG, Newcomb RW, Beem MO. Pulmonary assessment of children after chlamydial pneumonia of infancy. J Pediatr 1986; 108:659–64.

80. Brasfield DM, Stagno S, Whitley RJ et al. Infant pneumonitis associated with cytomegalovirus, chlamydia, pneumocystis and ureaplasma. Pediatr 1987; 79:76–83.

81. Schachter J, Sweet RL, Grossman M et al. Experience with the routine use of erythromycin for chlamydial infections in pregnancy. New Engl J Med 1986; 314:276–9.

82. Meheus A, Schulz KF, Cates W. Development of prevention and control programs for sexually transmitted diseases in developing countries. In: Holmes KK, Mårdh P-A, Sparling PF, Wiesner PJ et al., eds. Sexually transmitted diseases, New York: McGraw-Hill, 1990:1041–5.

83. Hammerschlag MR, Cummings C, Roblin PM et al. Efficacy of neonatal ocular prophylaxis for the prevention of chlamydial and gonococcal conjunctivitis. New Engl J Med 1989; 320:769–72.

84. Corey L, Spear PG. Infections with herpes simplex viruses. New Engl J Med 1986; 314:686–91.

85. McLung H, Seth P, Rawls WE. Relative concentrations in human sera of antibodies to cross reacting and specific antigens of herpes simplex virus 1 and 2. Am J Epidemiol 1976; 104:192–201.

86. Nahmias AJ, Josey WE, Naib ZM et al. Antibodies to Herpes virus hominis virus types 1 and 2 in humans. Am J Epidemiol 1970; 91:539–52.

87. Yeager AS, Arvin AM. Reason for the absence of a history of recurrent genital infections in mothers of neonates infected with herpes simplex virus. Pediatr 1984; 73:188–93.

88. Whitley RJ, Corey L, Arvin A, Lakeman F et al. Changing presentation of neonatal herpes simplex virus infection. J Infect Dis 1988; 158:109–16.

89. Tejani N, Klein SW, Kaplan M. Subclinical herpes simplex genitalis infections in the perinatal period. Am J Obstet Gynecol 1979; 135:547.

90. Bolognese RJ, Corson SL, Fuccillo DA et al. Herpes virus hominis type II infections in asymptomatic pregnant women. Obstet Gynecol 1976; 48:507–10.

91. Vontver LA, Hickok DE, Brown Z et al. Recurrent genital herpes simplex virus infections in pregnancy: infant outcome and frequency of asymptomatic recurrences. Am J Obstet Gynecol 1982; 143:75–84.

92. Nahmias AJ, Keyserling HL, Kerrick CM. Herpes simplex. In: Remington JS, Klein JO, eds. Infectious diseases of the fetus and newborn infant, Philadelphia: WB Saunders, 1983:638–43.

93. Prober GC, Sullender WM, Yasukawa LL et al. Low risk of herpes simplex virus infections in neonates exposed to the virus at the time of vaginal delivery to mothers with recurrent genital herpes simplex virus infections. N Engl J Med 1988; 316:240–4.

94. Nahmias AJ, Josey WF, Naib ZM et al. Perinatal risk associated with maternal genital herpes simplex virus infection. Am J Obstet Gynecol 1971; 110:825.

95. Hutto C, Arvin A, Jacobs R et al. Intrauterine herpes simplex virus infections. J Pediatr 1987; 110:97–101.

96. Corey L, Adams HG, Brown ZA et al. Genital herpes simplex virus infections: clinical manifestations, course and complications. Ann Int Med 1983; 98:958–72.

97. Stavraky KM, Rawls WE, Chiavetta J et al. Sexual and socioeconomic factors affecting the risk of past infections with herpes simplex virus type 2. Am J Epidemiol 1983; 118:109–21.

98. Whitley RJ, Arvin AM, Corey L et al. Vidarabine versus acyclovir therapy of neonatal herpes simplex virus infection. Pediatr Res 1986; 20:323.

99. Light IJ. Postnatal acquisition of herpes simplex virus by the newborn infant: a review of the literature. Pediatr 1979; 63:480–2.

100. Sullivan-Bolyai JKZ, Fife KH, Jacobs RF et al. Disseminated neonatal herpes virus type 1 from a maternal breast lesion. Pediatr 1983; 71:455–7.

101. Yeager AS, Ashsley RL, Corey L. Transmission of herpes simplex virus from the father to neonate. J Pediatr 1983; 103:905–7.

102. Hatherlay LI, Hayes K, Jack I. Herpes virus in an obstetric hospital: prevalence of antibodies in patients and staff. Med J Aust 1980; 2:325–9.

103. Sullivan-Bolyai J, Hull HF, Wilson C et al. Neonatal herpes simplex virus infection in King County, Washington: increasing incidence and epidemiologic correlates. JAMA 1983; 250:3059–62.

104. Adam E, Sharma SD, Zeigler O et al. Seroepidemiologic studies of herpes virus type 2 and carcinoma of the cervix. II. Uganda. J Natl Cancer Inst 1972; 48:65–72.

105. Templeton AC. Generalized Herpes simplex in malnourished children. J Clin Pathol 1970; 23:24–30.

106. Mosley RC, Corey L, Benjamin D et al. Comparison of viral isolation, direct immunofluorescence and indirect immunoperoxidase techniques for detection of genital herpes simplex virus infection. J Clin Microbiol 1981; 13:913–8.

107. Arvin AM, Yeager AS, Bruhn FW et al. Neonatal herpes simplex infection in the absence of mucocutaneous lesions. J Pediatr 1982; 100:715–21.

108. Whitley RJ and Hutto C. Neonatal herpes simplex virus infections. Pediatr Rev 1985; 7:119–26.

109. Whitley RJ, Yeager A, Kartus P et al. Neonatal herpes simplex virus infection: follow-up evaluation of vidarabine therapy. Pediatr 1983; 72:778–85.

110. Acyclovir dosage for neonatal herpes and duration for herpes encephalitis in adults. Med Lett Drugs Ther 1990; 32:90.

111. Gutman LT, Wilfert CM, Eppes S. Herpes simplex virus encephalitis in children: analysis of cerebrospinal fluid and progressive neurodevelopmental deterioration. J Infect Dis 1986; 154:415–21.

112. Whitley RJ, Arvin A, Prober C et al. Vidarabine versus acyclovir therapy of neonatal herpes virus infection. J Infect Dis 1988; 158:109–16.

113. Cibis A, Burde RM. Herpes simplex virus induced congenital cataracts. Arch Ophthalmol 1971; 85:220–3.

114. CDC. 1989 Sexually transmitted diseases treatment guidelines. MMWR 1989; 38(S8):16–8.

115. Benitz WE, Tatro DS. The pediatric drug handbook, Chicago: Year Book Medical Publishers, 1988:635.

116. CDC. Progress towards achieving the 1990 objectives for pregnancy and infant health. MMWR 1988; 37:405–8, 413.

117. Rush RW, Keirse MJ, Howat P et al. Contribution of preterm delivery to perinatal mortality. Br Med J 1976; 2:965–8.

118. Barns TEC. Obstetrics in the third world with particular reference to field research into delivery of maternal care to the community. In: Stallworthy J, Bourne G, eds. Recent advances in obstetrics and gynaecology, New York: Churchill Livingstone, 1979:109–36.

119. Majr A, Aggarival V, Sanghir H et al. The Nairobi birth survey I: the study design, the population and outcome results. J Obstet Gynecol East Centr Africa 1982; 1:132–9.

120. Puffer RR, Serrano CV. Patterns of birth weight, Washington, DC: Pan American Health Organization, 1987 (scientific publication no. 504).

121. Handsfield HH, Hodson WA, Holmes KK. Neonatal gonococcal infections: orogastric contamination with Neisseria gonorrhoeae. JAMA 1973; 225:697–701.

122. Elliott B, Brunham RC, Laga M, Piot P et al. Maternal gonococcal infection as a preventable risk factor for low birth weight. J Infect Dis 1990; 161:531–6.

123. Amstey MS, Sleedman KT. Symptomatic gonorrhea and pregnancy. J Am Vener Dis Assoc 1976; 3:14–6.

124. Armstrong JH, Zacarias F, Rein MR. Ophthalmia neonatorum: a chart review. Pediatr 1976; 57:884–92.

125. Edwards LE, Barroda MT, Hamann AA et al. Gonorrhoeae in pregnancy. Am J Obstet Gynecol 1978; 132:637–41.

126. Spence MR: Gonorrhea in a military prenatal population. Obstet Gynecol 1973; 42:223.

127. Stamm WE, Guinan ME, Johnson C et al. Effect of treatment regimen for Neisseria gonorrhoeae on simultaneous infection with Chlamydia trachomatis. New Engl J Med 1984; 310:545.

128. Schachter J, Holt J, Goodner E et al. Prospective study of chlamydial infection in neonates. Lancet 1979; 2.377–80.

129. Frommell GT, Rothenberg R, Wang S et al. Chlamydial infection of mothers and their infants. J Pediatr 1979; 95:28–32.

130. Heggie AD, Lumicao GG, Stuart LA et al. Chlamydia trachomatis infection in mothers and infants. Am J Dis Child 1981; 135:507–11.

131. Martin DH, Koutsky L, Eschenbach DA, et al. Prematurity and perinatal mortality in pregnancies complicated by maternal Chlamydia trachomatis infections. JAMA 1982; 247:1585–8.

132. Harrison HR, Alexander ER, Weinstein L. Cervical epidemiology and outcomes: chlamydia trachomatis and mycoplasma infections in pregnancy. JAMA 1983; 250:1721–7.

133. Gravett MG, Nelson HP, DeRouen T et al. Independent association of bacterial vaginosis and Chlamydia trachomatis infection with adverse pregnancy outcome. JAMA 1986; 256:1899–903.

134. Sweet RL, Londus DV, Walker C et al. Chlamydia trachomatis infection and pregnancy outcome. Am J Obstet Gyecol 1987; 156:824–33.

135. Hillier S, Holmes KK. Bacterial vaginosis. In: Holmes KK, Mårdh P-A, Sparling PF, Wiesner PJ et al. Sexually transmitted diseases, New York: McGraw-Hill 1990:553.

136. Gravett MG, Hummel D, Eschenbach DA et al. Preterm labor associated with subclinical amniotic fluid infection and with bacterial vaginosis. Obstet Gynecol 1986; 67:229–37.

137. Martius J, Krohn MA, Hillier SL et al. Relationships of vaginal lactobacillus species, cervical Chlamydia trachomatis and bacterial vaginosis to preterm birth. Obstet Gynecol 1988; 71:89–95.

138. Berg AO, Heidrich EF, Fihn SD et al. Establishing the cause of genitourinary symptoms in women in a family practice. JAMA 1984; 251:620–5.

139. Amsel R, Totten PA, Spiegel CA et al. Nonspecific vaginitis: diagnostic criteria and microbial and epidemiologic associations. Am J Med 1983; 74:14–22.

140. Hallen A, Pahlson C, Forsum U et al. Bacterial vaginosis in women attending STD clinic: diagnostic criteria and prevalence of Mobiluncus spp. Genitourin Med 1987; 63:386–9.

141. Eschenbach DA, Hilliers S, Critchlow C et al. Diagnosis and clinical manifestations of bacterial vaginosis. Am J Obstet Gynecol 1988; 158:819–28.

142. Hill LH, Ruparelia H, Embil JA. Nonspecific vaginitis and other genital infections in three clinic populations. Sex Transm Dis 1983; 10:114–8.

143. Hill LV, Luther ER, Young P et al. Prevalence of lower genital tract infections in pregnancy. Sex Transm Dis 1988; 15:5–10.

144. Shafer MA, Sweet RL, Ohm-Smith MS. Microbiology of the lower genital tract in postmenarchal adolescent girls: differences by sexual activity, contraception, and presence of nonspecific vaginitis. J Pediatr 1985; 107:974–81.

145. Cassell GH, Waites KB, Gibbs R et al. Role of Ureaplasma urealyticum in amnionitis. Pediatr Infect Dis 1986; 5:S247–52.

146. Mason PR, Katzenstein DA, Chimbira THK et al. Vaginal flora of women admitted to hospital with signs of sepsis following normal delivery, caesarian section or abortion. Centr Afr J Med 1989; 35:344–51.

147. Krohn MA. Bacterial vaginosis and amniotic fluid infection among women delivering at term. Presented at the International Conference on Antimicrobial Agents and Chemotherapy, Atlanta, October 1, 1990.

148. Cotch MF. Carriage of trichomonas vaginalis is associated with adverse pregnancy outcome. Presented at the International Conference on Antimicrobial Agents and Chemotherapy, Atlanta, October 1, 1990.
149. Iwasaka T, Wada T, Kidera Y, Sugimori H. Genital mycoplasma colonization in neonatal girls. Acta Obstet Gynecol Scan 1986; 65:269–72.
150. Klein JO, Buckland D. Finland M. Colonization of newborn infants by mycoplasmas. N Engl J Med 1969; 280:1025–30.
151. Braun P, Lee YH, Klein JO et al. Birth weight and genital mycoplasmas in pregnancy. N Engl J Med 1971; 284:167–71.
152. Sanchez PJ, Regan JA. Vertical transmission of Ureaplasma urealyticum in full term infants. Pediatr Infect Dis 1987; 6:825–8.
153. Iwasaka T, Wada T, Kidera Y et al. Hormonal status and mycoplasma colonization in the female genital tract. Obstet Gynecol 1986; 68:263–6.
154. McCormack WM, Rosner B, Lee Y et al. Colonization with gential mycoplasmas in women. Am J Epidemiol 1973; 97:240–5.
155. Naessens A, Cammu H, Foulon W et al. Epidemiology and pathogenesis of Ureaplasma urealyticum in spontaneous abortion and early premature labor. Acta Obstet Gynecol Scand 1987; 66:513–6.
156. Harrison HR. Cervical colonization with Ureaplasma urealyticum and pregnancy outcome: prospective studies. Pediatr Infect Dis 1986; 5:S266–9.
157. Munday PE, Porter R, Falder PF et al. Spontaneous abortion: an infectious etiology? Br J Obstet Gynecol 1984; 91:1177–80.
158. Thomsen AC, Taylor-Robinson D, Brogaard HK et al. The infrequent occurrence of mycoplasmas in amniotic fluid from women with intact fetal membranes. Acta Obstet Gynecol Scand 1984; 63:425–9.
159. Robertson JA, Honore LH, Stemke GW. Serotypes of Ureaplasma urealyticum in spontaneous abortion. Pediatr Infect Dis 1986; 5:S270–2.
160. Kundsin RB, Driscoll SG, Pelletier PA. Ureaplasma urealyticum incriminiated in perinatal morbidity and mortality. Science 1981; 213:474–5.
161. Quinn PA. Evidence supporting the role of genital mycoplasma infections in habitual spontaneous abortions. In: Proceedings of the third meeting of the International Organization for Mycoplasmology, Custer, SD, September 1980.
162. Stray-Pederson B, Eng J, Reikvam TM. Uterine T-mycoplasma colonization in reproductive failure. Am J Obstet Gynecol 1978; 130:307–11.
163. Shurin PA, Alpert S, Bernard-Rosner BA et al. Chorioamnionitis and colonization of the newborn infant with genital mycoplasmas. N Engl J Med 1975; 293:5–8.
164. Hillier SL. The association of Ureaplasma urealyticum with preterm birth, chorioamnionitis, post partum fever, intrapartum fever and bacterial vaginosis. Pediatr Infect Dis 1986; 5:S349–54.
165. Gibbs RS, Blanco JD, St. Clair PJ et al. Mycoplasma hominis and intrauterine infection in late pregnancy. Sex Transm Dis 1983; 10:S303–6.
166. Lamont RF, Taylor-Robinson D, Newman M et al. Spontaneous early preterm labour associated with abnormal genital bacterial colonization. Br J Obstet Gynaecol 1986; 93:804–10.

167. Waites KB, Rudd PT, Crouse DT et al. Chronic Ureaplasma urealyticum and
     Mycoplasma hominis infections of central nervous system in preterm infants.
     Lancet 1988; 1:17–21.
168. Cassell GH, Crouse DT, Waites KB et al. Does Ureaplasma urealyticum cause
     respiratory disease in newborns? Pediatr Infect Dis 1988; 7:535–41.
169. Wang EEL, Frayha H, Watts J. et al. Role of Ureaplasma urealyticum and other
     pathogens in the development of chronic lung disease of prematurity. Pediatr
     Infect Dis 1988; 7:547–51.
170. Romero R, Mazor M, Oyarzun E et al. Is genital colonization with Mycoplasma
     hominis or Ureaplasma urealyticum associated with prematurity/low birth
     weight? Obstet Gynecol 1989; 73:532–6.

PART III
ACTIONS FOR CONSIDERATION

SEXUAL BEHAVIOR AS A RISK FACTOR FOR SEXUALLY TRANSMITTED DISEASE

Dr. Sevgi O. Aral
Division of STD/HIV Prevention
Centers for Disease Control
Atlanta, Georgia 30333

INTRODUCTION

Sexuality is an important aspect of human behavior. It is central to people's intimate personal lives and psychology. In addition, gender is a pivotal factor in personal identity; it determines the subjective experience of life and one's options in life both biologically and socially. Sexuality is also of fundamental significance to society, since it is the mechanism of societal survival. Consequently, all cultures have well-established, elaborate, and firm rules and norms regulating sexual behavior and all aspects of social conduct related to sexual behavior. The norms and values surrounding sexuality may vary greatly across cultures. What behaviors are allowed, who can have sexual intercourse with whom, to what extent sexuality is an appropriate subject matter for social discussion, and among which members of society are all specified by culture and tend to vary across societies. Yet, some behavioral proscriptions are similar across societies. For example, in many cultures, sexual unions between older men and younger women are acceptable, while unions between older women and younger men are not condoned. Similarly, in many societies, having multiple sex partners is an acceptable, even desirable behavior for men, while the same behavior is considered unacceptable for women.

Perhaps because of its central importance for individuals and society, sexuality tends to be a very complex and sensitive issue in most populations. Often, there is great distance between normative proscriptions regarding sexual behavior and sexual practice. As a result, the socialization process of initiating the young into sexual activity is often awkward. Everyday practice determines the sexual behaviors that place individuals at risk of reproductive tract infections (RTIs), while normative proscriptions define what messages can be delivered about those behaviors and by whom. The distance between normative proscriptions and everyday practice is important to consider in developing prevention programs and policy.

Gender, in addition to being a pivotal factor in individual identity, is a major axis of social organization in most societies. Even the simplest forms of social organization differentiate individuals by age and gender. Perhaps the most primitive social stratification system is the difference between men and women with regard to social status, material resources, and power. Gender power relations are related to issues of sexuality and sexual behavior in complex ways. Often, women's place in society is defined in terms of their sexual or reproductive relationships to men. A woman may be someone's (some man's) daughter, wife, mistress, or mother; alternatively, she may be related to many men, as in the case of commercial sex workers. These relationships set severe limitations on the extent to which women can control their own sexuality. Thus, gender and sexuality have different meanings for men and women biologically, psychologically, and socially. These different meanings are reflected in powerful gender differentials in sexual behavior.

RTIs, especially sexually transmitted diseases (STDs), also have different meanings for men and women. First, STDs place a greater burden on women biologically. Infections are more often asymptomatic in women than in men. These infections therefore may not be diagnosed and treated. Diagnosis may also be more difficult in women, especially in less-developed countries, where syndromic and clinical methods may be the only available diagnostic techniques. Women also suffer worse sequelae—including pelvic inflammatory disease (PID), ectopic pregnancy, infertility, and cervical cancer—following sexually transmitted infections (STIs). Second, STDs constitute a more negative social experience for women than for men because the stigma associated with STDs is much greater for women. In fact, in some societies, these infections may be status- and image-enhancing for men, while they are stigmatizing for women. Such stigma constitutes a barrier to seeking health care and thus promotes increased incidence of sequelae among women and further spread of STDs.

In what follows, we discuss specific dimensions of sexual behavior that are associated with risk of STDs, and the relationships among them. We describe the sexual/health behaviors that influence STD risk, and the nonbehavioral characteristics of the individual that influence risk of infection and sexual behavior (Figure 1). Finally, we briefly discuss variations in STD rates across populations (Figure 2). We conclude with a consideration of research needs in the area of sexual behavior and its determinants as they relate to prevention and control of STIs.

DIMENSIONS OF SEXUAL BEHAVIOR AND RISK FOR STDs

Sexual behaviors have multiple dimensions that influence risk of STDs and their sequelae. These dimensions include age at sexual debut; number of sex partners accumulated over one's lifetime; number of sex partners over a specific recent time period (e.g., past month, past three months—the more partners one has, the greater the likelihood of infection); how one recruits sex partners (i.e., whether one is discriminating in the recruitment of partners); demographic characteristics of partners; behavioral characteristics of partners; frequency and timing of intercourse; sexual practices (e.g., oral, vaginal, anal intercourse and masturbation); and sexual/health practices and related aspects (e.g., use of vaginal douches, use of contraceptive methods, male circumcision, and coinfection with other STDs).

An individual's risk of acquiring an STI or developing STI sequelae can be viewed as consisting of five components. These components are the risk of interaction with an infected person who may become a sex partner, exposure to the infection of that partner, acquisition of the STI when exposed, development of a symptomatic STD if infected, and development of sequelae following the STI or STD. Each of these components is closely associated with at least one of the multiple dimensions of sexual behavior.[1] An individual's likelihood of exposure to an infected partner depends on the number of sex partners she has, the demographic and behavioral characteristics of the partners, and the manner in which she recruits sex partners.[2] Individuals who recruit sex partners indiscriminately on the streets or in bars have a higher likelihood of running into an infected partner than individuals who recruit people they already know through other connections as their sex partners.[3] Whether or not a person actually gets exposed to the infection of the infected partner depends on sexual practices and condom use. In addition, frequency of intercourse may affect the number of repeated exposures.

Acquisition of an STI during sexual intercourse with an infected partner is further affected by the presence or absence of coinfections with other sexually transmitted pathogens. Following infection, development of a symptomatic STD depends mainly on immunologic factors, a discussion of which is beyond the scope of this paper. Although we now know little about the determinants of symptom status, it may be important to examine this as a separate component of risk of acquiring an STD because symptom status is often a critical cue to action for seeking diagnosis and therapy. Particularly in women, many infections are asymptomatic. For example, 25 percent of the American population is infected with herpes virus type 2,[4] and three out of four infected persons are not aware of their infection.[5]

Whether or not an individual develops STD sequelae—such as PID, infertility, or ectopic pregnancy—and infects others in the community is influenced by her likelihood of receiving early and appropriate diagnosis and therapy. Diagnosis and therapy are affected by the individual's (and, indirectly, the community's) behaviors in seeking health care and by the availability and accessibility of STD services. In the case of asymptomatic infections, the relative importance of seeking STD-specific health care diminishes. For these cases, availability of STD services through integrated primary health care is more important; also, behaviors of health care providers carry greater significance. Compared with men, women tend to have a greater proportion of asymptomatic STIs. Thus, for example, STD screening for women during family planning, antenatal, and maternal-child health visits are strongly recommended.[6]

Available evidence linking each dimension of sexual behavior to specific infections is variable in quality and reflects the history of our evolving understanding of the role of sexual behavior in STD epidemiology. Thus, for example, while we have conclusive evidence on the association between number of current partners and risk for bacterial infection, we are still dealing with educated conjecture regarding the associations between partners' behavioral characteristics and risk for viral infection.

■ *Early age at sexual debut* has been associated with increased risk of cervical cancer;[7,8] viral infections, including herpes simplex virus (HSV) infection[9,10] and human papilloma virus (HPV) infection;[11] and bacterial infections, including those with gonorrhea[12] and *Chlamydia trachomatis*.[13,14] In the United States (and perhaps other northern countries), persons who have their coital debut early in life have a longer period of exposure to different sex partners over their lifetime.[15] They also tend to have greater numbers of partners per unit of time[16] and tend to choose partners who are at higher risk for STDs.[17] In addition, among young women, the status of the epithelium in the uterine cervix during adolescence may be particularly important in risk of infection.[15] In early puberty, the

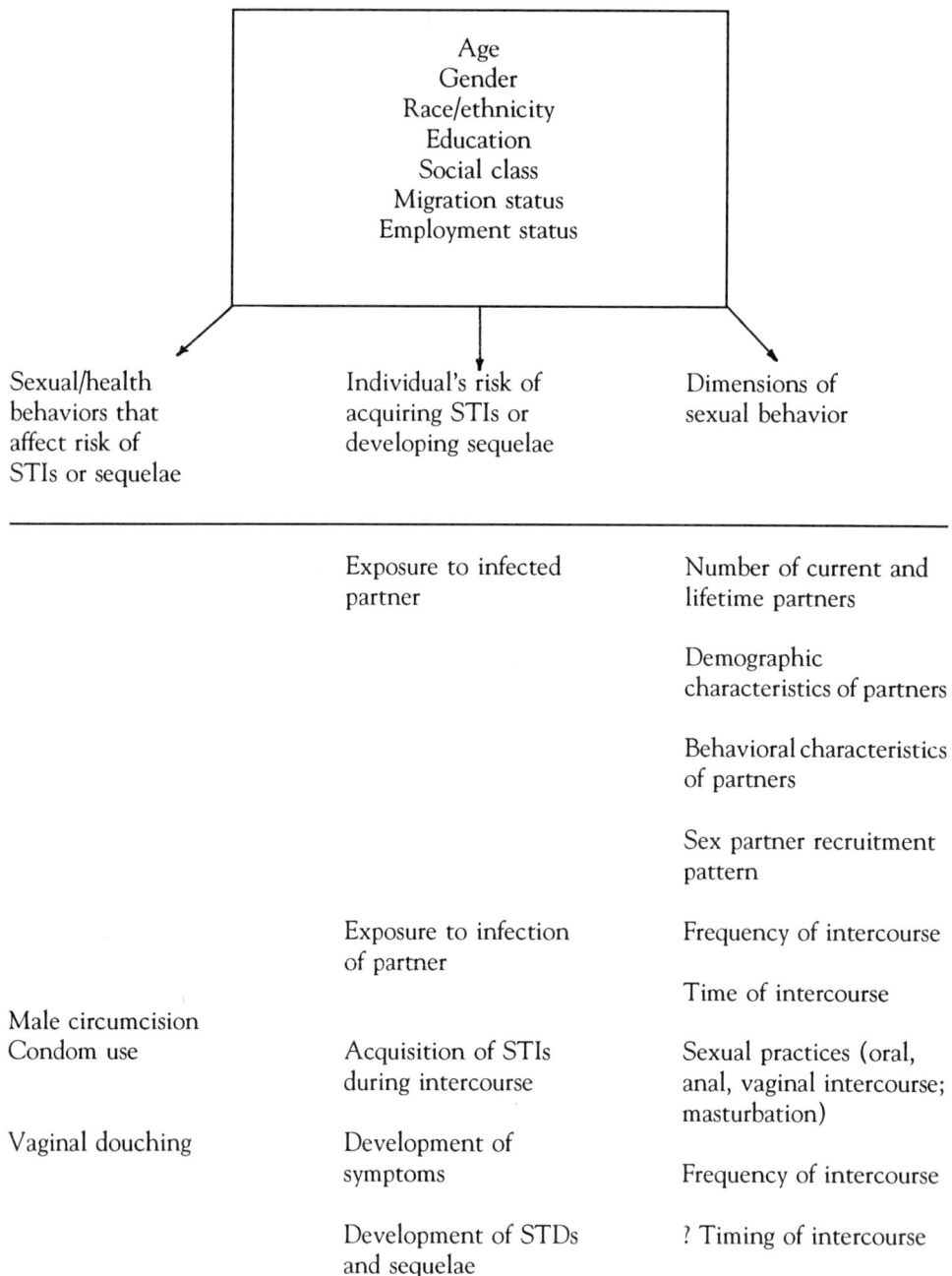

Figure 1. Behavioral and Nonbehavioral Characteristics
of the Individual that Affect STD Risk

columnar epithelium extends from the endocervical canal into the face of the cervix in the vagina, and thus is fully exposed to pathogens. This transformation zone of columnar epithelium is the primary site of invasion by both chlamydial and gonococcal organisms. In addition, HPV infection of the exposed area of the transformation zone at an early age results in cervical cytologic changes during the teenage years.[18] The columnar epithelium recedes into the endocervical canal with age, but it places the teenager at a biologically increased risk.[15] Thus, early age at sexual debut is associated with increased risk of STDs for both behavioral and biological reasons.

■ *Number of lifetime sex partners* is positively associated with increased cumulative risk for sexually transmitted conditions. This dimension of sexual behavior has been associated with STD sequelae such as cervical cancer,[10,19] PID,[20,21] ectopic pregnancy,[22] and tubal infertility;[23] with bacterial STIs such as chlamydial infection;[24,25] and particularly with viral STIs, including HSV infection,[10,26] HPV infection,[10,27] hepatitis B virus (HBV) infection,[28] and human immunodeficiency virus (HIV) infection.[29,30] The association between number of lifetime partners and viral STIs is simple and direct; since viral infections cannot be cured, risk for these infections is accumulated throughout one's lifetime. The association between number of lifetime partners and bacterial STI is based in part in the colinearity among various dimensions of sexual behavior. Bacterial STIs are curable; thus, risk for these infections is not cumulative and is not necessarily related to number of past sexual partners. However, since individuals who have large numbers of lifetime partners also tend to have large numbers of current partners, and since having large numbers of current partners increases one's risk for bacterial STIs, having large numbers of lifetime partners tends to be a marker for bacterial, as well as viral, STIs.

■ *Numbers of current sex partners* (e.g., partners over the most recent one, three, six, or 12 months) is positively associated with risk for bacterial STIs, including chlamydial infection,[24,31,32] gonorrhea,[33] syphilis,[34] and chancroid.[35] The time period specified in questions about current partners is variable. A recently emerging pattern is to inquire about the past three and 12 months. This combination minimizes recall bias (especially relevant for individuals with many partners) and allows for sufficient variability in the measure.

■ *Frequency of sexual intercourse* has not received much attention as a risk factor for STDs. Few studies have included questions about this dimension of sexual behavior. Thus, the limited available evidence points to frequency of sexual intercourse as a risk factor for PID[36-39] and acquisition of HIV infection.[40] The probability of transmission during a single episode of sexual intercourse is variable for different pathogens and is not 100 percent for any of them.[41] Thus, given that an individual has an infected sex partner, we would expect the risk of acquiring infection to be directly associated with frequency of intercourse with that partner.

■ *Timing of intercourse* within the woman's menstrual cycle is another dimension of sexual behavior that may be associated with risk of infection. Sexual intercourse during menses is a risk factor for female-to-male transmission of HIV.[42] It has been hypothesized to affect risk of developing PID, but data showing such an association are scarce.[43,44]

■ *Specific sexual practices* constitute a discrete sexual behavior dimension. Anal intercourse, particularly receptive anal intercourse, is associated with the acquisition of HIV infection[45,46] and HBV infection.[47] Oral-genital contact is associated with pharyngeal gonorrhea.[48] Conversely, masturbation is protective against all STDs.

■ A nondiscriminating *sex partner recruitment pattern* (as reflected in having intercourse with anonymous partners, having intercourse within 24 hours of meeting a person, or having intercourse with any partner only once) increases the risk of being infected with gonorrhea[49,50] and syphilis.[51] Lack of empirical evidence linking sex partner recruitment patterns to risk of other STIs perhaps reflects investigators' failure to address this issue rather than a lack of association.

■ Finally, *characteristics of sex partners*, including sociodemographic characteristics (e.g., age, race, socioeconomic status) and behavioral characteristics (e.g., number and type of partners, circumcision status), constitute an important dimension of sexual behavior. While closely related to sex partner recruitment patterns, sex partner characteristics make up a distinct dimension, which may be the most important factor influencing STD risk for most women who tend to have a limited number of lifetime partners. Sex partner characteristics, particularly partners of partners, emerge as an important risk factor for cancer of the cervix.[52,53] Having intercourse with intravenous drug users or bisexual men increases a woman's risk for HIV infection.[54] In addition, one predictor of STIs among commercial sex workers (CSWs) is the price for services, which is an indicator of the socioeconomic status of sex partners.[55] Workers who charge higher prices for their services tend to have fewer infections. This finding is complicated by the fact that women who charge lower fees also have more clients during fixed time periods. Given the high correlation between numbers of clients and socioeconomic status of clients, it may be impossible to separate the distinct effects of each of these sexual behavior dimensions on infection risk.

The recognition of many of the above dimensions of sexual behavior is quite recent. Thus, relevant data are limited. Moreover, many of these dimensions of sexual behavior are highly correlated with each other.[49] As a result, specifying the role of each in determining the risk of STIs is difficult.

SEXUAL/HEALTH BEHAVIORS AND RISK FOR STDs

In addition to the dimensions of sexual behavior discussed above, sexual/health, behaviors, including condom use, vaginal douching, and male circumcision, influence risk of STIs or their sequelae. Use of condoms, particularly consistent use of condoms, can be protective against bacterial infections such as gonorrhea and chlamydial infection, and against viral infections, including HSV, HPV, and HIV.[56] Vaginal douching appears to be associated with increased risk for PID,[57,58] ectopic pregnancy,[59,60] and cervical cancer.[61] However, the role of confounding in these associations and the mechanism through which vaginal douching affects STD sequelae are not yet clear. Male circumcision appears to protect against acquisition and transmission of STIs. This apparent protective effect is observed for genital herpes,[62] syphilis,[63] chancroid,[64] and HIV infection.[64,65]

Just as the various dimensions of sexual behavior are highly correlated with each other, they tend to be correlated with the sexual/health behaviors discussed above. Moreover, as indicated above, some sexual behaviors are strongly associated with the likelihood of being infected with a sexually transmitted pathogen, and infection with one of these pathogens appears to increase the risk of acquiring others.[66,67,68] Thus, often it is difficult to differentiate between sexual behavior as a confounder in associations among biologic risk factors and sexual behavior itself as risk factor for STDs.

NONBEHAVIORAL FACTORS AFFECTING RISK FOR STDs

Characteristics of the Individual

Behavioral factors do not account for all of the interindividual variability in STD risk.

Sociodemographic characteristics of individuals—including age, gender, race/ethnicity, education, social class, migration status, and employment status—influence the risk for STIs independently of their effect on currently recognized dimensions of a person's sexual behavior. Young age, male gender, minority race/ethnicity, lower levels of education and socioeconomic status, unemployment, and migrant status are associated with higher incidence of STDs.[69,70] These individual characteristics determine the social environments in which the individual circulates. Thus, they are associated with the prevalence of infection in the group, the group's access to and utilization of health care services, and the likelihood that a particular sex partner one chooses from the group is infected.

Characteristics of the Aggregate

Just as the risk of STDs varies across individuals, STD rates vary across societies and across social groups within a society. Characteristics of the population such as age

Age composition

Sex ratio

Geographic mobility

Women's status

Sexual norms

Accessibility of health services

Adequacy of aggregate health-care seeking

Figure 2. Characteristics of the Aggregate that Affect STD Rates

composition, sex ratio, geographic mobility, status of women, sexual norms, accessibility of health services, and adequacy of health-care seeking in the population account for most of the intersocietal or intergroup variability in STD rates.

Youthful age composition (i.e., a situation in which the number of infants, children, and young adults exceeds the population of older adults) influences STD rates in several ways. First, it implies a large and increasing sexually active population. Second, the burden of socializing the upcoming generation is greater in populations with youthful age composition, and this may result in greater differences in normative expectations and values between generations. Third, the relative scarcity of older men may increase promiscuity among this group because of the almost universal acceptance and practice of sexual unions between older men and younger women. Perhaps more important, youthful age composition is indicative of a high birthrate, which emphasizes women's reproductive role, often to the exclusion of any other roles.

A sex ratio imbalance (i.e., an excess of men or women) contributes to increased promiscuity among members of the relatively scarce gender. Such imbalance is common in southern countries as a result of gender-specific labor migration and long periods of political and social unrest or war, which often result in higher mortality rates among men. Where women are the scarce gender and economic resources are extremely limited, the social context may be conducive to exchanging sex for needed or desired resources. Even when resources are not so limited, sex may be exchanged for money. For example, CSWs tend to establish business around military bases or mining towns. Where men are scarce, their relatively more promiscuous behavior may place all their female sex partners at increased risk for STIs.

The heterogeneity of economic growth rates and the decline in the relative importance of agriculture have led to high levels of geographic mobility in southern countries. Men and women move from rural to urban areas, and from countries with lower economic growth rates to those with higher rates of growth. Often, these labor migrations select for either men or women, thereby creating important imbalances in the sex ratio. Even where the sex ratio in the aggregate does not deviate much from unity, gender-specific geographic mobility disrupts specific sexual unions, and thus contributes to higher rates of sex partner change. Women themselves may recruit additional partners, or their male partners may do so. Both of these behavior patterns increase women's risk for STIs.

The predominant norms and values regarding sexuality in a society obviously influence sexual behavior and STD rates. An oversimplified classification scheme would include a minimum of three distinct society types in this regard: societies where both men and women have few lifetime sex partners, and sexual unions are characterized mostly by mutual monogamy; societies where both men and women have relatively large numbers of sex partners; and societies marked by a double standard, where men have large numbers of sex partners, but women do not. For Sub-Saharan Africa, two prototypes of heterosexual networking have been described.[69] In one prototype, social structure is patrilineal, women tend to be dependent on men and have few partners, and men often have sex with a relatively small number of women (CSWs), who themselves have very large numbers of partners. In the second prototype, women are more independent and tend to be better educated; both men and women tend to have multiple sexual partnerships. Prevalence of STIs tends to be higher in countries that resemble the first prototype than in those resembling the second prototype.[70] In many societies in Asia, Latin America, North Africa, and the Middle East, there are marked double standards of sexual activity. Often, these societies develop well-established national sex industries (India, Japan, and Indonesia are examples) or international sex industries (e.g., Thailand, Taiwan, Hong Kong, and the Philippines), which are conducive to the spread of STIs.

The social status of women in a society and the predominant gender power relations influence sexual behavior and STD rates in very important ways. In societies where a woman's status is defined only in terms of her relationships to men—as daughter, sister, wife, mother, and sexual partner—women tend to be less educated, economically and socially dependent on men, and lack power in interpersonal relationships. The sexual double standard tends to prevail in such societies, and an overwhelming majority of women are at risk for STDs because of the sexual behaviors of their partners.

This social and sexual structure has two important implications for the prevention of STDs. First, in the short run, behavioral interventions focusing on men are more important than those focusing on women, since it is men's behaviors that create the elevated infection risk and since the existing power inequalities between men and women make it more difficult for women to implement preventive behavior change. This is particularly valid for societies in which the sexual double standard prevails. Second, in the long run, enhancing women's social status—through increased literacy, education, labor force participation, and economic independence, and changes in the normative structure—will have great positive impact on the prevention of STDs. In fact, we would expect behavioral interventions focusing on men and those aimed at enhancing women's social status to interact, further magnifying their synergistic impact.

Another characteristic of the aggregate that influences STD rates is availability and accessibility of health services for STDs. The absence or inaccessibility of such services, whether offered through specialized STD clinics or through integrated primary care programs, makes both treatment of bacterial infections and delivery of focused behavioral interventions difficult at best. In the context of southern countries and resource-poor settings, innovative reproductive health programs that link child survival with family planning and with prevention and control of STDs would result in preservation of fertility and improved health for women.[70] Such programs would render delivery of therapy for bacterial STIs relatively independent of STD-related health-care seeking. This is an important advantage, since STIs in women often tend to be asymptomatic and since STD-related health-care seeking is rather inadequate among women, particularly among those who are not knowledgeable about STDs, who view these infections as stigmatizing, or who are prevented from seeking health care.

IMPLICATIONS FOR RESEARCH

Our knowledge of sexual behavior and its determinants is limited. Our understanding of the dimensions of sexual behavior that are relevant to prevention and control of STDs and RTIs is still evolving. In addition, the limited available data do not evenly represent sexual experience in all countries. The paucity of data from southern countries is remarkable. Research priorities in the area of sexual behavior need to be defined in each country locally with the participation of epidemiologists and persons responsible for developing programs and policies to prevent and control RTIs. Nevertheless, some research questions appear to have almost universal relevance. These include the following:

1. What are the prototypical aggregate sexual behavior patterns associated with high STD rates?

2. What are the societal health service accessibility and aggregate health-care-seeking patterns associated with high STD rates?

3. In societies marked by high STD rates, what are the characteristics of women's social status?

4. What are the determinants of sexual behavior patterns and women's social status?

5. What are the implications of women's social status and its determinants for preventive interventions at the individual and aggregate levels?

An additional concern is related to the inadequacy of available methodologies for data collection and analysis in the area of sexual behaviors that place women at risk for STIs. More specifically, collection of data on sensitive subjects, such as private sexual behaviors, may require special techniques. Validity and reliability of such data may be questionable, and these issues warrant further methodological research. Integrating biomedical measures may be particularly helpful in establishing the validity and reliability of sexual behavior measures. Also, a number of factors create difficulties in the analysis of data on sexual behavior as a risk factor for STIs: the high correlations among different dimensions of sexual behavior; between sexual behavior and STIs; between risk of acquiring one infection and the presence of other infections; and among sexual behavior, STIs, and sexual/health behaviors such as circumcision and condom use. Thus, we need methodological research on different ways of analyzing data marked by colinearity.

While research needs in the area of sexual behavior are great, the need for timely interventions is even greater. Thus, the challenge is to develop an agenda that will allow us to bring about preventive behavior change as we keep on gathering data and learning about behaviors.

ACKNOWLEDGMENTS

I am grateful to Robert Brunham, Willard Cates, King Holmes, Mary Lewis, and Judith Wasserheit for their help in the preparation of this manuscript.

REFERENCES

1. Aral SO, Cates W. The multiple dimensions of sexual behavior as risk factor for sexually transmitted disease: the sexually experienced are not necessarily sexually active. Sex Transm Dis 1989; 12:173–7.

2. Aral SO, Holmes KK. Epidemiology of sexual behavior and sexually transmitted diseases. In: Holmes KK, Mårdh PA, Sparling PF, Wiesner PJ, eds. Sexually transmitted diseases, second edition, New York: McGraw-Hill 1990:19–36.

3. Hearst N, Hulley SB. Preventing the heterosexual spread of AIDS: are we giving our patients the best advice? JAMA 1988; 259:2428–32.

4. Johnson RE, Nahmias A, Magder LS et al. A seroepidemiologic survey of the prevalence of herpes simplex virus type 2 infection in the United States. N Engl J Med 1989; 321:7–12.

5. Nahmias A. Prevalence of herpes infections in a health maintenance organization. Presented at the International Society for STD Research, Brighton, England, August 2, 1985.

6. Ronald A, Aral SO. Interactions for the prevention and control of reproductive tract infections in developing countries. Presented at the Conference on Reproductive Tract Infections in the Third World: National and International Policy Implications, Bellagio, Italy, April 29–May 3, 1991.

7. Edebiri AA. Cervical intraepithelial neoplasia: the role of age at first coitus in its etiology. J Reprod Med 1990; 35:256–9.

8. Herrero R, Brinton LA, Reeves WC et al. Sexual behavior, venereal diseases, hygiene practices, and invasive cervical cancer in a high-risk population. Cancer 1990; 65:380–6.

9. Stavraky KM, Rawls WE, Chiavetta J, Donner AP, Wanklin JM. Sexual and socioeconomic factors affecting the risk of past infections with herpes simplex virus type 2. Am J Epidemiol 1983; 118:109–21.

10. Kjaer SK, Engholm G, Teisen C et al. Risk factors for cervical human papilloma virus and herpes simplex virus infections in Greenland and Denmark: a population-based study. Am J Epidemiol 1990; 131:669–82.

11. Reeves WC, Caussy D, Brinton LA et al. Case-control study of human papilloma viruses and cervical cancer in Latin America. Int J Cancer 1987; 40:450–4.

12. Phillips RS, Hanff PA, Wertheimer A, Aronson MD. Gonorrhea in women seen for routine gynecologic care: criteria for testing. Am J Med 1988; 85:177–82.

13. Shafer MA, Beck A, Blain B et al. Chlamydia trachomatis: important relationships to race, contraception, lower genital tract infection, and Papanicolaou smear. J Pediatr 1984; 104:141–6.

14. Li DK, Daling Jr, Wang SP, Grayston JT. Evidence that chlamydia pneumoniae, strain TWAR, is not sexually transmitted. J Infect Dis 1989; 160:328–31.

15. Cates W Jr. The epidemiology and control of sexually transmitted diseases in adolescents. In: Adolescent medicine: state of the art reviews, vol. 1, no. 3, Philadelphia: Hanley and Belfuy, 1990.

16. CDC, Premarital sexual experience among adolescent women, United States, 1970–1988. MMWR 1990; 39(51,52):929–32.

17. Greenberg J, Aral SO, Magder L. Age at sexual debut: a marker for risky sexual behavior. Poster presented at the 12th Annual Meeting of the Society for Behavioral Medicine, Washington DC, March 22, 1991.

18. Moscicki A-B, Winkler B, Irwin CE Jr, Schachter J. Differences in biologic maturation, sexual behavior, and sexually transmitted disease between adolescents with and without cervical intraepithelial neoplasia. J Pediatr 1989; 115:487–93.

19. Kjaer SK, Teisen C, Haugaard BJ et al. Risk factors for cervical cancer in Greenland and Denmark: a population-based cross-sectional study. Int J Cancer 1989; 44:40–7.

20. Cates W Jr, Rolfs RT Jr, Aral SO. Sexually transmitted diseases, pelvic inflammatory disease, and infertility: an epidemiologic update. Epidemiol Rev 1990; 12:199–220.

21. Marchbanks PA, Lee NC, Peterson HB. Cigarette smoking as a risk factor for pelvic inflammatory disease. Am J Obstet Gynecol 1990; 162:639–44.

22. Chow JM, Yonekura L, Richwald GA, Greenland S, Sweet RL, Schachter J. The association between Chlamydia trachomatis and ectopic pregnancy: a matched-pair, case-control study. JAMA 1990; 263:3164–7.

23. Brunham RC, Maclean JW, Binns B et al. Chlamydia trachomatis: its role in tubal infertility. J Infect Dis 1985; 152:1275–82.
24. Schachter J, Stoner E, Moncada J. Screening for chlamydia infections in women attending family planning clinics. West J Med 1983; 138:375–9.
25. Handsfield HH, Jasman LL, Roberts PL, Hanson VW, Kothenbeutal RL, Stamm WE. Criteria for selective screening for Chlamydia trachomatis in women attending family planning clinics. JAMA 1986; 255:1730–4.
26. Breinig MK, Kingsley LA, Armstrong JA et al. Epidemiology of genital herpes in Pittsburgh: serologic, sexual, and racial correlates of apparent and inapparent herpes simplex infections. J Infect Dis 1990; 162:299–305.
27. Koutsky LA, Galloway DA, Holmes KK. Epidemiology of genital human papilloma virus infection. Epidemiol Rev 1988; 10:122–63.
28. Alter MJ, Ahtone J, Weisfuse I, Starko K, Vacalis TD, Maynard JE. Hepatitis B virus transmission between heterosexuals. JAMA 1986; 256:1307–10.
29. Darrow WW, Echenberg DF, Jaffe HW et al. Risk factors for human immunodeficiency virus (HIV) infections in homosexual men. Am J Public Health 1987; 77:479–83.
30. Hunter D, Maggwa A, Mati J et al. Risk factors for HIV infection among women in a low risk population in Nairobi, Kenya. Sixth International Conference on AIDS, Abstract No. Thc.573, Vol. 1, San Francisco, June 21, 1990.
31. Harrison HR, Costin M, Meder JB et al. Cervical Chlamydia trachomatis infection in university women: relationship to history, contraceptive, ectopy, and cervicitis. Am J Obstet Gynecol 1985; 153:244–51.
32. Johnson BA, Poses RM, Fortner CA, Meier FA, Dalton HP. Derivation and validation of a clinical diagnostic model for chlamydial cervical infection in university women. JAMA 1990; 264:3161–70.
33. Pederson AHB, Bonin P. Screening females for asymptomatic gonorrhea infection. Northwest Med 1971; 70:255–61.
34. Rothenberg R. The geography of syphilis: a demonstration of epidemiologic diversity. In: Morriset R, Kurstak E, eds. Advances in sexually transmitted diseases, Utrecht, Netherlands: VNU Science Press, 1986:125–33.
35. Schmid GP, Sanders LL, Blount JH et al. Chancroid in the United States: re-establishment of an old disease. JAMA 1987; 258:3265–68.
36. Lee NC, Rubin GL, Boruck R. The intrauterine device and pelvic inflammatory disease revisited: new results from the Women's Health Study. Obstet Gynecol 1988; 72:1–6.
37. Marchbanks PA, Lee NC, Peterson HB. Cigarette smoking as a risk factor for pelvic inflammatory disease. Am J Obstet Gynecol 1990; 162:639–44.
38. Wølner-Hanssen P, Eschenbach DA, Paavonen J et al. Decreased risk of symptomatic chlamydial pelvic inflammatory disease associated with oral contraceptive use. JAMA 1990; 263:54–9.
39. Lee NC, Rubin GL, Grimes DA. Measures of sexual behavior and the risk of pelvic inflammatory disease. Obstet Gynecol 1991; 77:425–30.
40. Padian NS, Shibaski SC, Jewell NP. Heterosexual HIV transmission and frequency of intercourse. J Infect Dis 1990; 161:883–7.

41. Jones R, Wasserheit JN. Introduction to the biology and natural history of sexually transmitted diseases. In: Wasserheit JN, Aral SO, Holmes KK, eds. Research issues in human behavior and sexually transmitted diseases in the AIDS era, American Society of Microbiology Publications.
42. De Vincenzi J, Ancelle-Park R, for the European Community Study Group. Heterosexual transmission of HIV: a European study. II, Female-to-male transmission. Fifth International Conference on AIDS, Abstract No. Th.A.0.20, Montreal, June 4–9, 1989.
43. Eschenbach D, Harnich JP, Holmes KK. Pathogens of acute pelvic inflammatory disease: role of contraception and other risk factors. Am J Obstet Gynecol 1977; 128:838.
44. Sweet R, Blankford-Dayle M, Robbie MO et al. The occurrence of chlamydial and gonococcal salpingitis during the menstrual cycle. JAMA 1985; 255:2062.
45. Kingsley LA, Detels R, Kaslow R et al. Risk factors for seroconversion to human immunodeficiency virus among male homosexuals. Lancet 1987; 1:345–9.
46. European Study Group. Risk factors for male to female transmission of HIV. Br Med J 1989; 298:411–5.
47. Schreeder MT, Thompson SE, Hadler SC et al. Hepatitis B in homosexual men: prevalence of infection and factors related to transmission. J Infect Dis 1982; 146:7–15.
48. Sackel SG, Alpert S, Fiumara NJ, Donner A, Laughlin KA, McCormick WM. Orogenital contact and the isolation of Neisseria gonorrhoeae, mycoplasma hominis, and ureaplasma urealyticum from the pharynx. Sex Transm Dis 1979; 6:44.
49. Aral SO, Soskolne V, Joesoef RM, O'Reilly KR. Sex partner selection as risk factor for STDs: clustering of risky modes. Sex Transm Dis 1991; 18:10–7.
50. Upchurch DM, Brady WE, Reichart CA, Hook EW. Behavioral contributions to acquisition of gonorrhea in patients attending an inner city sexually transmitted disease clinic. J Infect Dis 1990; 161:938–41.
51. Rolfs RT, Goldberg M, Sharrar RG. Risk factors for syphilis: cocaine use and prostitution. Am J Public Health 1990; 80:853–7.
52. Peters RK, Thomas D, Hagan DG, Mack TM, Henderson BE. Risk factors for invasive cervical cancer among Latinas and non-Latinas in Los Angeles County. J Natl Cancer Inst 1986; 77:1063–77.
53. Harris RW, Brinton LA, Cowdell RH et al. Characteristics of women with dysplasia or carcinoma in situ of the cervix uteri. Br J Cancer 1980; 42:359–69.
54. Chu SY, Peterman TA, Doll LS, Buehler JW. Bisexual men with AIDS in the United States: epidemiology and their role in the AIDS epidemic in women. Amer J Public Health 19912, Vol. 82, No. 2; 220–4.
55. Day S. Prostitute women and AIDS: anthropology. AIDS 1988; 2:421.
56. Stone KM, Grimes DA, Magder LS. Personal protection against sexually transmitted diseases. Am J Obstet Gynecol 1986; 155:180–8.
57. Forrest KA, Washington AE, Daling JR, Sweet RL. Vaginal douching as a possible risk factor for pelvic inflammatory disease. J Natl Med Assoc 1989; 81:159–65.
58. Wølner-Hanssen P, Eschenbach DA, Paavonen J et al. Association between vaginal douching and acute pelvic inflammatory disease. JAMA 1990; 263:1936–41.

59. Chow W-H, Daling JR, Weiss NS, Moore DE, Soderstrom R. Vaginal douching as a potential risk factor for tubal ectopic pregnancy. Am J Obstet Gynecol 1985; 153:727–9. (Also see reference 22.)

60. Aral SO, Mosher WD, Cates W Jr. Vaginal douching among reproductive age women in the United States: 1988. Am J Public Health 1992, Vol. 82, No. 2; 210–4.

61. Gardner JW, Schuman KL, Slattery ML, Sanborn JS, Abbott TM, Overall JC. Is vaginal douching related to cervical carcinoma? Am J Epidemiol 1991; 133:368–75.

62. Taylor PK, Rodin P. Herpes genitalis and circumcision. Br J Vener Dis 1975; 51:274.

63. Parker SW et al. Circumcision and sexually transmissible disease. Med J Aus 1983; 2:288.

64. Cameron DW, Lourdes JD, Gregory MM et al. Female-to-male transmission of human immunodeficiency virus type I: risk factors for seroconversion in men. Lancet 1989; 2:403–7.

65. Fischl M, Fayne T, Flanagan S et al. Seroprevalence and risks of HIV infections in spouses of persons infected with HIV. Fourth International Conference on AIDS, Abstract No. 4060, Stockholm, 1988.

66. Wasserheit JN. Epidemiological synergy: inter-relationships between HIV infection and other STDs. Presented at the International Workshop on AIDS and Reproductive Health, Bellagio, Italy, October 29–November 2, 1990.

67. Simonsen JN, Cameron DW, Gakinya MN et al. Human immunodeficiency virus infection among men with sexually transmitted diseases. N Engl J Med 1988; 319:274–8.

68. Aral SO, Holmes KK. Epidemiology of sexual behavior and sexually transmitted diseases. In: Holmes KK, Mårdh PA, Sparling PF, Wiesner PJ, eds. Sexually transmitted diseases, second edition, New York: McGraw-Hill 1990:19–36.

69. Larson A. Social context of human immunodeficiency virus transmission in Africa: historical and cultural cases of East and Central African sexual relations. Rev Infect Dis 1989; 11:716–31.

70. Holmes KK, Aral SO. Behavioral interventions in developing countries. In: Wasserheit JN, Aral SO, Holmes KK eds. Research issues in human behavior and sexually transmitted diseases in the AIDS era, American Society of Microbiology Publications, 1991.

ASSESSMENT AND PRIORITIZATION OF ACTIONS TO PREVENT AND CONTROL REPRODUCTIVE TRACT INFECTIONS IN THE THIRD WORLD

Allan Ronald, M.D.
Professor and Head
Department of Internal Medicine
Health Science Centre, Room GC430
700 William Avenue
Winnipeg, Manitoba
Canada R3E OZ3

Sevgi O. Aral, Ph.D.
Division of STD/HIV Prevention
Centers for Disease Control
Atlanta, GA 30333

INTRODUCTION

The World Health Organization (WHO) estimates that over 200 million reproductive tract infections (RTIs) due to sexually transmitted pathogens occur each year among women in developing countries. Some 3–5 million women are seropositive for human immunodeficiency virus (HIV) in developing countries, millions have unsafe abortions that result in infections, and each year, uncounted numbers incur infection because of inadequately performed family planning, prenatal, delivery, and postnatal services. About 500,000 women die of pregnancy-related causes,[1] primarily infections. Despite the immensity of these problems and their significance to the health of women and their offspring, RTIs have received low priority in most developing countries. However, the HIV epidemic and the recognition of preventable morbidity and mortality associated with pregnancy and contraception have recently drawn attention to RTIs as an important area for interventions.

Vertical programs are being implemented in most countries in the areas of family planning, maternal and child health (MCH, consisting of improved antenatal care, immunization, and oral rehydration, among other services), and AIDS control. These programs are variably effective. In most countries, they have contributed little to strengthening the basic, primary health infrastructure. Also, the efficiency of many of these initiatives in delivering cost-effective programs has not been carefully evaluated.

Reproductive Tract Infections, Edited by A. Germain *et al.*
Plenum Press, New York, 1992

Interventional research is poorly developed and has a low status in Western academic medicine. We have usually initiated and promoted "medical interventions" without much consideration as to their effectiveness or efficiency. This, along with entrenched interests, has often resulted in an expensive, discontinuous health care system that is refractory to well-designed intervention studies. In developing countries, these problems are exacerbated by weak health research infrastructure in which epidemiology, health economics, and health policy analysis are often not well represented either in ministries of health or in universities. Balancing this pessimistic scenario are recent observations that may allow substantial improvements to women's reproductive health, including the following:

- The realization that RTIs not only are a significant health problem but have serious social and economic consequences[1]
- The changing view of women in society; an increasing number of initiatives to improve the legal, economic, and social welfare of women throughout the world; and the expanding organizational capacity among women
- The very substantial allocation of funds for the control of AIDS, which may have a favorable impact on other RTIs
- A nascent realization that programs already in place in MCH, family planning, and sexually transmitted diseases (STDs) can achieve a synergy that would markedly improve women's health
- An increasing appreciation for the role of health research as a strategy to improve health.[2] For example, vaccines will become available over the next 5–10 years for several STDs.
- The recognition that primary health care must be developed within community structures, that new programs must be integrated horizontally into these systems, and that these all must be well managed for optimal efficiency

For most potential interventions, there is little scientific evidence for effectiveness in preventing or controlling specific RTIs in developing countries. However, precedents with other infections, common sense, and careful surmise lead us to contend that many interventions not only are worthwhile but should be urgent priorities. These initiatives must be carefully documented and evaluated as they are implemented, to build a base for strategic planning and further program implementation. Most societies are experiencing a period of restrained growth in health and social services. Although we recognize that new funds may not be available, it is our considered opinion that within existing budgets, a great deal can be done through resource reallocation and program alteration.

We identify about 40 possible interventions and summarize the evidence that supports each of these. The interventions are organized into those that can occur within the health care system, those that are primarily educational or behavioral, and those that are directed to improving the overall status of women in society. To our knowledge, no one has previously identified or ranked a compendium of possible interventions for RTIs in developing countries. This initial attempt specifies general principles, defines a ranking system, and outlines the scope of the interventions.

RTIs, particularly STDs, occur in society because of a complex, poorly understood cascade of causes. Prevention strategies can be developed at several levels:

- Efforts to alter the status of women in society with programs to improve literacy, economic well-being, marital fulfillment, and justice

- Interventions designed to provide individuals and groups with specific educational and health promotion messages with regard to sexuality, RTIs, and motherhood that allow women to make better choices about their health
- Interventions to increase the program expertise and resources for women during routine care, in contraceptive services, during pregnancy, and at delivery.
- Public health initiatives designed to reduce the reservoir for STDs through improved case management, screening programs, treatment of partners, and targeting of high-risk groups
- Interventions to increase the health-seeking behavior of individuals and the ability of health providers to manage infections before complications occur

ASSESSING INTERVENTIONS

General Principles

To implement interventions, the following factors are considered:

- Health issues addressed by interventions must be perceived to be significant by the societies in which the illness is occurring, as well as being shown by the scientific community to be an essential health priority.[2]
- Most interventions must be delivered within the existing structures in the society. In most developing countries, this means integrating interventions into the primary care system, building whenever possible on existing resources, health providers, and programs.
- Technologies and strategies appropriate for the society must be developed and used. "Small," perhaps incomplete solutions may often be preferable to comprehensive interventions, especially where human, financial, and institutional resources are limited.
- Infrastructures for research and evaluation of interventions must be strengthened, and their autonomy facilitated.
- Interventions must be efficient. This implies that any intervention must be shown to be worth doing, given the competing priorities for resources and the logistical difficulties inherent in its implementation.
- Ultimately, strategies to improve women's leadership role in societies, literacy, and control of their own choices will, we believe, be more important than specific targeted biomedical programs in improving their reproductive health.

The Ranking of Interventions

We have used four categories to define the present status of interventions:

Reject: These interventions should not be considered further. In our opinion, they will not reduce the disease burden of RTIs in women in developing countries, either because there is no scientific evidence or consensus supporting them, because they are culturally inappropriate, or because they address problems that have not been shown to be significant.

Investigate: Although there are no published studies that show these interventions can be implemented effectively in most developing countries, they should be addressed as research priorities.

Field-test: Although efficacy studies have shown in some countries that these interventions can work, effectiveness studies showing that they work outside of a research milieu and efficiency studies showing that they are worth doing are necessary before they are more widely introduced in developing countries.

Implement: These are interventions that do not require further investigation; they are proven to be worth doing.

The scientific evidence for an intervention can be categorized within three levels of certainty:

Proven: The intervention has been shown to be worthwhile by prospective, randomized, controlled, and, if possible, community-based studies. Few interventions in RTIs in developing countries meet this standard of excellence.

Tentative: Uncontrolled or nonrandomized, often retrospective studies suggest that the intervention might work.

Assumed: Although little or no scientific evidence exists, individuals with expertise from personal experience agree that the intervention is worthwhile. Interventions based on this premise often turn out not to work.

The Politics of Interventions

For interventions to succeed, profound changes are required in political will of nations, in societal norms and attitudes about sexual behavior, and in the status of women. It seems clear that gender power relations are key both at the level of the individual couple and at the societal level. Changing gender power relations so that women can protect themselves and their children against infection requires strategies to improve women's leadership role, literacy, and control of their own choices. These societal changes are probably far more important than specific biomedical interventions.

In developing countries, most interventions are defined and implemented through government policies and agencies. These initiatives are often undertaken for political reasons, including as a response to international pressure or indigenous lobby groups, as well as through democratic processes. Roemer and Roemer have reviewed the role of government in global health and concluded that its contributions can be described in three categories.[3] First, economic and social advancement, particularly egalitarian social policies, are changing the developing world. For instance, in the least developed countries, adult literacy rose from 19 percent in 1970 to 32 percent in 1980, and the proportion of children enrolled in primary schools increased from 39 percent in 1970 to 54 percent in 1984.[4] The ratio of females to males in primary schools rose from 53:100 to 74:100.[4] Tragically, many of these gains may be in jeopardy because of the debt crisis, structural adjustment, and inadequate ongoing management.

Second, international communications, measured by several parameters, increased severalfold from 1970 to 1986.[5] We are increasingly a global village. Worldwide affirmation of human rights, including the right to health services as a social entitlement, has also become ascendant in much of the developing world. Although these international statements may be seen as "mere paper" that has no relationship to reality, they ultimately do shape political strategies and influence health systems. The 1978 Alma Alta Declaration is an outstanding example of the influence of international agencies on health priorities.

Third, the commitment of national wealth to the health care system doubled between 1960 and 1980 as a proportion of the gross national product.[6] However, health allocations have been curtailed, particularly in Africa, during the past decade because of structural adjustment, and the resulting health implications are alarming.[7]

INTERNATIONAL HEALTH INTERVENTIONS

The control of RTIs requires global initiatives. In societies where resources are very limited, the design and evaluation of programs, the development of specific products, and the generation and dissemination of knowledge can be carried out most efficiently with international resources and leadership.

Intervention: To establish an international coordinating agency for the control of RTIs. WHO has at least four programs that could be concerned with RTIs in women in developing countries. These are the Programme for Sexually Transmitted Diseases, the Global Programme on AIDS, the Population Control Programme, and the Maternal and Child Health Programme. These programs all have track records. A careful critique of their strengths and weaknesses in the control of RTIs should be carried out with the intent to learn from their successes in mobilizing world opinion and national program activity. Should the mandate of any of these programs be expanded to meet more effectively the need for liaison and coordination of global RTI control programs? Do national control programs in RTIs require global leadership? Are there global priorities for research? Is an ongoing advocacy role necessary?

Recommendation: None, pending future review.

(Rank: investigate. Evidence: assumed. Priority: high.)

Intervention: To encourage the pharmaceutical industry and the scientific community to develop more effective, more easily administrated, less-expensive treatment options for individuals with RTIs in developing countries. Available treatment regimens are less than ideal for most RTIs. Several bacterial STDs are difficult to treat because of increasing antibacterial resistance.

Recommendation: Well-designed trials in the environment in which the drugs used are necessary. Pharmaceutical companies could be encouraged to become involved on altruistic and commercial grounds.

(Rank: implement. Evidence: assumed. Priority: high.)

Intervention: To develop management guidelines for RTIs. WHO develops management guidelines for most RTIs. At present, these have not been validated through critical, well-executed field studies.

Recommendation: WHO should develop and publish guidelines for the management of RTIs and update these at least every 2–3 years. These guidelines and accompanying algorithms should be validated to ensure they meet appropriate standards of efficiency—that is, they achieve reasonable therapeutic outcomes at an affordable cost.

(Rank: implement. Evidence: assumed. Priority: high.)

Intervention: To develop simple, specific, sensitive, inexpensive diagnostic tests that can be performed in clinic settings with limited quality control. Rapid improvement in diagnostic tests is occurring with advances in molecular biology.[8] Nonetheless, many technologies require venipuncture, shipping specimens, mailing reports, and recalling patients. These are certain to be ineffective in most developing countries, where logistical support systems are inadequate to complete the circle and sustain the intervention. As they are developed, tests should be evaluated for sensitivity, specificity, simplicity, and cost. These must be balanced within a decision analysis that also recognizes the disease burden and the effectiveness of interventions. Consensual decisions should be made by national health care providers and, if possible, the involved community, following well-designed field tests that establish the efficiency of the laboratory procedure in "real" environments.

Recommendation: International leadership should be provided to develop new technologies for diagnosis with guidelines for their evaluation and distribution.

(Rank: investigate. Evidence: assumed. Priority: very high.)

Intervention: To identify areas in which common strategies can be shared and multiplied throughout the world and effectively used to control RTIs. Numerous interventions can be identified in which sharing of resources, either regionally or globally, will improve effectiveness and reduce cost. These might include the training of leaders and managers, and the development and dissemination of educational programs, surveillance techniques, and computer software. Information-sharing opportunities should be considered, particularly workshops in which participants have an opportunity to address and solve real problems and review the "pilot" interventions. Furthermore, governments in countries that make wise decisions with regard to the health of women should be recognized and acclaimed. Specific awards could be identified and recipients honored. Increasingly, it is recognized that the celebration and sharing of success is good management practice and a useful educational strategy.

Recommendation: Interventions should be made to assist national RTI programs and recognize innovative, creative government initiatives in women's health.

(Rank: implement. Evidence: assumed. Priority: high.)

NATIONAL HEALTH POLICY AND CAPACITY

Intervention: To develop a national strategic plan with a national director coordinating a multilevel, multidisciplinary program to control RTIs. We believe that effective national leadership with delegation to appropriate individuals is a cost-effective way to administer a national plan for the control of RTIs. An identified individual should have the programmatic responsibility for surveillance and training activities, integrating care at the community level, liaising with all programs relevant to women's health (including HIV control programs), facilitating drug supplies, ongoing review of management protocols, ensuring both continuous and intermittent program reviews, and identifying research needs and facilitating clinical epidemiological investigation.

A strategic plan must be developed in consultation with community representatives and "front-line" health care providers. Specific targets should be set within the context of the strategic plan as a means to justify and assess the use of resources for the control of RTIs and provide necessary reinforcement to the decision makers and politicians. In order to be successful, it is essential that this program be developed as a multisectoral collaborative effort and avoid the vertical "top-down" features of many externally imposed programs.

Recommendations: Each country should consider the appointment of a national RTI/STD program director with a small central support staff to develop and implement a strategic plan for the prevention and management of all RTIs.

(Rank: implement. Evidence: assumed. Priority: high.)

Intervention: To integrate family planning, HIV/AIDS control, antenatal care, and MCH with programs for the prevention, diagnosis, and treatment of RTIs within the primary care system. Primary care should be the centerpiece of national health care programs; in most countries, between 30 percent and 70 percent of the population now have access to primary care systems with varying efficiency and effectiveness. Within or adjacent to these care systems are programs to deliver immunization, well-baby care, family planning, and antenatal care. These programs are often funded by external donors, and reasonably well organized, coordinated, and delivered by nurses or less-trained individuals with specific skills. Women with proven or suspected RTIs are often shunted away from these organized prevention programs. In some areas, they may be referred to a remote STD clinic, sent to the "curative arm" of the primary system, or left to fend for themselves. Can primary care systems, currently serving mothers and their children, be expanded to include prevention, diagnosis, and treatment programs for RTIs? Could this strengthen their existing mandate and serve the interests of their clients?

Two main issues would need to be addressed: First is the development of human resources through training, motivation, and attitudinal changes necessary to deliver new services such as sexual health promotion, sexual risks assessment, and RTI management. Second is the increased resources needed within current structures for an expanded RTI program. Benefits that would accrue to this service reorganization would be a renewed emphasis on reproductive health as it relates to pregnancies, family planning, and sexuality; more efficient health care delivery for women; multiple opportunities for reinforcing educational messages to prevent RTIs; and shared ownership of essential programs that require further strengthening. Despite these presumed advantages, this intervention remains controversial among professionals concerned with population control, MCH, and child survival, and has not been critically evaluated. Routinely incorporating RTI control programs into these health care services will require the leadership of international and national agencies to facilitate and encourage program synergy, as well as operations research to develop the appropriate training material. Careful program evaluation of the original program mandates and effects on RTIs are required.

Recommendations: Each country should consider strategies to integrate the prevention, diagnosis, and treatment of RTIs into existing programs in family planning, safe motherhood, and child survival within the primary care system.

(Rank: field-test. Evidence: tentative. Priority: very high.)

Intervention: To develop and implement treatment guidelines that are scientifically sound, cost-effective, and incorporated into the health care system through well-designed algorithms with ready access to the appropriate drugs. Substantial evidence proves that well-designed treatment guidelines developed through scientific studies, consensus, and experience lead to improved therapeutic outcomes throughout the health care system. For developing countries, treatment guidelines must be put into appropriate management algorithms. Additionally, drugs must be made available through an Essential Drug Program to the primary health care provider. Too frequently, inappropriate drugs are provided for the management of RTIs, or if drugs are provided, they are used for the management of other illnesses. In Zambia, this has been resolved through a special drug kit provided to health units and designated only for STDs and RTIs.[8] This also permits the cost of treatment for RTIs to be monitored.

Recommendation: Each country should consider adopting WHO guidelines and algorithms for the management of RTIs as appropriate and ensure their communication to all primary care givers through newsletters, educational programs, and posters. Drugs for RTIs should be clearly identified, perhaps within a special kit, and used solely for management of patients with RTIs.

(Rank: implement. Evidence: assumed. Priority: high.)

Intervention: To train professionals. Professionals with varying expertise and skills are essential in order to develop, staff, and administer programs to prevent and manage RTIs.

(1) *Scientists.* In order to develop research capacity for RTIs in Third World societies, independent investigators in behavioral sciences, epidemiology and health systems research, microbiology, infectious diseases, and obstetrics and gynecology are required. Women in particular should be recruited. Scientists are essential to undertake operations research appropriate to the culture, as well as more formal prospective interventional trials. Program evaluation depends upon their expertise. An appropriate target for "RTI research scientists" would be at least one per million of population. Most scientists should be employed in a milieu where they are integrated with strategic planning groups in the ministry of health and have educational contact with students. Those who are physicians should have limited, defined access to patient responsibilities. Interdisciplinary research should be a major goal. Strategies are needed not only to train individuals to be independent investigators, but to ensure successful careers. Scientists must be able to maintain their creativity through networking, peer review, and other means to ensure reasonable productivity for 10–15 years following training.

(2) *Health care professionals.* A small cadre are needed to provide appropriate care for more difficult illnesses. Traditionally, these individuals have been physicians who have trained in obstetrics and gynecology or in genitourinary medicine and venereology. We encourage programs to train nurse clinicians or other personnel in reproductive health and RTIs with the goal to determine if individuals with more limited clinical backgrounds can provide referral care and organize educational programs. This could mean important alternate ways to provide leadership for the care of RTIs in developing countries.

(3) *Managers.* Coordination and management of health care systems are deficient in many societies. We need to determine the expertise at the managerial level needed to ensure that the care system operates efficaciously for RTIs in the context of the overall health of women. We do not have models, but would urge that this be seen as a priority.

(4) *Epidemiologists.* Active surveillance of RTIs, analysis of the data, and development of policy and control strategies based on this information are essential to any RTI program. Epidemiologists need to be strategically placed in ministries of health in order to influence decision makers. The recent experience of the Global Epidemic Intelligence Training Program suggests that a strategy to recruit and train health ministry physicians in epidemiology leads to improved health outcomes.[9]

Recommendation: Human resources need to be determined and programs developed to prepare individuals for work on RTIs with ongoing career support.

(Rank: implement. Evidence: assumed. Priority: very high.)

Intervention: To ensure that a national reference laboratory and designated regional laboratories can provide the necessary support for the diagnosis of RTIs. Some common RTIs can be diagnosed only by the laboratory. Serologic screening for syphilis and HIV, culture or gram stain for gonococci, and direct microscopic examinations for *Trichomonas vaginalis* are some examples. Although laboratory expertise for these procedures has been introduced in most developing countries, performance is variable and the vast majority of patients with RTIs do not have access to laboratory diagnosis. The reasons for this include inadequate training, poor supervision, lack of reagents, lack of equipment maintenance, and absence of quality control. Despite the difficulties, RTI control programs will require some laboratory support.

One feature of such support might be a national laboratory with a mandate to supervise and train personnel in provincial, district, or hospital laboratories; maintain a national quality control system; act as a reference laboratory; tabulate surveillance activities that originate from the laboratory; and monitor antibacterial resistance of selected pathogens. Another feature might be province, hospital, or clinical laboratories to carry out the five or six essential procedures required to diagnose RTIs for which syndromic diagnosis is inadequate. Ultimately, these technologies must become sufficiently simple so that care providers in the clinic setting can perform simple diagnostic tests for important RTIs.[10]

Recommendation: All countries should establish, within existing laboratory systems, the diagnostic procedures necessary for the management of RTIs that cannot be diagnosed adequately with clinical criteria.

(Rank: implement. Evidence: assumed. Priority: medium.)

Intervention: To establish surveillance. Surveillance is a powerful tool to convince decision makers of the overall contribution of RTIs to women's health. It can be used to deploy resources for both control and treatment interventions appropriately, to show the effectiveness of specific interventions, and to establish and achieve specific control targets. Despite its proven validity in many societies for a variety of disease states, it is rarely used in the campaign against women's RTIs to any extent in developing countries other than in HIV/AIDS control programs. Even when information is laboriously collected from care givers, it is then stored without analysis or incorporation into subsequent decision-making processes. Reasons for this presumably include lack of expertise in data analysis and information systems, as well as lack of epidemiological skills. We would suggest that the following be considered by all countries as appropriate subjects for surveillance:

- Prevalence of ophthalmia neonatorum and congenital syphilis
- Prevalence of positive syphilis serology in pregnant women
- Prevalence of gonococcal cervicitis in pregnant women or women who are seeking contraceptive advice (occasional surveys)
- Prevalence of genital ulcer disease, HIV, gonococcal cervicitis, and syphilis in selected, sentinel, high-frequency transmitter populations
- Prevalence of primary and secondary infertility
- Sexual behavior surveys
- Condom use
- Cervical neoplasia
- Bacterial and antibacterial antimicrobial susceptibility (periodic assessment)

This intervention requires careful analysis with regard to its cost-benefit ratio in particular settings. If established, it should be carried out so that data will be comparable within countries over time and between countries. Extensive coordination and considerable effort will be required to ensure that surveillance systems are set in place in a way that will yield useful information. Surveillance also requires infrastructure for computer technologies and biostatistics. Surveillance of diseases or pathogens needs to be integrated into behavioral surveillance systems—identifying epidemiological associations between individual RTIs, as well as between RTIs and sexual behavior data, can become a significant way to design educational and behavioral interventions and also to understand the varying epidemiology of RTIs within different societies.

Recommendation: Surveillance systems, including analysis and effective use of data collected, should be implemented in all societies.

(Rank: implement. Evidence: assumed. Priority: high.)

Intervention: To update health care providers through regional and national workshops, symposia, and meetings, and to provide appropriate books and journals. Lack of access to information is a significant impediment to health improvement in developing countries. This fact applies both to technical details in specific areas of expertise and to an awareness of new developments and ideas that should circulate through communities of scientists, administrators, and health care providers. Multiple information systems are accessible to individuals in the industrialized world. In developing countries, textbooks 10–20 years out-of-date are often the only materials available. How can learning remain exciting for the many individuals involved in the control and management of RTIs? Perhaps lessons learned from other areas of adult education could be applied to this area to provide individuals, particularly educators and health care providers, access to appropriate information for continuous learning throughout life.

Recommendation: Continuing adult education programs need to be designed and implemented for health care providers in each country.

(Rank: implement. Evidence: assumed. Priority: medium.)

HEALTH SERVICES FOR WOMEN

This category includes services for pregnant women (MCH clients); family planning clients; and nonpregnant, noncontracepting women who use primary health centers.

MCH Clients (Pregnant Women)

Intervention: To train traditional birth attendants (TBAs) and improve their skills to prevent RTIs during pregnancy and at delivery, and to educate women about STDs and sexual health. A large proportion of pregnant women are cared for and delivered by TBAs. Many of these attendants have developed culturally accepted indigenous practices that have a major influence on the women receiving care. Initiatives are being taken to focus attention on the role and potential of TBAs within the health system. This has included government recognition of TBAs, additional training and ongoing education, development of specific kits for improved delivery, and ongoing supervision by trainers. To our knowledge, no programs have attempted to use TBAs to promote sexual health or to reduce unsafe sexual practices.

Recommendation: The role of TBAs in the prevention of RTIs and the promotion of sexual health should be evaluated.

(Rank: investigate. Evidence: assumed. Priority: medium.)

Intervention: To routinely test women for HIV during pregnancy or at term, counsel HIV-positive women to avoid subsequent pregnancies, offer appropriate care for their children, and enter both the women and their spouses into an ongoing support program to avoid further transmission of HIV. The cost of a program to screen all pregnant women in Kinshasa, Zaire (population 3.5 million), is estimated to be $1 million annually.[11] In Kinshasa, a prospective study found that there was no "high-risk" profile with adequate sensitivity to identify women who would likely be infected. Also, symptoms identified only about one third of the prenatal women who actually had HIV infection. The investigators concluded that HIV screening programs are prohibitively expensive and that other strategies to identify HIV-infected pregnant women were insufficiently sensitive to be of value.[11] They suggested that programs to control perinatal acquired HIV should continue to focus on vigorous prevention campaigns targeted at all sexually active women. Similarly, in a prospective study from Nairobi, postpartum counseling of women found to be infected with HIV at term usually failed to reduce the likelihood that the women would have subsequent pregnancies or share information with their spouse.[12] No studies have shown that infant survival can be significantly improved if knowledge about HIV serostatus is available to care givers of infants during early life.[18]

Recommendation: Routine testing for HIV during pregnancy or at term is not worthwhile.

(Rank: reject. Evidence: tentative. Priority: low.)

Intervention: To screen, diagnose, and treat gonococcal infection during pregnancy. The burden of gonococcal disease is substantial. The prevalence of gonococcal infection in pregnancy varies from 1 percent to 8 percent in developing countries. Gonococcal infection during pregnancy is associated with premature birth, neonatal ophthalmia, and postpartum endometritis.[13,14,15] In industrial countries, screening for gonococcal infection in pregnancy is cost-effective in populations in which the prevalence exceeds 1 percent. No prospective study to date in developing countries has shown that cost-effective intervention during pregnancy will prevent these complications.

Recommendation: More efficient, inexpensive strategies to diagnose and treat gonococcal infection during pregnancy should be a research priority.

(Rank: investigate. Evidence: proven. Priority: high.)

Intervention: To screen pregnant women for syphilis and treat those with positive serology. The prevalence and incidence of syphilis vary considerably. However, in some countries, the prevalence of positive serology exceeds 10 percent and congenital syphilis is responsible for as much as 30 percent of perinatal mortality.[16] Over one half of mothers with untreated syphilis will have an adverse outcome. In Zambia, a prospective intervention study has shown that the programmatic cost of preventing an adverse outcome is about US$12.00.[16] However, many factors curtail the efficiency of syphilis control programs in pregnancy. These include inadequate, simple diagnostics (the rapid plasma reagin, RPR, has a sensitivity of about 90 percent); the requirement for technical accuracy and quality control of serology; late attendance for prenatal care; failure to treat sexual partners; acquisition of infectious syphilis during pregnancy after treatment; and lack of benzathine penicillin in the clinic setting.

Recommendation: All pregnant women should be screened for syphilis and treated if serologically positive. Additional investigation is required to identify tests with increased sensitivity and specificity that can be performed by the health care provider; to ensure that 80 percent or more of pregnant women with positive serology, and their sexual partners, receive treatment within the first 20 weeks of pregnancy; and to develop education and risk assessment programs to reduce the acquisition rate of syphilis during pregnancy.

(Rank: implement. Evidence: proven. Priority: very high.)

Intervention: To screen for chlamydial infections during pregnancy or at delivery in order to diagnose and treat these infections and prevent complications during and following pregnancy in women and their newborns. The morbidity of *Chlamydia trachomatis* infection in mothers and their infants has been shown in numerous studies in both the industrialized and developing worlds over the past five years.[17] Interventions are now considered to be cost-effective in populations where the prevalence of *Chlamydia trachomatis* exceeds 6 percent. Presumably, this prevalence is commonly exceeded in pregnant women throughout the developing world.[14] However, the diagnosis and management of chlamydial infections in pregnancy is impractical in most of the developing world because technologies for diagnosis of chlamydial infection are expensive and too complicated for widespread introduction in primary care settings; algorithms to diagnose chlamydial infection without laboratory support are both insensitive and nonspecific and have not been adequately field-tested;[17] and proven, well-tolerated, inexpensive regimens that can be prescribed during pregnancy for women and their sexual partners to predictably cure 90 percent of women are not available. Despite this pessimistic scenario, we predict that within five years, appropriate interventions will be developed to reduce the morbidity of *Chlamydia trachomatis* infections by early diagnosis and treatment as follows:

- The morbidity of *Chlamydia trachomatis* infection in the upper genital tract of women and in the respiratory tract of infants will be shown to be substantial in studies from numerous Third World societies.
- Prospective community-based studies will show that simple technologies or "risk identification" can recognize *Chlamydia trachomatis* with sufficient sensitivity and specificity to make routine treatment possible.
- Affordable treatment regimens will be shown to be effective in at least 90 percent of women.
- A vaccine will be discovered to prevent upper tract infection or prevent transmission from mothers to their newborns.

In the meantime, primary prevention strategies to reduce occurrence of all STDs, particularly during pregnancy, will have some impact on prevalence of *Chlamydia trachomatis* infection.

Recommendation: The diagnosis and treatment of *Chlamydia trachomatis* infection in pregnancy should not be attempted in most developing countries until simpler diagnostics and appropriate treatment regimens are possible.

(Rank: investigate. Evidence: proven. Priority: high.)

Intervention: To institute routine ophthalmic prophylaxis in all newborns. Ophthalmia occurs in 1–10 percent of infants in developing societies. Among those born to mothers with gonococcal infection, the risk of ophthalmia is about 50 percent; among those born to mothers with chlamydial infection, the risk exceeds 30 percent.[14] Routine prophylaxis at birth with silver nitrate, tetracycline, or erythromycin reduces the incidence of ophthalmia by over 80 percent.[19]

Recommendation: Routine ophthalmic prophylaxis at birth is a cost-effective intervention that should be introduced into all settings in which births occur.

(Rank: implement. Evidence: proven. Priority: very high.)

Intervention: To reduce iatrogenic RTIs by introducing and strengthening safe motherhood programs in primary care systems. Safe motherhood programs have been introduced in several countries, and they will have significant impact on illness and death due to RTIs, because these infections are currently the most common cause of death during pregnancy.[20] National interventions to reduce all RTIs during pregnancy and at delivery require a continuing focus on iatrogenic RTIs. Training of midwives and TBAs, provision of kits, and early access to antibiotics are the primary strategies.[21]

Recommendation: Prevention of iatrogenic RTIs should be implemented through safe motherhood programs throughout the primary care system.

(Rank: implement. Evidence: assumed. Priority: high.)

Intervention: To immunize all infants during the first year of life against hepatitis B, to prevent later acquisition, and thus, transmission.[22] In developing countries with high endemicity of hepatitis B, most infections occur through vertical transmission at birth or during early childhood. By contrast, in industrialized countries, heterosexual spread accounts for 20–50 percent of incident cases. Universal immunization of infants at birth may be the most effective strategy for preventing hepatitis B. It will target the presumably common modes of transmission and ultimately prevent heterosexual transmission.[22]

Recommendation: Universal rather than targeted hepatitis B immunization policy should be considered in developing countries in order to provide immunity before heterosexual transmission occurs.

(Rank: field-test. Evidence: proven. Priority: high.)

Family Planning Clients

Intervention: To prevent pelvic infection associated with IUD insertion or use. During the first four months after IUD insertion, women are about 1.5 times more likely to develop pelvic inflammatory disease (PID) than are women using no contraception.[23] The excess risk of PID in IUD users appears to be due in part to sexually transmitted RTIs.[23] Presumably, this is because of the spread of infection during insertion or subsequent spread of STD pathogens from the lower genital tract. Providers should be supported to screen clients carefully for contraindications to IUD use, including multiple partners (and partners' multiple partners), and to use aseptic techniques. It is not cost-effective to screen women for *Neisseria gonorrhoeae* or *Chlamydia trachomatis* before insertion of an IUD, but if risk factors or symptoms are present that suggest an STD, empiric treatment should be provided. Administering antibacterial treatment just prior to insertion of the IUD may decrease subsequent PID.[24] If an individual is at risk of STDs, she should be encouraged not to use an IUD or, at least, to use condoms concurrently with the IUD. STDs acquired subsequent to IUD insertion can invade the upper tract. At IUD insertion, clients need to be educated about the importance of avoiding STDs and urged to return to the clinic if they change partners.

Recommendation: Further research is required before any treatment recommendations can be given for prophylaxis with IUD insertion. However, all clients should be carefully screened for contraindications and educated about the risk of STDs at IUD insertion.

(Rank: field-test. Evidence: tentative. Priority: high.)

Intervention: To provide access to simple, safe technology for terminating pregnancy. Low-cost, simple technologies for ending pregnancy are available.[25] Although there are legal and ethical questions in many societies with regard to pregnancy termination, the RTIs responsible for much of the illness and death associated with unsafe abortions must be addressed by all societies.

Recommendation: Safe abortion services should be available.

(Rank: field-test. Evidence: proven. Priority: high.)

Intervention: To develop and market contraceptives that can prevent both infection and pregnancy. Spermicides that are also very effective against all potential STDs, particularly viruses, can be designed. They need to be incorporated into vehicles for use, field-tested, and marketed. Inexpensive barrier methods that women can use with or without their partner's knowledge and consent are an equally important priority.[26]

Recommendation: The highest priority should be given to introducing and field-testing a variety of products for women to use and control to prevent both pregnancy and RTIs.

(Rank: field-test. Evidence: proven. Priority: very high.)

Intervention: To improve understanding of the link between infertility and RTIs through educational programs for both the public and health care givers, and to target resources for infertility management to prevent RTIs. Infertility is a significant public health problem in many developing countries: prevalence of primary infertility ranges between 5–20 percent, and for secondary infertility prevalence ranges between 1–25 percent.[27] In these countries, 50–75 percent of infertility is due to RTIs, predominately *Neisseria gonorrhoeae* and *Chlamydia trachomatis*. The relationship of RTIs to infertility is not appreciated by women or health care providers. In most developing societies, the "new reproductive technologies" are not available for the management of infertility. Promoting understanding of the causative links between RTIs and the ability to conceive and deliver a healthy baby may encourage women to reduce risky sexual practices.

Recommendation: Health promotion and educational efforts to link infertility with RTIs should be developed within all health care settings in which women receive care, particularly family planning clinics.

(Rank: implement. Evidence: proven. Priority: high.)

Nonpregnant, Noncontracepting Women Using Primary Health Centers

These women are more difficult to access than women attending MCH or family planning clinics. However, many of them will irregularly attend primary care settings for treatment of a variety of illnesses. Interventions need to be developed and tested in order to identify strategies to prevent RTIs in these women.

Intervention: To give women an opportunity during routine primary care to discuss briefly their concerns with regard to sexual health, and to undergo a risk assessment. Women who feel they are at increased risk because of their own or their partner's sexual activity should be given additional information. Risk assessment and programming for sexual health are largely undeveloped. Perhaps self-help groups can be formed within the community health care system or elsewhere (religious, educational institutions) in which women can learn together.

Recommendation: Women who are neither pregnant nor seeking family planning need to be routinely assessed for sexual risks; appropriate educational strategies are needed.

(Rank: field-test. Evidence: tentative. Priority: medium.)

Intervention: To provide women with a female-controlled protective technology against infection, which need not be a contraceptive. Although most women presumably will accept combined spermicides and anti-infective agents, a proportion want only to be protected from infections. Anti-infective substances must be inexpensive, easy to use, and not associated with local adverse reactions.

Recommendation: Topical regimens that will kill viruses and bacteria and are not spermicidal should be developed, tested, and marketed.

(Rank: investigate. Evidence: assumed. Priority: medium.)

Intervention: To regularly screen to identify and treat cervical neoplasia early. Cervical cancer ranks among the top three cancers in most developing countries.[28] In industrialized societies, epidemiological and biological evidence links carcinoma of the cervix to infections with human papilloma virus. Cervical screening programs and the treatment of abnormal lesions require substantial infrastructure and technical expertise. At present, there is no evidence to suggest that these programs can be incorporated into the primary care systems in most developing countries. Additional studies are needed on the causality of cervical cancer in developing countries, for further understanding of the biology and epidemiology of the causal agent.

Recommendation: Programs to prevent cervical cancer through cervical cytology screening at present should not be developed in most developing country settings. However, investigation into simpler diagnostic technologies to recognize early cervical neoplasia and studies into the etiology and epidemiology of cervical neoplasia is a high priority.

(Rank: investigate. Evidence: tentative. Priority: medium.)

Intervention: To screen women for HIV infection on request (with the diagnosis of other STDs or high-risk behavior, or with the diagnosis of HIV infection or AIDS in family members) in order to provide appropriate education and counseling, to identify discordant couples, and to offer support and preventive counseling. Programs in developing countries to inform women about their HIV status are controversial.[29] Unresolved issues include lack of resources for testing and for counseling in most developing countries, lack of evidence that education and counseling at the time of screening change behavior, and lack of access to useful therapy for HIV-positive patients.[30] The diagnosis of HIV infection in one member of a couple may be the start of a useful intervention. Preliminary information suggests that with counseling and support, couples can be encouraged to remain together as a family, and that with precaution, the uninfected partner may delay or prevent seroconversion.[31]

Recommendation: Research on the usefulness of HIV screening for appropriate target groups is a priority in order to deliver effective educational and counseling messages. In particular, further studies of discordant couples to determine effective strategies to maintain the family unit and prevent further HIV transmission should be an urgent priority.

(Rank: investigate. Evidence: tentative. Priority: very high.)

CORE GROUP (HIGH-FREQUENCY) TRANSMITTERS

Core groups are the reservoir for many STDs. Their frequent change of partners permits STD pathogens to persist in a community or, in some instances, to increase rapidly through continuous dissemination from this reservoir. The reservoir consists of female commercial sex workers (CSWs), their clients and their partners, and others in society who have multiple partners and unprotected intercourse. The number of partners required to belong to this group is not defined, but 5–10 new sexual partners each year would put an individual at markedly increased risk of acquiring and transmitting STDs.[32] Perhaps 2 percent of sexually active women and 20 percent of sexually active men in some urban African societies meet this criterion and would be appropriate targets for core group control.[33] Programs designed to reduce STDs in this population will be cost-effective and logistically possible within societies where core groups can be identified and accessed.[34] Some STDs, particularly genital ulcer disease, remain endemic in populations only if core groups are significant contributors to "at-risk" individuals. Heterosexual HIV epidemics in most societies require participation of large core groups in order to develop explosive increases in prevalence of 1 percent or more annually in sexually active adults. Many members of high-risk groups are infected with multiple pathogens; frequently, they transmit two or more pathogens during an intercourse episode. For example, genital ulceration increases HIV excretion through the genital tract, and men who acquire chancroid have a twofold increase of also acquiring HIV.[35,36]

Intervention: To reduce the spread of STDs to and from CSWs, two strategies are needed. First, develop regulations to require periodic examination and testing for STDs and HIV. This strategy has been used in the Philippines and Thailand, as well as in European countries. *Second, provide ready access to care and treatment programs to reduce this reservoir of STDs.* Efforts to improve the health of CSWs and reduce their risk of transmitting STDs or HIV to their clients can be very effective through self-motivated, relatively inexpensive efforts that emphasize ready access to health care, provision of free condoms, and peer education. An economic analysis in Nairobi of the benefits suggests that the cost of preventing a case of HIV ranges between US$7.00 and $11.00, depending on the assumptions chosen.[37]

Recommendation: First, for prevention and control of RTIs in CSWs and their clients, a strategic plan should be integrated within the national STD control program. Second, CSWs should be encouraged to become involved in their own health and that of their clients. Third, health care providers should be encouraged to offer empathy and support to CSWs. Fourth, research into the significance of CSWs as a reservoir for STDs and the efficiency of interventions is urgently required.

(Rank: implement. Evidence: proven. Priority: very high.)

Intervention: To understand the role of men with multiple sex partners in the epidemiology of STDs and the efficacy of interventions, including strategies to reduce high-risk behavior. Interventions are being developed for men in occupational categories considered to place them at high risk of STDs. However, risk assessment and appropriate, cost-effective interventions are needed for all men. The health-seeking behavior that results in men's obtaining treatment for STDs has not been studied adequately in developing countries. Male promiscuity is accepted in many societies. Society tends to be far less judgmental toward men who are within the core group and who are also reservoirs for STDs. To our knowledge, no prospective studies have seriously addressed the issue of "socially sanctioned male promiscuity" or attempted to determine whether any generally acceptable interventions would address it. Should the male stereotype in a society undergo significant change in the era of HIV? What are the strategies that would permit various societies to examine this issue?

Recommendation: Behavioral studies to determine the motivation for men to become members of the core group or to purchase sex are necessary. Also needed are identification and study of interventions to reduce this reservoir, including consideration of screening with simple, inexpensive technologies to identify subclinical infection; more ready access to treatment; and more effective social marketing of condoms.

(Rank: field-test. Evidence: tentative. Priority: very high.)

Intervention: To control and, if possible, eradicate genital ulcers due to Haemophilus ducreyi (chancroid) in order to reduce HIV transmission. Control of chancroid is possible in industrialized societies. Chancroid has no proven asymptomatic subclinical reservoir and appears to flourish as an endemic disease only in societies in which men use CSWs, a significant proportion of men are uncircumcised, and no effective control programs are in place. No sustained effort has been made to control genital ulcers in any developing country. Evidence from Sub-Saharan Africa suggests that a significant proportion (10–30 percent) of HIV heterosexual transmission can be attributed to genital ulcers in women.[34,35] This intervention would include general and targeted education to high-risk groups about the significance of genital ulcers and their relationship to AIDS; programs to provide a regular examination, effective treatment, and condoms to CSWs; and treatment programs within the primary care system to treat genital ulcer disease.

Recommendation: This intervention should be implemented now, with operations research to acquire knowledge on its widespread implementation.

(Rank: implement. Evidence: tentative. Priority: high.)

Intervention: To encourage public health authorities and specific population groups to consider widespread pubertal and adult circumcision to reduce the incidence of STDs, particularly HIV, in men, and thereby reduce the opportunity for transmission to their female sexual partners. The male foreskin markedly increases the risk of men's acquiring several STDs. Uncircumcised men appear to have 5–10 times the risk of HIV acquisition as circumcised men, and about twice the risk of chancroid and syphilis.[35,38-41] This is presumptive evidence that these men will more likely infect their partners. Although unproven, it can be assumed that widespread circumcision will markedly reduce the opportunity for STDs, including HIV, to spread rapidly in communities.[41]

Recommendation: Male circumcision should be promoted for public health.

(Rank: field-test. Evidence: tentative. Priority: very high.)

BEHAVIORAL AND EDUCATIONAL INITIATIVES

Interventions can be undertaken to change behaviors to interrupt the chain of events that lead to new STDs in women. In general, new STDs and their sequelae develop as a result of three consecutive steps: being exposed to infection through intercourse with an infected sex partner; acquiring infection during sexual intercourse with an infected partner; and failing to have the infection diagnosed and treated in a timely manner. Additionally, in the aggregate, infected women contribute to the development of further incident cases of RTIs in other women by transmitting their infection to men, who may in turn infect other women. Thus, behavioral interventions may aim at changing behaviors to avoid women's exposure to infected partners; preventing infection after exposure to an infected partner; and promoting early diagnosis and therapy to avoid secondary infections, sequelae of infections, and further transmission.

Behaviors that put women at risk for exposure to and acquisition of STDs are not confined to women's own behaviors. The majority of women in both industrialized and developing societies are monogamous. These women are placed at risk for sexually transmitted infections because of their sexual partners' behaviors. Thus, behavioral interventions to reduce the risk of exposure to and acquiring RTIs, must be targeted to men as well as women. In fact, if all behavioral interventions were equally and perfectly successful, interventions aimed at men would prevent greater numbers of women from developing RTIs than would similar interventions aimed at women, since each man engaging in preventive behavior would protect more than one woman against STDs.[42]

In addition, behaviors of health care providers are associated with women's risk for developing RTI sequelae. Health care providers' failure to diagnose and treat an existing infection in a man or woman allows the development of new cases of STDs and sequelae in women. Similarly, health care providers' failure to counsel men and women on risk reduction allows new cases of STDs to be transmitted to women. Furthermore, health care providers' failure to implement preventive protocols in their health care practice leads to iatrogenic infections following deliveries, abortions, IUD insertions, and other procedures. Thus, behavioral interventions must also be targeted to health care providers to encourage them to provide risk reduction counseling, implement preventive protocols in their health care practice, and improve the diagnosis and treatment of RTIs. Provision of health care services is often inadequate, especially in the STD area. Behavioral interventions focusing on health care providers will be more effective in the context of improved and expanded health care services. Such services may focus differentially on men and women. Specifically, services for symptomatic individuals may focus on men, whereas services for asymptomatic individuals may focus on women, since women tend to be asymptomatic more often than men. Population impacts of behavioral interventions targeting health care providers depend largely on the opportunities for interaction between the general public and health care providers. For example, risk reduction counseling provided during family planning visits can reach only that segment of the female population that receives family planning services.

Core groups of high-frequency transmitters, such as CSWs, are important in the prevention of STDs, since they tend to be easy to identify and are marked by a high prevalence of infection. These groups play an important role in the transmission dynamics of STDs, particularly bacterial infections with short durations of infectiousness and low transmissibility.[42] Since the livelihood of CSWs depends on maximizing exposure to sex partners, behavioral interventions aimed at minimizing exposure to infected partners are less appropriate for this group. Interventions aimed at avoiding acquisition of infection during exposure to a potentially infected partner, and interventions aimed at improving early diagnosis and treatment of STDs, can be effective and markedly reduce STD transmission.[34,43]

Distinct behavioral interventions have synergistic effects, magnifying each other. For example, interventions to increase women's awareness of RTI symptoms and interventions to increase availability and accessibility of health care services reinforce each other. Synergy can be achieved between interventions targeting different groups. For example, interventions aimed at men to increase their sense of responsibility for protecting their female partners and interventions aimed at women to increase their symptom recognition and health-care seeking, condom use, and avoidance of acquisition of infection if exposed, can facilitate each other. Synergistic effects can also be achieved between different channels of communication. For example, similar condom use messages communicated through television and in the context of risk reduction counseling during family planning visits reinforce each other. Synergistic effects among behavioral interventions, health services interventions, and interventions targeting groups of high-frequency transmitters will help produce a net public health impact that is greater than the sum of the parts.[34,44]

While it has not been studied systematically, responsiveness of populations to preventive behavioral interventions appears to be variable. Several parameters of social context may be associated with such responsiveness. Educational levels of target groups affect the ease with which public health messages are understood; gender power relations influence the extent to which women are able to implement suggested behavioral changes, especially if their male partners oppose the change; and employment demands dictated by the economic structure may render some messages impossible to implement. For example, monogamy may be particularly difficult if spouses are separated for extended periods.[45] Thus, it may be important to facilitate some basic social change process, such as increasing educational levels and empowering women, to increase the effectiveness of behavioral interventions. In situations where women's social status is defined *only* vis-á-vis that of men—that is, as daughter, wife, mother, or "prostitute"—it is unrealistic to expect women to be able to implement any changes in behavior against the desires of the men in question.[46,47] Nonetheless, in many societies where women's social status is defined predominantly on the basis of their relationship to men, women have been organized and have effectively implemented many changes.

Experience with behavioral interventions is limited, especially in developing countries. Hardly any information is available on their efficacy in different societal contexts. Systematic evaluation of behavioral interventions and their population impact has not been a priority. Most behavioral intervention programs to prevent the transmission of HIV have consisted of mass media campaigns with the goal of enhancing information. We do not have adequate systematic data on different types of behavioral interventions and their relative effectiveness with different target groups and in different societies. Nevertheless, there are many interventions that have no potential adverse effects and that, on the basis of expert judgment, would be expected to have a favorable impact in many societies. These interventions should be implemented as soon as possible simultaneously. They should be evaluated, and information about the experience should be disseminated.

In initiating behavioral interventions, it is essential to get the attention and commitment of decision makers nationally and in local communities. Nongovernmental organizations with similar values should also be recruited.

Intervention: To further develop mass media campaigns. Campaigns targeted to the general population to address issues related to STDs, their symptoms, and their sequelae, integrated with programs to prevent HIV, should be effective. This information should encourage avoidance of sexual intercourse with individuals at increased risk of infection, urge consistent use of condoms, and educate about RTIs.

Recommendation: All governments and a variety of nongovernmental organizations should be encouraged to launch frequent, well-designed mass media campaigns.

(Rank: implement. Evidence: tentative. Priority: very high.)

Intervention: To further educate health care providers and motivate them to educate their clients. Risk reduction counseling provided while other health care services are delivered is effective in industrialized societies. In order to be effective, health care providers need to know the role of risk assessment, early diagnosis and treatment, and counseling in avoiding STDs. They also need to learn how to recognize, care for, and counsel individuals who are members of core groups of transmitters. Simple management algorithms need to be learned and used correctly.

Recommendation: Governments and professional organizations should encourage and support health care workers to acquire the knowledge, skills, and attitudes to enable them to be more effective care givers in the prevention and management of RTIs.

(Rank: implement. Evidence: tentative. Priority: very high.)

Intervention: To develop programs within the primary, secondary, and postsecondary educational systems to increase the knowledge of STDs and their sequelae, ensure that all individuals know how they can be prevented, and introduce individuals to the concept of sexual health. Adolescents in most countries are at considerable risk of STDs and their sequelae. Information about sexuality is often communicated poorly within the home environment. Properly designed and taught curricula may be very effective in altering sexual behavior and reducing STDs among youth.

Recommendation: Incorporation of material on sexual health and STDs into school curricula is an urgent priority in all societies.

(Rank: implement. Evidence: tentative. Priority: very high.)

IMPROVEMENT OF WOMEN'S STATUS

Intervention: To ensure that national legal codes provide women with rights in the workplace, in marriage relationships, in the educational system, in inheritance, and in other areas where gender discrimination against women exists. Throughout the world over the past century, increased legal rights have been slowly granted to women in most societies. Evidence that this has improved the well-being of women as well as society is substantial. Lack of entitlement and resultant lack of authority and power are principal causes of many women's health problems, including RTIs.

We would urge individuals everywhere to further the legal and social arguments to facilitate legal and judicial change that will ensure that women are equal before the law and in the courts. We would suggest that this would be an appropriate area for the international donor community and international organizations such as the World Bank and the International Monetary Fund to address in the context of ongoing discussions on national priorities. We would also urge governments to continue to review these issues through diplomatic channels and other venues. Courageous political leadership will be required within all societies for this to occur. However, in the absence of change, most other interventions will be wholly or partially ineffective.

Recommendation: Legal and judicial changes must be implemented in all societies to ensure equal rights for women.

(Rank: implement. Evidence: assumed. Priority: very high.)

Intervention: To reduce the supply of CSWs by addressing issues of poverty and discrimination that force women to choose this means of survival, by launching efforts to reduce the demand. Innovative strategies to provide alternate income sources for women in order to reduce the likelihood of their beginning or continuing to work as CSWs have not been studied in any effective manner. Interventions to reduce the demand side have also not been investigated. In many societies, a significant proportion of women are now HIV-infected and presumably are the source of a significant proportion of new HIV infections in the community.

Recommendation: Governments need to review their policies with regard to discrimination, stigmatization, and harassment of CSWs. This review needs to be combined with programs to prevent women from becoming CSWs and to rehabilitate existing workers. Additional creative strategies are necessary to determine how the demand for CSWs can be reduced within society through interventions with clients.

(Rank: field-test. Evidence: assumed. Priority: high.)

Intervention: Encourage employment and housing policies to ensure that couples remain together. Spousal separation occurs very frequently in developing countries for a variety of reasons. In most instances, men migrate to work sites, particularly mines, or to cities to seek work without their spouses. Extramarital sexual encounters ensue, with risks of STDs, and these diseases often are secondarily spread to the spouse when the marital sexual relationship is resumed.[39] In many towns in rural Africa, most of the initially HIV-infected men were individuals who had spent periods of time in town without their spouses.

Recommendation: Government and businesses should have employment policies to facilitate couples' remaining together. When this is not possible, employees should be provided with specific educational information about "safer" sexual practices and the risks of STDs and HIV.

(Rank: implement. Evidence: assumed. Priority: high.)

CONCLUSIONS

The psychological and physical health of women can be very significantly improved by interventions that prevent and more effectively manage RTIs. The issues relating to RTIs are inordinately complex and cannot always be brought into a clear focus for targeted interventions. Poorly understood intricate interactions occur between RTIs and long-standing behavioral patterns and cultural traditions.

As a result, the broad area of women's health cannot be addressed without moving on many fronts to identify both general and specific issues. We would encourage the development of forums for a continuing dialogue between women from developing countries and their political representatives, international funding bodies, and scientists in order to increase the understanding of the disease burden of RTIs and to identify the interventions that may be successful.

TABLE 1: A SUMMARY OF INTERVENTIONS FOR RTIs

TYPE OF INTERVENTION	RANK	EVIDENCE	PRIORITY
International health interventions			
Global coordinating body	Investigate	Assumed	High
Improved treatment options	Implement	Assumed	Medium
Simple diagnostic techniques	Investigate	Assumed	Very high
Development of "intellectual capital"	Field-test	Assumed	Medium
Disseminate information	Implement	Assumed	High
National health policy and capacity			
National strategic plan	Field-test	Assumed	High
Integrated services	Field-test	Tentative	Very high
Treatment guidelines and drug availability	Implement	Assumed	High
Training of professionals	Implement	Assumed	Very high
Reference and regional laboratories	Implement	Assumed	Medium
Surveillance	Implement	Assumed	High
Information sharing	Implement	Assumed	Medium
Health services for women			
Routine risk assessment	Field-test	Tentative	High
Female-controlled condoms	Investigate	Assumed	High
Cervical cancer screening	Investigate	Tentative	High
Traditional birth attendant training	Field-test	Assumed	Medium
Routine HIV screening in pregnancy	Reject	Tentative	Low
Routine gonococcal screening in pregnancy	Investigate	Proven	High
Routine syphilis screening in pregnancy	Implement	Proven	Very high
Routine chlamydial screening in pregnancy	Investigate	Proven	High
Prophylaxis for neonatal ophthalmia	Implement	Proven	Very high
Preventing iatrogenic RTIs in pregnancy	Implement	Assumed	Medium
Immunization against hepatitis B	Field-test	Proven	High
Safe IUD insertion	Field-test	Tentative	High
Safe abortion	Field-test	Tentative	Very high
Contraceptives that prevent RTIs	Field-test	Proven	Very high
Linking of RTIs and infertility	Implement	Tentative	High
Screening and counseling on request women who are at increased risk for HIV	Investigate	Tentative	Very high

TABLE 1: A SUMMARY OF INTERVENTIONS FOR RTIs

TYPE OF INTERVENTION	RANK	EVIDENCE	PRIORITY
Core group transmitters			
CSW programs	Implement	Proven	Very high
Men with multiple sex partners	Field-test	Tentative	High
Genital ulcer control	Implement	Tentative	High
Male circumcision	Field-test	Tentative	Very high
Behavioral and educational initiatives			
Mass media campaign	Implement	Tentative	Very high
Health provider education	Implement	Tentative	Very high
Youth education	Implement	Tentative	Very high
Improvement of women's status			
Development and implementation of legal codes	Implement	Assumed	Very high
Alternatives to prostitution	Field-test	Assumed	High
Prevent separation of spouses	Implement	Assumed	High

TABLE 2: SUMMARY OF INTERVENTION PRIORITIES

Essential to implement immediately
  National strategic plan with leadership
  Integration of RTI services into existing programs
  Provision of treatment guidelines and drugs
  Training of professionals and leaders
  Surveillance with appropriate analysis and use of data
  Ophthalmia prophylaxis
  Mass media communications
  Youth-targeted prevention
  Prevention of syphilis in pregnancy
  Health provider education and motivation
  CSW care and infection prevention
  Genital ulcer disease control
  Equity gender issues
  Establish reference and regional laboratory services

Important but less essential to implement immediately
  Link infertility to RTIs both educationally and programmatically
  Prevent iatrogenic infections during pregnancy
  Prevent spousal separation through employment opportunities
  International information sharing
  International improved treatment options

Essential to field-test
  HIV screening initiatives
  IUD infection prevention
  Improved strategies for condom use
  Routine risk assessment by health providers
  Reduce male promiscuity
  Safe abortion technologies
  Hepatitis B immunization
  Develop nongovernmental organizations for RTI prevention
  Male circumcision

Essential to investigate
  Global RTI control coordination
  Develop global "intellectual capital"
  Develop simple diagnostic technologies
  Develop economic alternatives to prostitution
  TBA training for RTI prevention
  Understand sexual behavior
  Develop local anti-infective controlled by women
  Cervical cancer screening
  Gonococcal screening in pregnancy
  Chlamydia screening in pregnancy

It is our conclusion that significant efforts need to be expended to improve the status of women everywhere and to increase the preventive expertise and ability to provide improved care within primary health systems. These two major ongoing initiatives in every society are essential as the framework within which the development of specific interventions that will lead to specific targeted accomplishments in the control of RTIs should occur. In the meantime, national and international research initiatives can redirect existing knowledge to improve and simplify diagnostic technologies, treatment regimens, and control strategies. Behavioral and anthropological studies can increase our knowledge of the value of the potential interventions. Existing effective programs can become models for replication throughout the developing world. Realistic targets can be set for demonstrated progress in the control of RTIs in most societies.

Some initial successes in this area are only the "end of the beginning." We should forecast rapid progress and work to ensure that it occurs. Few, if any, insurmountable obstacles now impede progress in this area. The reproductive health and well-being of many millions of women is a very significant goal. Within the context of limited resources and difficult choices, many of the interventions identified by this exercise can occur and will be very worthwhile.

REFERENCES

1. Wasserheit J. The significance and scope of reproductive tract infections among Third World women. Int J Gynecol Obstet 1989; Supp 3:145–68.
2. Evans J. Health research and development, Boston: Oxford University Press, 1990.
3. Roemer M, Roemer R. Global health, national development and the role of government. Am J Pub Health 1990; 80:1188–90.
4. United Nations Conference on Trade and Development. The least developed countries in 1987, Geneva, 1987.
5. United Nations. 1985/86 Statistical Yearbook, New York, 1988: Table 13.
6. World Bank. Financing of health services in developing countries: an agenda for reform, Washington, DC, 1987.
7. Structural adjustment and health in Africa (editorial). Lancet, 1990; 1:885–6.
8. Hira SK. STD patient management: policies and procedures in Zambia. Presented at the Seventh International Conference on AIDS, Florence, Italy, June 16–21, 1991.
9. Morrow RH Jr., Lansang MA. The role of clinical epidemiology in establishing essential national health research capabilities in developing countries. Infect Dis Clin North Am 1991; 5:235–46.
10. Hitchcock PJ, Wasserheit JN, Harris JR, Holmes KK. Sexually transmitted diseases in the AIDS era: development of STD diagnostics for resource limited settings is a global priority. Sex Transm Dis 1991; 18:133–5.
11. Hassig SE, Kinkela N, Nsa W et al. Are there alternatives to pregnancy serological screening in Kinshasa, Zaire? AIDS 1990; 4:913–6.
12. Temmerman M, Moses S, Kiragu D, Fusallaus, Wamola IA, Piot P. Impact of single session post partum counselling of HIV infected women on their subsequent reproductive behavior. AIDS Care 1990; 2:247–52.
13. Elliot B, Brunham RC, Laga M et al. Maternal gonococcal infection as a preventable risk factor for low birth weight. J Infect Dis 1990; 161:531–6.

14. Fransen L, Nsanze H, Klauss V et al. Ophthalmia neonatorum in Nairobi, Kenya: the roles of Neisseria gonorrhoeae and Chlamydia trachomatis. J Infect Dis 1986; 153:862–9.

15. Plummer FA, Laga M, Brunham RC et al. Postpartum upper genital tract infections in Nairobi, Kenya: epidemiology, etiology and risk factors. J Infect Dis 1987; 156:92–8.

16. Hira SK, Bhat GJ, Chikamata DM et al. Syphilis interventions in pregnancy: Zambia demonstration project. Genitourin Med 1990; 66:159–64.

17. Datta P, Laga M, Plummer FA et al. Infection and disease after perinatal exposure to Chlamydia trachomatis in Nairobi, Kenya. J Infect Dis 1988; 158:524–8.

18. Braddick MR, Kreiss JK, Embree JE et al. Impact of maternal HIV infection on obstetrical and early neonatal outcome. AIDS 1990; 4:1001–5.

19. Laga M, Plummer FA, Piot P et al. Prophylaxis of gonococcal and chlamydial ophthalmia neonatorum: a comparison of silver nitrate and tetracycline. N Engl J Med 1988; 318:653–7.

20. Chi IC, Whatley A, Wilkens L, Potts M. In hospital maternal mortality risk by caesarean and vaginal deliveries in less developed countries—a descriptive study. Int J Gynecol Obstet 1986; 24:121–31.

21. Simpson-Hebert M, Christie LS, Streich J. Traditional midwives and family planning. Popul Rep 1980; 8:447–91.

22. Maynard JE, Kane MA, Alter MJ et al. Control of hepatitis B by immunization: global perspectives. In: Zuckerman AJ, ed. Viral hepatitis and liver disease, New York: Alan R. Liss, 1988: BD 967–9.

23. Grimes DA. Intrauterine devices and pelvic inflammatory disease: recent developments. Contracept 1987; 36:97.

24. Sinei SK. Preventing IUD related pelvic infections: the efficacy of prophylactic antibiotics at insertion. Personal communication.

25. Kay B, Kabir S. A study of costs and behavioral outcomes of menstrual regulation services in Bangladesh. Soc Sci Med 1988; 26:597–604.

26. Stein ZA. HIV prevention: the need for methods women can use. Am J Public Health 1990; 80:460–2.

27. World Health Organization Task Force on Infections, Pregnancies and Infertility. Perspectives on prevention. Fertil Steril 1987; 47:964–8.

28. Parking DM, Stjern J, Muir CS. Estimates of the world wide frequency of twelve major cancers. Bull WHO 1984; 62:163–82.

29. Goodgame RW. AIDS in Uganda—clinical and social features. New Engl J Med 1990; 323:383–9.

30. Lindan C, Allan S, Carael M et al. Knowledge, attitudes, and perceived risk of AIDS among urban Rwandan women: relationships to HIV infection and behavior change. AIDS 1991; 5:993–1002.

31. Feldblum OJ, Hira SK, Mukololo P et al. Anti-HIV efficacy of barrier contraceptives in HIV discordant couples. Personal communication.

32. Brunham RB, Plummer FA. A general model of sexually transmitted disease epidemiology and its implications for control. Med Clin North Am 1990; 74:1339–52.

33. Ngugi EN. Unpublished data.

34. Moses S, Plummer FA, Ngugi EN, Nagelkerke NJD, Anzala AO, Ndinya-Achola JO. Controlling HIV in Africa: effectiveness and cost of an intervention in a high frequency STD transmitter core group. AIDS 1991; 5:407–11.

35. Cameron DW, Simonsen JN, D'Costa LJ et al. Female to male transmission of human immunodeficiency virus type 1: risk factors for seroconversion in men. Lancet 1989; 2:403–7.

36. Plummer FA, Wainberg MA, Plourde P et al. Detection of HIV-1 in genital ulcer exudate of HIV-1 infected men by culture and gene amplication. J Infect Dis 1990; 161:810–1.

37. Plummer FA, Simonsen JN, Cameron DW et al. Co-factors in male-female sexual transmission of HIV. J Infect Dis 1991; 163:233–9.

38. Simonsen JN, Cameron DW, Gakinya MN et al. Human immunodeficiency virus infection among men with sexually transmitted diseases: experience from a center in Africa. N Engl J Med 1988; 319:274–8.

39. Pepin J, Plummer FA, Brunham RC, Piot P, Cameron DW, Ronald AR. The interaction of HIV infection and other sexually transmitted diseases: an opportunity for intervention. AIDS 1989; 3:3–9.

40. Hart G. Venereal disease in a war environment: incidence and management. Med J Aust 1975; 1:808–11.

41. Moses S, Bradley JE, Nagelkerke NJD, Ronald AR, Ndinya-Achola JO, Plummer FA. Geographical patterns of male circumcision practices in Africa: association with HIV seroprevalence. Int J Epidemiol 1990; 19:693–7.

42. Holmes KK, Aral S. Behavioral interventions in developing countries. In: Wasserheit, Aral, Holmes, Hitchcock, eds. Research issues in human behavior and STDs in the AIDS era, Washington, DC: American Society for Microbiology, 1991.

43. Plummer FA, Ngugi EN. Prostitutes and their clients in the epidemiology and control of sexually transmitted diseases. In: Holmes K, Mårdh P-A, Sparling F et al., eds. Sexually transmitted diseases, second edition, New York: McGraw-Hill, 1990; 71–6.

44. Llosa MV. The storyteller. Lane H, trans. Penguin Books; 1989.

45. Standing H, Kisekka MN. Sexual behavior in Sub-Saharan Africa—a review and annotated bibliography. London: Overseas Development Administration, 1989.

46. Sivard RL. Women: a world survey, Washington, DC: World Priorities, 1987.

47. Larson A. Social context of human immunodeficiency virus transmission in Africa: historical and cultural bases of East and Central African sexual relations. Rev Infect Dis 1989; 11:716–31.

ECONOMIC IMPACT OF REPRODUCTIVE TRACT INFECTIONS AND RESOURCES FOR THEIR CONTROL

Peter Piot
WHO Collaborating Centre on AIDS
Department of Microbiology
Institute of Tropical Medicine
Nationalestraat 155
2000 Antwerp, Belgium

Jane Rowley
Department of Pure and Applied Biology
Imperial College, University of London
Prince Consort Road, London SW7 2BB
United Kingdom

INTRODUCTION

There is little doubt that the various reproductive tract infections (RTIs) and their complications and sequelae are a significant public health problem in terms of morbidity and, common opinion among the medical profession notwithstanding, mortality.[1-6] This paper reviews the economic burden of RTIs in the developing world, as well as resources available and needed for their prevention and control. Since data on these topics are scarce to nonexistent, we are by necessity quite vague in many sections of this paper, and we do not quantify resources needed to control RTIs.

THE ENVIRONMENT FOR RTI CONTROL

Control of RTIs has not been a popular topic with governments or the medical establishment. The reasons for this are multiple, including a lack of knowledge of the scope of the problem and societal and technical factors. However, several factors are contributing to an increased global awareness of the importance of RTIs. These include the emergence of human immunodeficiency virus (HIV) infection and AIDS as a major public health problem, better documentation of the social and economic impacts of sexually transmitted diseases (STDs), the identification of several STDs as risk factors for the spread of HIV, and a growing recognition of the disease burden in *adults*, particularly women, in developing

Reproductive Tract Infections, Edited by A. Germain *et al.*
Plenum Press, New York, 1992

countries, as compared with a fairly exclusive attention to childhood diseases up to now.[7,8] Some of the more general obstacles to RTI control and prevention are listed below:

1. The generally disadvantaged situation of women in terms of education, nutrition, health, and labor
2. Existing attitudes and cultural and religious beliefs about sex, reproduction, and women's right to protect themselves
3. Poor access of women to health and social services, which are often poorly developed or weak
4. National public health authorities' and international agencies' neglect of RTI control
5. Insufficiently developed control and prevention strategies

The first three obstacles concern the status of women in general. In many parts of the developing world, where the health systems are of poor quality, and have even severely deteriorated, as in Africa, women's access to health and social services has been consistently less than that of men. This disparity often starts at birth, as illustrated by the higher infant and under-five mortality of girls than boys in several Asian countries.[9] Whereas Western women have a higher life expectancy at birth than their male counterparts, the reverse is true for many women in the Third World, as in Bangladesh, China, Bhutan, Nepal, India, and Pakistan. The cumulative lifetime risk of maternal mortality reaches one in 20 in some of the lowest-income countries—such as Ethiopia and Benin—compared with one in 6,000–10,000 in the United States and Europe. Educational opportunities are also less for women than for men, which has serious implications for health. It is estimated, for example, that one year of mother's education is associated with a 9 percent decrease in under-five mortality,[9] but the literacy rate for women is only 52 percent of that for men in South Asia, 57 percent in the Middle East, and 61 percent in Sub-Saharan Africa.

A second set of obstacles is the reluctance of public health policymakers to address STDs and RTIs. J. Wasserheit quotes four common arguments for not dealing with RTIs: they are not fatal; they are too expensive and too complicated to treat; they are related to sexual behavior, which is difficult to change; and they are likely to stigmatize programs such as family planning and maternal and child health (MCH).[2] Furthermore, public health and research professionals have been clearly inadequate in their response to these arguments, and clear control strategies have not been communicated to policymakers or have still to be developed. Research on the economic and social impacts of RTIs, and on the cost-effectiveness of interventions to prevent them, should contribute to the allocation of more resources for RTI control.[5,8,10]

ECONOMIC AND SOCIAL CONSEQUENCES ASSOCIATED WITH RTIs

The major goals of RTI control include the prevention of infection and the prevention of complications and sequelae of RTIs such as infertility, maternal mortality, ectopic pregnancy, and congenital infection. Traditional strategies for RTI control and prevention are listed below:[10–13]

1. Providing adequate diagnostic and treatment facilities for STD patients
2. Limiting complications by early detection and adequate treatment

3.   Reducing the risk of infection during genital tract procedures by making medically safe delivery and interruption of pregnancy available
4.   Reducing exposure to infection by offering health education and promoting condom use
5.   Limiting further transmission by counseling and partner referral
6.   Imposing regulations and taxes (such measures as prohibiting commercial sex, imposing a tax on alcohol, and establishing legal closing hours of bars have not proved effective for STD control, but they are very common throughout the world).

Research on the economic consequences of STDs is still very limited. Only one study has attempted to quantify the economic costs of RTIs and their complications and sequelae in developing countries,[5] and only a few studies have attempted to quantify RTI costs in developed countries. However, these studies have shown that the economic costs associated with RTIs and their complications and sequelae are substantial. For example, E. Washington, S. Hira, G. Morris, S. Moses, and colleagues[10] estimated that in 1990, the direct and indirect costs of pelvic inflammatory disease (PID) and its sequelae in the United States would reach US$3.5 billion. M. Over and P. Piot concluded that STDs, excluding HIV infection, account for 5 percent of the total discounted healthy life years lost in Sub-Saharan Africa, and HIV infection for 10 percent.[5] Figure 1 shows the contribution of STDs to healthy life lost, as compared with the contribution of other diseases in Sub-Saharan African urban populations.

In the next sections, we review the limited information available on the various costs associated with RTIs and their complications and sequelae in developing countries. We have opted not to address the economic consequences of HIV infection. (See D. Nabarro and C. McConnell[8] for a recent review.)

Direct Costs

The direct costs of RTI include the costs of diagnosing and treating the disease and of preventing its spread. Prevention costs are discussed in the next section.

In estimating the direct costs of a disease, it is important to consider the access an individual has to health care, the resources available for health care, and the quality of the care available. Per capita expenditure on health care in developing countries is a fraction of the sum spent in developed countries (see Table 1); as a result, many treatment procedures carried out in developed countries are not financially feasible in developing countries (e.g., in vitro fertilization of infertile women). The situation is further complicated by the inequitable distribution of health resources within countries.[15] Shortages of drugs, equipment, laboratory facilities, and health care personnel also constrain the type of diagnostic and treatment procedures that can be used.[16]

The diagnosis of RTIs in women is complicated by the fact that these infections are frequently asymptomatic in women. While data on the cost of diagnosing RTIs in Third World countries are not available, there are some estimates of the cost of diagnosing different STDs. Table 2 records, for a hypothetical Third World country, estimates of the cost of screening a woman for various STDs using different diagnostic techniques, and the sensitivity and specificity of these techniques. Clinical diagnosis is the cheapest and quickest to carry out, but also the least sensitive and specific. For instance, the clinical diagnosis of chlamydial infection, while costing approximately US$0.17 in our example, is only 40 percent sensitive and 70 percent specific. The alternative diagnostic techniques involve antigen detection or culture and are estimated to cost US$5.08–$12.08, a sum substantially greater than per capita national health care budgets in many low-income developing countries (see Table 1). Research efforts need to be directed toward the development of simple, inexpensive, and rapid diagnostic tests for use in clinical settings.

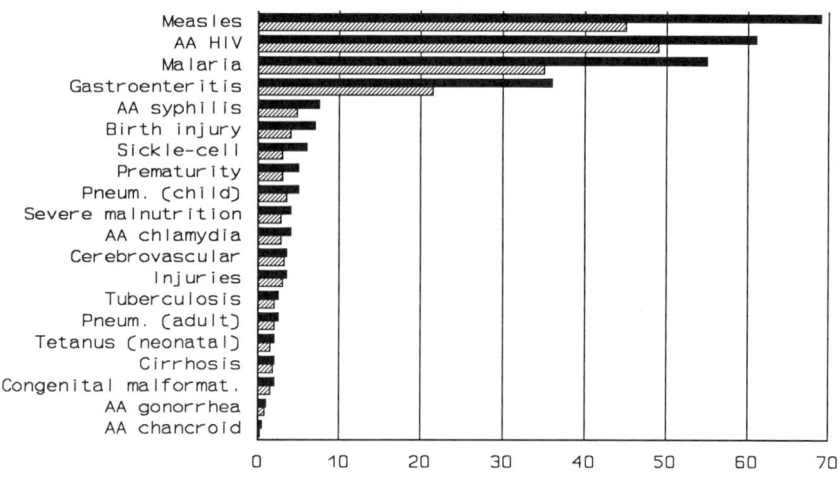

Percentage of healthy life years lost

*HIV seroprevalence of 5 percent.
Discount rate of 3 percent.

**Figure 1. Static Burden of STDs Relative to Other Diseases
in a High-Prevalence African City:*
Healthy Life Days Lost per Capita†**

Information on the cost of treating RTIs is also very limited. The only published estimates available are of the cost of treating a woman with an STD (see Table 3). These figures suggest that the cost of treating a woman for syphilis, chlamydial infection, gonorrhea, or chancroid is less than US$1.50. A comparison of the cost of diagnosing and treating STDs suggests that in some circumstances (e.g., high prevalence of an STD, insufficient or nonexistent laboratory facilities), the mass treatment of those population groups at risk may be a cost-effective alternative to screening prior to treatment.

Table 1. Government Health Expenditure (1988) and Percentage of Population with
Access to Health Services (1980–87) for Countries with a per Capita Gross National
Product below US$500 in 1988 and for the United Kingdom and United States

Country	Government expenditure on health as % of total government expenditure, 1988	Per capita government expenditure on health, 1988 (US$)	% of population with access to health services, 1980–87
Ethiopia	1.3	1.5	46
Malawi	1.9	3.2	80
Nepal	0.8	1.5	NA
Burkina Faso	0.9	1.8	49
Mali	0.7	1.7	15
Uganda	0.2	0.7	61
Nigeria	0.2	0.6	40
Zambia	1.2	3.5	75
India	0.3	1.1	NA
Pakistan	0.2	0.7	55
Kenya	1.7	6.5	NA
Togo	1.7	6.3	61
Ghana	1.3	5.0	60
Sri Lanka	1.7	7.1	93
Indonesia	0.4	1.8	75
United Kingdom	NA	602.1	NA
United States	NA	929.3	NA

Note: NA = not available.
Sources: references 8 and 18.

Table 2. Cost, Sensitivity, and Specificity of
Screening Techniques for STDs in Women

Disease	Type of screening technique	Cost per test (US$)	Cost of clinic/lab* (US$)	Total cost of diagnosis (US$)	Sensitivity (%)	Specificity (%)
Syphilis	Serology	1.5	0.08	1.58	95	95
Chlamydia	Clinical	0.0	0.17	0.17	40	70
	Culture	12.0	0.08	12.08	80	99
	Antigen detection	5.0	0.08	5.08	75	95
Gonorrhea	Clinical	0.0	0.17	0.17	40	70
	Culture	5.0	0.08	5.08	95	100
	Microscopy	1.0	0.17	1.17	50	70
Chancroid	Clinical	0.0	0.17	0.17	80	60
	Culture	5.0	0.08	5.08	70	100

* Cost per clinic or lab hour is assumed to be $1.00.
Source: reference 5.

Table 3. Cost of Treating a Case of STD, and Treatment Effectiveness in Women

Disease	Drug cost (US$)	Cost of clinic* (US$)	Cost per case (US$)	Treatment effectiveness (%)
Syphilis	0.80	0.25	1.05	99
Chlamydial infection	0.25	0.25	0.50	90
Gonorrhea	1.00	0.20	1.20	95
Chancroid	0.15	0.17	0.32	90

* Cost per clinic hour is assumed to be $1.00.
Note: Development of drug resistance will change drug cost, cost per case, and treatment effectiveness.
Source: reference 5.

Table 4 shows estimates of the costs of screening and treating 1,000 women for four STDs, assuming prevalence rates of 1–25 percent. Given the high costs of laboratory tests for the diagnosis of STDs, treating all women is less expensive than diagnosis followed by treatment at virtually all levels of infection. However, important potential drawbacks of such mass treatment should also be considered, but are much more difficult to cost. These include side effects of drugs for the women and eventual fetus, more rapid emergence of antimicrobial resistance, and lack of possibility of partner notification.

Table 4. Cost of Screening and Treating 1,000 Women for
STDs at Different Prevalences of Infection

Disease	Type of screening technique	Cost of screening (US$)	Cost of screening and treating (US$) at following seroprevalences:				Treatment effectiveness (%)
			1%	5%	10%	25%	
Syphilis	Serology	1,580	1,640	1,680	1,730	3,370	94
	Treat everyone	0	1,050	1,050	1,050	1,050	99
Chlamydia	Clinical	170	570	560	540	1,110	18
	Culture	12,080	12,090	12,100	12,120	24,210	72
	Antigen	5,080	5,110	5,120	5,140	10,250	68
	Treat everyone	0	500	500	500	500	90
Gonorrhea	Clinical	170	300	340	380	680	18
	Culture	5,080	5,090	5,140	5,190	10,290	90
	Microscopy	1,170	1,190	1,240	1,290	2,490	45
	Treat everyone	0	1,200	1,200	1,200	1,200	95
Chancroid	Clinical	170	300	300	310	610	72
	Culture	5,080	5,080	5,090	5,100	10,180	63
	Treat everyone	0	320	320	320	320	90

Note: Estimates of screening and treating costs as in Tables 3 and 4.

Costs of Treating RTI Sequelae. Few data are available on the complications and sequelae of RTIs (adverse outcomes of pregnancy, maternal mortality, cervical cancer, ectopic pregnancy, infertility, and chronic pelvic pain). Complications and sequelae occur more often in developing countries than in developed countries because of cultural barriers to seeking care, restricted access to health care, insufficient diagnostic facilities, and antibiotic resistance patterns,[1] among other factors.

The cost of treating these complications and sequelae are almost certainly much greater than the costs of treating the infection itself. While no quantitative data are readily available, hospital admission records from gynecology wards suggest that the opportunity costs of these preventable complications are substantial. For instance, the treatment of PID in Sub-Saharan Africa accounts for 1–44 percent of admissions to gynecology wards;[17,21] in

Benin City, Nigeria, ectopic pregnancies account for 15 percent of all gynecology admissions.[18]

Several reports document the considerable numbers of women admitted to hospitals in the developing world for treatment of "incomplete abortion"—a euphemism for illegally induced abortion—and its complications.[19,20,21] Such women require longer hospitalization, more blood units, and more anesthesia and surgical interventions (including hysterectomy) than women admitted for other reasons. Thus, incomplete abortion drains considerably on hospital resources, and if the expenditures made for treating complications of unsafe abortions went instead to family planning programs, the latter could provide better services (including contraception and safe abortions) to more people. The cost of treating complications of induced abortions may account for up to 50 percent of the resources of some hospitals, according to a World Health Organization report.[22,23,24]

Programs to reduce the incidence of RTIs in the female population and to administer early treatment of RTIs will substantially reduce the development of complications and sequelae, and have a major impact on the costs of RTIs.

Indirect Costs

The indirect costs of a disease include the value of the labor lost from morbidity, debility, and premature mortality, as well as the value of any labor diverted from other productive uses to care for the ill.

Recognition has only recently grown that RTIs are an important cause of morbidity and mortality in women and in children born to infected women. While there are no estimates of the indirect costs of RTIs, Over and Piot[5] have estimated the average annual number of discounted healthy (or productive) days of life lost per capita by women with STDs in an urban area in Africa. Their estimates range from 0.25 days for chancroid to 15.9 days for syphilis and 60.6 days for HIV infection, assuming a discount rate of 3 percent. Table 5 shows the benefit of preventing STDs in men and women in the same setting, expressed as discounted healthy life years (DHLYs) saved per case prevented. These figures suggest that preventing STDs results in considerable health gain.

These figures, however, do not fully include the impact of STDs on infant morbidity, debility, and mortality. Estimates of the incidence of STD complications in infants born to infected women suggest that STDs are substantial causes of infant morbidity, debility, and mortality. For example, it is estimated that 50–80 percent of pregnant women with syphilis whose pregnancies extend beyond 12 weeks have an adverse outcome: 30–40 percent have spontaneous abortions, 10–20 percent experience perinatal or infant deaths, and 10–20 percent bear infants with congenital syphilis.[14] Thus, in a country where the prevalence of syphilis in pregnant women is 10 percent, some 5–8 percent of all pregnancies that extend beyond 12 weeks have an adverse outcome from syphilis.[25]

The economic and social consequences of RTIs extend beyond these indirect costs. A number of studies have shown that the illness or death of a productive member of a household can have a substantial negative impact on the welfare of the other members of the household.[26-28] Infertility due to RTIs also has serious consequences for the individual woman, the marriage, and sometimes the community as a whole. Infertile women, but not usually men, can suffer severe personal and social stigma.

Table 5. Average Number of DHLYs Saved
per Case Prevented in a High-Prevalence Urban Area*

Disease	Women	Men
Syphilis	3.9	3.7
Chlamydial infection	1.3	0.8
Gonorrhea	1.0	0.7
Chancroid	0.2	0.2
HIV infection	19.5	19.5

* Includes years lost because of debility and premature
mortality, assuming a discount rate of 3 percent.

THE NEED FOR DATA

The lack of data on the economic consequences of RTIs in developing countries urgently needs to be remedied. Results of the few existing studies suggest that there are substantial economic costs associated with RTIs and their complications and sequelae. Before more comprehensive analyses of their economic consequences can be carried out, more data are required. Information on the economic consequences of RTIs will be of use to health care planners for allocating resources to the treatment and control of RTIs. The present lack of data may certainly be a key reason that so little attention is given to the treatment and prevention of RTIs.[29]

SELECTED INTERVENTIONS AND AFFORDABLE OPTIONS

Unfortunately, there is little information available on the effectiveness and costs of the currently available interventions against RTIs in the developing world, though data are increasingly being collected on the cost-effectiveness of AIDS-directed interventions (mostly those dealing with the prevention of blood-borne infections).[5,30]

There are even fewer data on the benefit of averting a case of STD (such as discounted healthy life days saved). It should be stressed that each case of STD prevented will also prevent additional cases. This effect is even more difficult to estimate, but it means that weighing only the benefits of preventing a single case against the cost of preventing a case is not sufficient; the so-called external benefits that accrue to persons other than the immediately affected individual must also be included.[5] Together with the cost of averting a case, information on potential healthy life days saved from each averted case provides powerful arguments to decision makers to allocate resources for RTI control.

Over and Piot[5] tried to calculate the cost per DHLY saved from case management for selected STDs in the developing world. Curing a case of syphilis resulted in "purchasing" a DHLY for US$0.1–$40, depending on the prevalence of disease and the case detection strategy used. Case management of chlamydial infection and gonorrhea is also highly cost-effective, especially if the intervention is targeted at a high-prevalence (core) group, with dollar costs per DHLY saved ranging from \$10 to \$41. The authors concluded that a program of STD treatment is highly cost-effective if it is targeted at high-prevalence groups. Outside such groups, case management strategies should focus on improved case finding in order to reduce the cost per case identified. Women who attend prenatal and family planning clinics, or who are seen at primary health care facilities, are a prime target group for such a case-finding program.

As compared with other interventions to improve adult health, the management of chlamydial infection, gonorrhea, and syphilis in populations with moderate prevalence rates ranked among the 10 most cost-effective interventions in a recent World Bank[32] study (Figure 2). It was preceded in cost-effectiveness only by blood screening for HIV, rehabilitation for leprosy, short-course chemotherapy for leprosy, antismoking campaigns plus tobacco taxes, and cataract surgery plus spectacles. We discuss briefly below selected interventions, and explore affordable options that are available and can make a difference.

Early Disease Detection and Treatment

Because of the complexity of etiologic diagnosis and the expense of recommended antibiotics, RTI interventions are often seen as impossible or as a bottomless financial pit.[2] However, recently proposed alternatives that simplify case management of RTIs may make this approach feasible and affordable at the primary health care level.[31] In addition, the cost of averting RTIs by early diagnosis and treatment should be compared with that of treating complications and sequelae of RTIs. It is remarkable that individuals and societies are often more readily willing to pay astronomical bills for in vitro fertilization than more modest sums for uncomplicated RTI control.

The primary goal of early case detection and treatment is the prevention of complications and sequelae of a particular RTI. In addition, treatment limits the spread of infection to others. Examples of this intervention strategy include case detection and treatment of gonococcal and chlamydial infection in pregnant women, nonpregnant women, or both, and screening and treatment based on serological evidence of syphilis to cure the women and to prevent congenital syphilis.

To the best of our knowledge, no reports (in contrast to simulations, such as in Table 4) are available on the effectiveness or costs of syndrome-oriented or simplified case management methods for detecting lower reproductive tract infections in women in the developing world. Such studies are urgently needed. Cost-effectiveness data from the United States are emerging for *Chlamydia trachomatis*. Studies in high-risk populations, such as STD patients, suggest that generalized treatment may be the most cost-effective approach.[33] Studies from low-risk populations, however, are nonconclusive. A study in California suggested that at a prevalence of 2 percent, it is cost-effective to detect and treat chlamydial infection in sexually active women.[34] In another study, however, screening for *Chlamydia trachomatis* was not found to be cost-effective in women with a probability of infection of less than 7 percent.[35] From these apparently contradictory data, it is clear that much remains to be done in this field.[36]

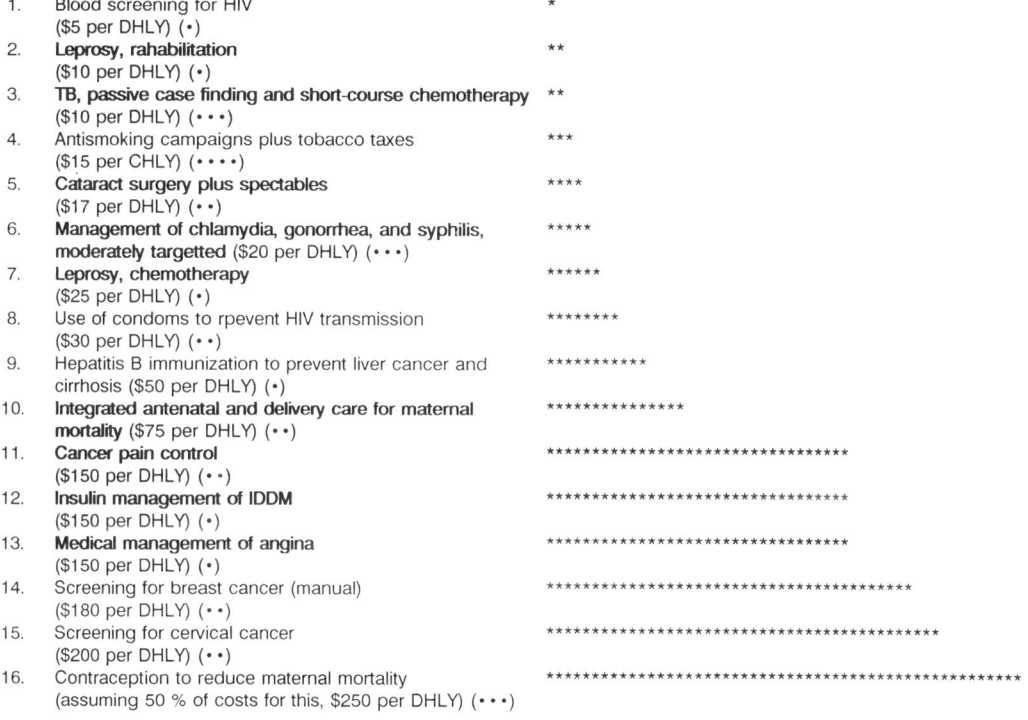

1. Blood screening for HIV   *
    ($5 per DHLY) (•)
2. **Leprosy, rahabilitation**   **
    ($10 per DHLY) (•)
3. **TB, passive case finding and short-course chemotherapy** **
    ($10 per DHLY) (• • •)
4. Antismoking campaigns plus tobacco taxes   ***
    ($15 per CHLY) (• • • •)
5. **Cataract surgery plus spectables**   ****
    ($17 per DHLY) (• •)
6. **Management of chlamydia, gonorrhea, and syphilis,**   *****
    moderately targetted ($20 per DHLY) (• • •)
7. **Leprosy, chemotherapy**   ******
    ($25 per DHLY) (•)
8. Use of condoms to rpevent HIV transmission   ********
    ($30 per DHLY) (• •)
9. Hepatitis B immunization to prevent liver cancer and   ***********
    cirrhosis ($50 per DHLY) (•)
10. **Integrated antenatal and delivery care for maternal**   ***************
    mortality ($75 per DHLY) (• •)
11. **Cancer pain control**   **********************************
    ($150 per DHLY) (• •)
12. **Insulin management of IDDM**   **********************************
    ($150 per DHLY) (•)
13. **Medical management of angina**   **********************************
    ($150 per DHLY) (•)
14. Screening for breast cancer (manual)   **
    ($180 per DHLY) (• •)
15. Screening for cervical cancer   ***
    ($200 per DHLY) (• •)
16. Contraception to reduce maternal mortality   **
    (assuming 50 % of costs for this, $250 per DHLY) (• • •)

Legend: (i)   Preventive interventions are in males, case management interventions are in **boldface** type.

(ii)   The number of heavy circles beside each intervention indicates how major is the burden of the
        condition(s) it addresses.

        Limited •
        Moderate • •
        Substantial • • •
        Very substantial • • • •   Figure continues on next page.

Figure 2. Improving Adult Health—The Cost-effectiveness of Interventions

17. **Management for selected opportunistic AIDS infections**
($300 per DHLY) (•)

18. Control of onchocerciasis vector to prevent blindness
($300 per DHLY) (•)

19. **Oral hypoglycemic management of NIDDM**
($330 per DHLY) (••)

20. Public preventive campaigns to prevent CVD
($600 per DHLY) (••)

21. **Tertiary management of colorectal and nasopharangeal cancer** (about $800 per DHLY) (•)

22. Screening for breast cancer (mammography)
($1800 per DHLY) (•)

23. Medical management of moderate to severe hypertension
($2000 per DHLY) (••)

24. **Mitral valve replacement for RHD**
(>$2000 per DHLY) (•)

25. Medical management of hypercholesterolemia
($4000 per DHLY) (•)

26. **Tertiary management of lung, liver, esophageal and stomach cancer** (over $4000 per HDLY) (••)

27. **AZT management of AIDS**
($5000 per DHLY) (•)

28. **Coronary artery bypass surgery**
($5000 per DHLY) (•)

x $330
x $600
x $800
x $1800
x $2000
x>$2000
x $4000
x $4000
x $5000
x $5000

0   50   100   150   200   250   300
Cost per discounted healthy life year gained (DHLY) in 1989 U.S. $

Legend: (i)   Preventive interventions are in males, case management interventions are in **boldface** type.

(ii)   The number of heavy circles beside each intervention indicates how major is the burden of the condition(s) it addresses.

Limited •
Moderate ••
Substantial •••
Very substantial ••••

Figure 2. Improving Adult Health—The Cost-effectiveness of Interventions (continued)

Somewhat more operational experience exists on the prevention of congenital syphilis by identifying and treating pregnant women with syphilis. In Norway, such a screening program is cost-effective, even at a very low prevalence rate of 0.01 percent.[37] This is mainly because of the high costs of medical, educational, and institutional care for handicapped children in industrialized countries. Almost no such data are available for a developing country. Syphilis screening is officially recommended in most developing countries. However, this intervention is implemented very inconsistently, even in countries with a prevalence of active syphilis of over 20 percent among pregnant women. Reasons for this include little or no political will, low awareness of the problem among health care providers, lack of hard currency, unavailability of serologic tests or penicillin, poor organization of the intervention, and low rates of antenatal clinic attendance during early pregnancy.

In an innovative demonstration project in Zambia, Hira and coworkers showed that it is possible to integrate congenital syphilis control into first-line antenatal care.[38] The program aims at increasing early attendance at antenatal clinics before 16 weeks of pregnancy, performance of an RPR (rapid plasma reagin test for syphilis) on-site, and prompt treatment of women with a reactive RPR. Although antenatal clinic attendance, screening, and treatment are still suboptimal, the intervention has reduced syphilitic adverse outcomes by two thirds (from 72 percent of adverse pregnancy outcome among seroreactive mothers at the control centers without intervention to 28 percent after the intervention). The cost of the intervention is shown in Table 6. The cost of averting each adverse outcome was $12. In Kenya, the cost of preventing one death from congenital syphilis was estimated at KSh1,200 (approximately $50).[39]

Efforts are also under way to make early detection of cervical cancer more accessible in the developing world. In a recent study in India, nearly half of all cases of early cervical cancer could be detected by clinical inspection.[40] However, more research is needed before this approach can be recommended, particularly because of its very low predictive value of an abnormal finding. Because of cervical cancer's high fatality rate, improvement of early detection and treatment should yield a substantial health benefit.

Antimicrobial Prophylaxis

The goal of antimicrobial prophylaxis is the prevention of infection itself (i.e., eye prophylaxis at birth) or the prevention of ascending infections and complications in women with uncomplicated RTIs (e.g., prophylaxis before introducing an IUD or during pregnancy termination). Eye prophylaxis at birth is highly effective to prevent gonococcal, but not chlamydial, ophthalmia neonatorum.[41] Introduction of this practice over a century ago led to the virtual elimination of blindness following neonatal gonococcal conjunctivitis in Europe.[42]

The cost of averting a case for two types of ocular prophylaxis, as compared with the cost of treating a case of gonococcal conjunctivitis, is shown in Table 7. At a maternal gonorrhea prevalence rate of 6 percent—a common prevalence in developing countries[3]— eye prophylaxis is cheaper than treating the cases that would occur in the absence of prophylaxis. This remains so until the maternal prevalence drops to 2 percent. The model does not take into account the direct and indirect costs of various degrees of visual impairment that are caused by delayed or ineffective treatment of gonococcal conjunctivitis.

Permanent visual impairment will occur especially and most severely among newborns not given prophylaxis.[43] The model also does not consider the risk that a case will not be detected and properly treated because diagnostic facilities and drugs are not available in most developing country settings. All these considerations make us believe that eye prophylaxis at birth is probably highly cost-effective at maternal gonorrhea prevalence rates well below 1 percent in a developing country context.

Table 6. Cost of Congenital Syphilis Intervention for 1,000 Women in Zambia

Component	Cost (US$)
Two tests per attendee (an initial visit and a repeated visit in last trimester) at $0.1 per test	200
Treatment of all reactors at first visit at $1 per treatment	100
Treatment of subsequent visit at $1 per treatment, assuming 20 percent will be re-treated	20
Treatment of spouses at $1 per treatment, assuming that 67 percent of the spouses of all reactors will be treated	80
Amortized cost for development and printing of behavioral and educational material	100
Amortized cost for microcentrifuges and lamps	100
Total	600

Source: reference 38.

Even if the economic benefit of averting a case is not known, the risk of blindness is an additional strong argument to administer ocular prophylaxis at birth in all developing countries, and to include it in traditional birth attendants' kits.

Some studies have shown that prophylactic use of inexpensive antibiotics, such as tetracycline, is effective for the prevention of PID after therapeutic abortion.[44,45] One study in Kenya also suggested that doxycycline prophylaxis for IUD insertion may decrease the incidence of PID and the number of post-IUD clinic visits by approximately one third.[46] However, there are no cost-effectiveness data on these interventions, and confirmation of these results is needed. As is the case for ocular prophylaxis at birth, antibiotic prophylaxis at IUD insertion or abortion is readily implementable.

Table 7. Cost of Ocular Prophylaxis for Gonococcal
Ophthalmia Neonatorum for 1,000 Newborns*

	Ocular prophylaxis		No ocular prophylaxis
	Silver nitrate	Tetracycline	
Cost per dose (US$)	$0.10 (single-dose vial)	$0.05 (multidose tube)	0
Cost for 1,000 newborns (US$)	$100	$50	0
% of exposed newborns with gonococcal conjunctivitis	7	3	47
Cost of treatment with centriaxone 125 mg IM (US$)	$21	$9	$141
Total cost (US$)	$121	$59	$141
Cost per case adverted (US$)	$4.3	$2.1	$5
% of cases with visual impairment	0.2–0.8	0.4–0.4	1.4–5.6

* Assumes 6 percent prevalence of maternal gonococcal infection.
Source: reference 42.

Behavioral and Societal Interventions

Both short-term and long-term behavioral interventions are available for the prevention of RTIs. They are reviewed elsewhere in this book. Analysis of their cost-effectiveness is hampered in the first place by lack of (hard-to-obtain) controlled data on their effectiveness and by scarce information on their costs.

Whereas condom use is at least partly effective in preventing acquisition of genital infections,[46] the effectiveness of other behavioral interventions aimed at reducing exposure to STDs in the developing world is less certain. The most promising results in the developing world appear to come from condom promotion activities, particularly by peer educators, among female commercial sex workers (CSWs) (e.g., in Kenya, Cameroun, and Ghana).[47,48] In the same World Bank exercise mentioned before, use of condoms to prevent HIV transmission ranked among the 10 most cost-effective interventions to improve adult health.[32] Social marketing of condoms, not free distribution, has been an impressively successful approach.[49] A financial and outcome evaluation of such programs should be feasible and should provide valuable information to estimate their cost-effectiveness. Such evaluations should cover the impact not only on HIV infection but also on the prevention of all RTIs.

G. Merritt and colleagues[50] estimated that the cost per couple of providing condoms in urban Africa greatly exceeds current government per capita health expenditures. It is clear that without added financial means, such as subsidies for condoms and their distribution, large-scale condom use by those at risk may not be feasible. Supply is also a problem, for both imported and locally produced condoms.

Family planning programs are a cornerstone in the control of RTIs, mainly by reducing the health risks of multiple closely spaced pregnancies and of complications of clandestine abortions (and sometimes by providing condoms and safe abortions). An estimated 20–40 percent of maternal deaths could be averted by avoiding unwanted pregnancies.[9] Another 25–50 percent could be prevented through safe abortion. The case of Romania illustrates the disastrous, but reversible, impact on maternal mortality in a developing country of criminalizing abortion.[51] In addition, improving skills of health care providers dealing with women's reproductive health may decrease the problem of postpartum, postabortion, and post-IUD insertion complications.

The relative costs, effectiveness, and benefits of STD control, family planning, and MCH to control RTIs remain to be explored. Questions that should be addressed include the following: How can the value of increased investment in STD control be compared with the value of ongoing investment in family planning and MCH? Is it likely that STD interventions are at least as significant and reasonable in cost as family planning and MCH initiatives? Are there synergies among the three that would increase their values? What are the dilemmas in trying to get these fields together?

The long-term impact of interventions for RTI prevention such as sex education in schools and increasing educational and job opportunities for women is unproven, but is likely, as such interventions have been associated with considerable improvement of other health indicators, such as under-five mortality.[5,9] Their implementation should be a priority in all countries, regardless of their impact on RTIs.

Targeting

Targeting of interventions for STD control is based on two major assumptions: first, that a relatively small proportion of the population is contributing to the maintenance of an endemic state of the infection (high-frequency transmitters or core groups); second, that the cost-effectiveness of an intervention increases if it focuses on groups with high rates of infection or reinfection, and such interventions may have an amplifying effect.[52] Thus, S. Moses and coworkers[53] estimated in 1990 that one female CSW with HIV infection in Nairobi was the source of 12 cases of HIV infection in the general population. If men utilizing commercial sex services used condoms in half of their sexual encounters with CSWs, over 5,000 cases of HIV infection per 1,000 CSWs per year would be prevented in the general population of Nairobi.

The impact of a targeted intervention is even more spectacular for STDs with a higher risk of transmission, such as gonorrhea. Figure 3 shows the dynamic effect of averting 100 cases of gonorrhea in a hypothetical core group, as compared with the effect of averting 100 cases in the noncore group only, following a onetime intervention. In this example, a policy of targeting a onetime intervention at a core population averts more than eight times as many case-years as a policy directed at the noncore population would have averted.

In Kenya, it was estimated that a condom promotion program among a population of CSWs resulted in a savings of US$350 per CSW on direct costs of gonococcal infection, disregarding savings on other STDs, such as HIV, chlamydial infection, syphilis, and chancroid.[39] However, in this calculation, capital costs and costs of information, education, and communication programs were not included. A similar cost-benefit would be obtained for targeted interventions in other core groups, such as the military, long-distance truck drivers, and of course, clients of CSWs. In addition, interventions targeted at partners of men and women belonging to such groups are probably indicated.

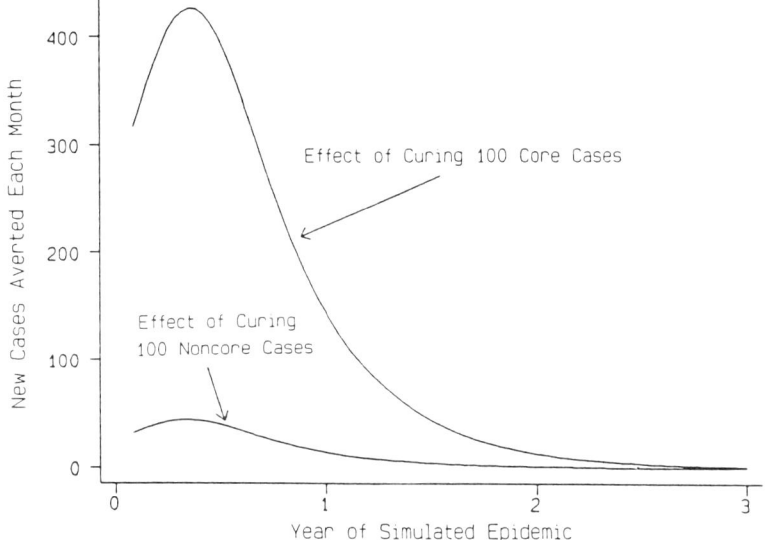

Source: reference 5.

Figure 3. Dynamic Benefit of Curing or Preventing 100 Cases of Gonorrhea in the Core and Noncore

Targeted interventions may be difficult to implement (e.g., how to reach high-frequency transmitters) and have undesirable side effects, particularly social stigmatization, that need to be addressed. These drawbacks should be considered in depth when planning is under way for interventions. Cost-effectiveness and cost-benefit are only two elements in selecting interventions. However, we suspect that interventions such as mass media campaigns aimed at the general public, as advocated and performed by many governments and international agencies, are not a cost-effective approach.

RESOURCES NEEDED TO IMPROVE INTERVENTIONS

The problem of RTIs seems overwhelming. Data on the costs of RTIs and on the cost-effectiveness of interventions are scarce, and information on current resources for RTI prevention and control is very limited. Below, we will discuss the types of resources that are required for RTI control, and urge that resources currently available be systematically mapped.

Institutional Resources Needed at the National Level

At the national level, the success of RTI control will depend mainly on political commitment; a well-functioning and effective primary health care system; the availability of a control and prevention strategy; a multisectoral approach, involving the health, education, and social departments; funds; and the availability of human and physical resources. There may be no need to create yet another national program, but depending on the size of the country, it seems essential that at least one high-level professional with expertise in RTI control and prevention serve as a liaison officer and technical advisor to programs that should incorporate RTI control in their activities—namely, primary health care services, MCH services, family planning services, AIDS/STD control programs, and ministries of education.

As a rule, a shift in the allocation of resources from higher level (reference) services to basic health services should promote a more efficient and equitable approach to RTI control in women. In addition, the emphasis on first-level referral possibilities for the management of obstetric problems should be complemented by improved means for diagnosis and treatment of genital infections in women at the primary health care level.

Finally, there is disappointingly little use made of the *complementarity* among existing programs, where the effectiveness of one program is enhanced by the implementation of another. The schism between AIDS and STD control programs in many countries is only one example but is being increasingly resolved.[54] For example, incorporating ophthalmia neonatorum and congenital syphilis control into MCH programs, and prevention of upper genital tract infections into family planning programs, is immediately feasible, without major new financial resources. A recent trial in Colombia demonstrated that AIDS prevention can be incorporated into a family planning program without harming the latter's functioning.[55]

Training

There is obviously a tremendous need for training health care providers and educators about RTIs. However, such training should not only aim at educating about the problems of RTIs, but emphasize the early diagnosis of RTIs and interventions designed to prevent the spread of RTIs. This implies that training modules be based on well-designed and cost-effective intervention models.

Priority should be given to training programs on management of ophthalmia neonatorum; prevention of congenital syphilis; prevention of puerperal and postabortion infection; prevention of infection following IUD insertion; management of genital ulcer disease; condom promotion among high-frequency transmitters and other individuals; and counseling, diagnosing, and treating women for STDs in primary health care, family planning, and MCH services. Modules for training and other educational materials (such as wall charts) should be developed to facilitate the programs.

Research

Data are urgently required on the prevalence of RTIs in women; the incidence of complications and sequelae in women and in children born to infected women; the medical costs associated with RTIs and their complications and sequelae; the implications of RTIs for morbidity and debility rates; and the broader economic and social consequences associated with a woman becoming ill, infertile, or dying.[56] Priority areas for support also include the following:

1. Development and evaluation of prevention technologies controlled by women, such as virucides and female barrier methods
2. Development of simplified approaches to case management
3. Development of simple and inexpensive tests for STDs in women
4. Evaluation of various interventions to control RTIs
5. Assessment of sexuality and gender power relations and the means to alter them

Resources for research on RTIs in the developing world are very limited, and not proportional to the impact of RTIs on the health of women and infants. Therefore, there is a case for a special fund managed by the above-mentioned RTI initiative or the World Health Organization to support such research.

Financial Resources

Where will the money come from to realize RTI control? How much money is needed to implement all these programs? It is clear that additional resources for the health sector and shifting resources from other sectors (especially the military) to health and social services will be necessary. However, instead of waiting for the unlikely financial resources, every effort should be made to adapt interventions to existing fiscal and other constraints and to optimize available resources. Finally, donors and governments will only be willing to contribute if they are convinced that proposed RTI programs will work and be effective.

CONCLUSIONS AND RECOMMENDATIONS

If RTI control and prevention have not been public health priorities until now, there must be reasons. As mentioned at the beginning of this paper, several of these reasons have to do with the status of women and with society's attitudes toward sexuality and reproductive health. However, it is our firm belief that the lack of a clear strategy, of well-founded priorities, and of effective and feasible interventions (in addition to the few established ones) has been at least as important a handicap as societal prejudices and political inertia.

As a research and public health community, we should stop limiting ourselves to carefully observing and elegantly analyzing the daily disasters of RTI-associated morbidity and mortality. Instead, we should resolutely take up the challenge to develop and evaluate interventions to identify, treat, and control RTIs—even if the scientific methodology to do this is often uncertain, and this kind of research is logistically and methodologically difficult. Until we do this, it will be difficult to estimate the resources that are needed and to raise the necessary funds.

The following priorities are proposed in order to better estimate the resources needed for RTI control and prevention in the Third World and to make the resources available:

1.   Development of strategies and priorities for RTI control, as well as a plan of action, by an ad hoc group drawn from donors, women's health advocates, and RTI and health system specialists, supported by a limited number of professional staff

2.   Sensitizing of policymakers in governments, donor agencies, and RTI-related programs to the problem of RTIs, presenting it as both a health and a development issue

3.   Immediate incorporation of selected interventions for RTI control into primary health care, family planning, MCH, safe motherhood, and AIDS control programs

4.   Development and evaluation of biomedical, behavioral, and societal interventions for RTI control and treatment in the developing world, as well as assessment of their cost-effectiveness

5.   Support of intervention-oriented research (as under the third recommendation) and the development of female preventive technology

REFERENCES

1. Wasserheit JN. The significance and scope of reproductive tract infections among Third World women. Int J Gynecol Obstet 1989; Suppl 3:145–68.

2. Wasserheit JN. Reproductive tract infections in Special challenges in Third World women's health. 117th Annual Meeting, American Public Health Association, October 1989, International Women's Health Coalition, New York, 1990.

3. Goeman J, Meheus A, Piot P. L' épidémiologie des maladies sexuellement transmissibles dans les pays en développement a l'ère du SIDA. Ann Soc Belge Méd Trop 1991; 71:81–113.

4. Brunham RC, Ronald AR. Comparative epidemiology of sexually transmitted diseases in industrialized and developing countries. In: Wasserheit JN, Aral SO, Holmes KK et al., eds. Research issues in human behavior and sexually transmitted diseases in the AIDS era, Washington, DC: American Society for Microbiology, 1991; 61–80.

5. Over M, Piot P. HIV infection and sexually transmitted diseases. In: Jamison DT, Mosley WH, eds. Disease control priorities in developing countries, New York: Oxford University Press for the World Bank, 1991.

6. Population Information Program. Complications of abortion in developing countries. Popul Rep 1980; 7:105–55.

7. Feacham RG, Jamison DT, eds. Disease and mortality in Sub-Saharan Africa, Oxford: Oxford University Press for the World Bank, 1991.

8. Nabarro D, McConnell C. The impact of AIDS on socioeconomic development. AIDS 1989; 3(Suppl 1):S265–72.

9. World Bank. World development report 1990, New York: 1990.

10. Washington AE, Arno PS, Brooks MA. The economic cost of pelvic inflammatory disease. JAMA 1986; 255:1732–5.

11. Piot P, Laga M. Current approaches to STD control in developing countries. In: Wasserheit JN, Aral SO, Holmes KK et al., eds. Research issues in human behavior and sexually transmitted diseases in the AIDS era, Washington, DC: American Society for Microbiology, 1991.

12. Piot P, Hira SK. Control and prevention of sexually transmitted diseases. In: Lamptey P, Piot P, eds. The handbook of AIDS prevention in Africa, Durham, NC: Family Health International, 1990.

13. Meheus A, Schulz KF, Cates W Jr. Development of prevention and control programs for sexually transmitted diseases in developing countries. In: Holmes KK, Mårdh P-A, Sparling PF et al., eds. Sexually transmitted diseases, second edition, New York: McGraw-Hill, 1990.

14. Fransen L, Van Dam CJ, Piot P. Health policies for controlling AIDS and STDs in developing countries. Health Policy Plann 1991; 6:148–56.

15. Rosenfield A. Maternal mortality in developing countries: an ongoing but neglected "epidemic." JAMA 1989; 262:376–9.

16. Foster SD. Improving the supply and use of essential drugs in Sub-Saharan Africa. Policy, Research, and External Affairs Working Paper 456, Washington, DC: World Bank, 1990.

17. Meheus A, Piot P. Provision of services for sexually transmitted disease in developing countries. In: Oriel JD, Harris JRW, eds. Recent advances in sexually transmitted diseases. Edinburgh: Churchill Livingstone, 1986.

18. Oronsaye AU, Odiase GI. Incidence of ectopic pregnancy in Benin City, Nigeria. Trop Doct 1981; 11:160–3.

19. Figà-Talamanca I, Sinnathuray TA, Yusof K et al. Illegal abortion: an attempt to assess its cost to the health services and its incidence in the community. Int J Health Serv 1986; 16:375–89.

20. Bongwele O, Nichols D, Miatudila M, Whatley A, Burton N, Janowitz B. Determinants and consequences of pregnancy wastage in Zaire, Research Triangle Park, NC: Family Health International, 1986.

21. Fortney JA. The use of hospital resources to treat incomplete abortions: examples from Latin America. Public Health Rep 1981; 96:574–9.

22. World Health Organization. Abortion. A tabulation of available data on the frequency and mortality of unsafe abortion, Geneva: World Health Organization, 1990.

23. Germain A. The Christopher Tietze International Symposium: an overview. Int J Gynecol Obstet 1989; Suppl 3:1–8.

24. Germain A, Ordway J. Women's health in the third world: balancing the scales. New York: International Women's Health Coalition, 1989.

25. Schulz KF, Cates W Jr, O'Mara PR. Pregnancy loss, infant death, and suffering: legacy of syphilis and gonorrhoea in Africa. Genitourin Med 1987; 63:320–5.

26. Evans T. The impact of permanent disability on rural households: river blindness in Guinea. IDS Bull 1989; 20:41–8.

27. Barnett T, Blaikie P. Community coping mechanisms in the face of exceptional demographic change. Report to the Overseas Development Administration.

28. Pryer J. When breadwinners fall ill: preliminary findings from a case study in Bangladesh. IDS Bull 1989; 20:49–57.

29. UNICEF. The state of the world's children 1989. Oxford: Oxford University Press, 1989.

30. Bertozzi SM. Economic research: its role in the fight against AIDS in Africa. AIDS 1991; 5(Suppl 1):845–54.

31. World Health Organization. Management of patients with sexually transmitted diseases, WHO Technical Reports, Series 810, Geneva: World Health Organization, 1991.

32. Jamison DT, Mosley WH. Selecting disease control priorities in developing countries. In: Jamison DT, Mosley WH, eds. Disease control priorities in developing countries, Washington, DC: World Bank, 1991 (in press).

33. Nettleman MD, Jones RB, Roberts SD et al. Cost-effectiveness of culturing for Chlamydia trachomatis. A study in a clinic for sexually transmitted diseases. Ann Intern Med 1986; 105:189–96.

34. Trachtenberg AI, Washington AE, Halldorson S. A cost-based decision analysis for chlamydia screening in California family planning clinics. Obstet Gynecol 1988; 71:101–8.

35. Phillips RS, Aronson MD, Taylor WC, Safran C. Should tests for Chlamydia trachomatis cervical infection be done during routine gynecologic visits? Ann Intern Med 1987; 107:188–94.

36. Handsfield HH, Jasman LL, Roberts PL, Hanson VW, Kothenbeutel RL, Stamm WE. Criteria for selective screening for Chlamydia trachomatis infection in women attending family plannning clinics. JAMA 1986; 255:1730–4.

37. Stray-Pedersen B. Economic evaluation of maternal screening to prevent congenital syphilis. Sex Transm Dis 183; 4:167–72.

38. Hira SK, Bhat GJ, Chikamata DM et al. Syphilis intervention in pregnancy: Zambian demonstration project. Genitourin Med 1990; 66:159–64.

39. National STD Control Programme. Two year plan for 1990–1991, Nairobi: Ministry of Health, 1990.

40. Sehgal A, Singh V, Bhamblani S, Luthra UK. Screening for cervical cancer by direct inspection. Lancet 1991; Vol. 1:282.

41. Laga M, Plummer FA, Piot P et al. Prophylaxis of gonococcal and chlamydial ophthalmia neonatorum: silver nitrate versus tetracycline. N Engl J Med 1988; 318:653–7.

42. Laga M, Meheus A, Piot P. Epidemiology and control of gonococcal ophthalmia neonatorum. Bull WHO 1989; 67:471–8.

43. Fransen L, Nsanze H, Klaus V et al. Ophthalmia neonatorum in Nairobi, Kenya: the roles of Neisseria gonorrhoeae and Chlamydia trachomatis. J Infect Dis 1986; 153:862–9.

44. Brewer C. Prevention of infection after abortion with a supervised single dose of oral doxycycline. Br Med J 1980; 281:780–1.

45. Grimes DA, Schulz KF, Cates W. Prophylactic antibiotics for curettage abortion. Am J Obstet Gynecol 1984; 150:689–99.

46. Sinei SKA, Schulz KF, Lamptey PR et al. Preventing IUD-related pelvic infection: the efficacy of prophylactic doxycycline at insertion. Br J Obstet Gynecol 1990; 97:412–9.

47. Lamptey P, Goodridge GAW. Condom issues in AIDS prevention in Africa. AIDS 1991; 5(Suppl 1) (in press).
48. Ngugi EN, Plummer F. Health outreach and control of HIV infection in Kenya. J AIDS 1988; 1:566–70.
49. Lamptey P, Potts M. Targeting of prevention programs in Africa. In: Lamptey P, Piot P, eds. The handbook of AIDS prevention in Africa, Durham, NC: Family Health International, 1990.
50. Merritt G, W Lyerly, J Thomas. The HIV/AIDS pandemic in Africa: issues of donor strategy. In: Miller N, Rockwell RC, eds. AIDS in Africa: the social and policy impact, Lewistown, NY: Edwin Mellen Press, 1988; 115–29.
51. Romania: on the road to success. Safe Motherhood 1990; no. 3:1–2.
52. Hethcote HW, Yorke JA. Gonorrhea transmission dynamics and control, Berlin: Springer Verlag, 1984.
53. Moses S, Plummer FA, Waiyaki P et al. Cost-effectiveness of an STD/AIDS control programme for high frequency transmitters in Nairobi, Kenya. Fifth International Conference on AIDS in Africa, Abstract T.RT.F.5, Kinshasa, 1990.
54. World Health Organization. Consensus statement from the consultation on global strategies for coordination of AIDS and STD control programmes. Geneva, 11–13 July 1990.
55. Vernon R, Ojeda G, Murad R. Incorporating AIDS prevention activities into a family planning organization in Colombia. Stud Fam Plann 1990; 21:335–43.
56. World Health Organization. Sexually transmitted diseases research needs, Geneva: World Health Organization, 1989.

PART IV
COUNTRY CASES

REPRODUCTIVE TRACT INFECTIONS IN BRAZIL: SOLUTIONS IN A DIFFICULT ECONOMIC CLIMATE

Aníbal Faúndes, M.D.
The University of Campinas
The Population Council
Caixa Postal 6181
13081 Campinas
São Paulo, Brazil

Dr. Ana Cristina Tanaka
Professor, Faculty of Public Health
University of São Paulo
Av. Dr. Arnaldo, 715
01255 São Paulo, Brazil

BACKGROUND

Brazil, a federal republic of 26 states, is heterogeneous in agroclimatic conditions, local economies, urban/rural distribution, culture, and social services. The population of 150 million is 68 percent urban. It is also young; 36 percent are 15 years old or younger. Women of fertile age (15–49) constitute 26 percent of the population.[1]

According to the 1988 Brazilian Constitution,[2] the public health sector should be unified and decentralized, and the private sector should be free to participate in health care. Brazil has a complex health system, with a range of public and private institutions providing services. The smallest administrative unit is the municipality, which has the theoretical mandate to provide direct curative care. Many municipalities have networks of health centers and even hospitals. The state and federal governments also must provide health care. Thus, a municipality may have a multiplicity of services, which does not necessarily mean good care, in either quantity or quality. In addition, in the absence of proper legislation, each level makes its own policy decisions.

During the 1980s, following the international trend toward focusing on primary health care, the federal Ministry of Health established norms for Integrated Assistance to Women's Health (Programa de Assistência Integral à Saúde da Mulher, or PAISM), including antenatal care, delivery and postpartum care, gynecologic and clinical assistance, prevention of gynecologic cancer, and provision of family planning. However, it has not had the capacity to fully implement PAISM.

Reproductive Tract Infections, Edited by A. Germain *et al.*
Plenum Press, New York, 1992

THE SCOPE OF REPRODUCTIVE TRACT INFECTIONS IN BRAZIL

Prevalence and Incidence

Sources of Information. In Brazil, there is no national system for collecting health information. Up to 1986, only infectious diseases, such as poliomyelitis, measles, and smallpox, had to be reported to the federal Ministry of Health. Since then, it has also become compulsory to report AIDS and congenital syphilis. An informal agreement between the federal government and the municipalities commits the latter to report registered deaths, including cause of death, age, sex, place of death, and residence; about 80 percent of the municipalities are reporting. With the exception of local death records, there is no source of reliable information that could provide an estimation of the prevalence or incidence of reproductive tract infections (RTIs). A few isolated studies allow a partial view of the situation in the country.

Sexually Transmitted Diseases (STDs), excluding AIDS. An extensive review of the national literature on STDs over the last 10 years reveals that 50 percent of reports discuss results of treatment or the use of new drugs, 15 percent describe new diagnostic and laboratory procedures or are theoretical texts, and 35 percent address the epidemiology of infection.

Most of these epidemiological studies refer to STDs, and only exceptionally to other RTIs. Most studies are based on information from clients attending specific clinics or from surveys of specific populations and simply describe the percentage distribution of all STDs diagnosed by disease. (Annex 1 is a summary of local studies.)

Table 1 shows the prevalence of four STDs in two dermatology clinics in university hospitals, in the cities of São Paulo and Fortaleza (State of Ceará). The São Paulo data show the percentage of all diagnosed STDs represented by each disease. The Fortaleza information is the number of diagnosed cases as a percentage of total number of individuals consulting the clinic. Data from São Paulo suggest a time trend in the percentage distribution of the STDs, with an increased proportion of condyloma, a decrease in gonorrhea, and stable levels of syphilis and nongonococcal urethritis. The data may indicate a tendency toward a dominance of viral infections among STDs.

Table 2 shows the incidence of selected STDs in the population of the Federal District, estimated as the number of cases diagnosed in health care services per 1,000 population. The sudden increase from 1981 to 1982 in the incidence of these three STDs may be related to better diagnosis and underscores the questionable reliability of the data. Several studies have shown that a large number of patients consult only a pharmacy, and they will never appear in the health statistics.[22,23]

AIDS. Compulsory reporting of the disease since 1986 makes data on AIDS better than data on other STDs. All the information is tabulated and analyzed by the Ministry of Health, and published periodically in the *Epidemiological Bulletin on AIDS*. In addition, during the last few years, narrower local studies have been presented at national and regional meetings on AIDS. Brazil is epidemiologically characterized as pattern I/II, indicating the transitional stage of the epidemic where more and more women begin to be affected.[24] Although the country has a relatively large number of reported AIDS cases, the first female with the disease was detected only in 1983; since 1985–86, a larger number of

Table 1. Prevalence of STDs among Patients Attending
Dermatology Clinics in São Paulo (SP)* and Fortaleza (For),† 1982–89

Year	Syphilis SP	Syphilis For	Gonorrhea SP	Gonorrhea For	Condylomata SP	Condylomata For	Urethritis SP	Urethritis For
1982	26.9	1.0	45.6	0.2	4.1	0.6	7.8	–
1983	23.0	2.0	37.5	0.2	8.0	0.7	19.6	0.3
1984	24.1	2.2	33.4	0.2	3.4	0.6	24.5	–
1985	24.5	1.6	28.9	0.3	7.6	0.5	20.7	0.2
1986	18.4	1.5	23.9	0.2	7.1	0.6	31.0	–
1987	21.6	–	10.5	–	7.5	–	26.5	–
1988	21.7	–	9.1	–	7.9	–	25.2	–
1989	18.7	–	9.3	–	11.5	–	21.3	–

* Percentage of all positive diagnoses of STD.
† Percentage of all persons assisted at the clinic.
Source: references 10, 19, and 21.

Table 2. Incidence of STDs in the Population of the Federal District,
1976–84 (per 1,000 Inhabitants)

STD	1976	1977	1978	1979	1980	1981	1982	1983	1984
Syphilis	0.35	0.19	0.40	0.34	0.50	0.55	2.36	1.26	2.1
Gonorrhea	0.08	0.09	0.12	0.28	0.79	0.55	3.12	2.60	5.9
Nongonococcal urethritis	–	–	–	–	0.00	0.38	0.88	1.36	1.8

Source: reference 10.

women have appeared in the statistics. The male-to-female ratio decreased from 35:1 in 1981–85 to 20:1 in 1986, and 11:1 in 1987. By March 1990, the reported male-to-female ratio for AIDS was 9:1 (11,070 men vs. 1,086 women).[25] Among women, 39 percent of cases are related to drug use, and 34 percent to heterosexual transmission. There is no information on nonsymptomatic human immunodeficiency virus (HIV) infection among women, though it is expected to be 50–100 times higher than confirmed AIDS cases.

Prevalence studies of HIV infection are limited: prevalence was 0.2 percent among blood donors in five hospitals in Goiania,[26] and 5 percent among patients who had received frequent hemodialysis in a hospital in São Paulo.[27] The prevalence was 11 percent among 148 prostitutes in Campinas, but rose to 53 percent for drug users and dropped to 6 percent among those who claimed not to use drugs.[28]

The Nucleus of Epidemiological Surveillance for AIDS, at the State University of Campinas, has tested a relatively large number of women for HIV: these women either use intravenous drugs, have multiple sexual partners, or have a male partner who is bisexual or a drug user. One in four HIV-positive women had some manifestation of the disease. Nevertheless, these results cannot be extrapolated to the universe of Brazilian women.

The prevalence among women receiving antenatal care in a clinic within the prostitution area in the city of Santos was 6 percent overall, and 24 percent among those who had two risk factors for AIDS.[29] In Ribeirão Preto, a city with a population of 200,000, about 300 miles northeast of São Paulo, nine of 1,006 pregnant women were HIV-positive; in five of these women, it was possible to identify risk factors.[30] In Campinas, among 132 women tested at the antenatal clinic who had risk factors for AIDS, 8 percent were positive.[31] Assuming no other women seen at that clinic during the same period were positive, the minimal prevalence would have been 0.5 percent.

Because the incidence of AIDS varies greatly from one region to another, these prevalence data cannot be considered representative of the whole country. According to the *Epidemiological Bulletin on AIDS*, Santos has the highest incidence (119 cases per 100,000 population), followed by the city of São Paulo (74 per 100,000). The incidence of AIDS in other cities varies: 42 per 100,000 in Ribeirão Preto, 41 per 100,000 in Rio de Janeiro, 21 per 100,000 in Campinas, 13 per 100,000 in Curitiba, 17 per 100,000 in Salvador, 13 per 100,000 in Goiania, and eight per 100,000 in Brasília. The regional differences are better illustrated by the fact that 63 percent of all AIDS cases in Brazil are found in the State of São Paulo.[32] That state has the busiest port in the country (Santos), which was likely the point of entrance of the disease into the country.

Puerperal Infections. Undoubtedly, postabortion and postpartum infections are important components of RTIs among Brazilian women. Unfortunately, though mass media often publish sensationalized information about abortion and on the importance given by women's organizations to this issue, few data exist on abortion and its complications.

Table 3. Number of AIDS Cases and Rate per 1,000,000 Population,
by Year of Diagnosis, 1985–1989

Measure	1985	1986	1987	1988	1989	Total
Number	473	928	2,077	3,314	3,706	11,070
Rate	3.6	6.8	14.9	23.3	25.6	–

Source: reference 25.

Similarly, the Brazilian medical literature has little information on postpartum infection except for references to the 10–24 percent of women who develop puerperal infections after cesarean section.[33,34] This information is relevant in a country with possibly a world-record cesarean section rate.[35]

Projections

It is practically impossible to make any projection, in view of the scarcity of historical series, the limited validity and reliability of the data, and the narrow scope of studies to date. The only data base with reasonable credibility refers to AIDS, which has shown a steady increase since the first case was identified in 1980. Table 3 shows a rapid increase in incidence up to 1988, but the number of new cases increased only moderately in 1989; apparently, the increase was also modest in 1990 (not shown). It is too early to say, but this may indicate a slowing in the spread of the disease.

Recommendations for Improving National Surveillance of RTIs

STDs. Most institutions presently providing health care for women collect some information on STDs, and on RTIs in general, and register them in routine clinical forms. Unfortunately, diagnosed cases are only a fraction of the total number of RTIs. Improvement in the local diagnostic capacity is thus a key element to achieve a minimal understanding of the dimension and evolution of RTIs in the country. In addition, a political decision is needed to institute an integrated system to record and transfer the collected data. To establish an appropriate national surveillance system, the federal government would have to enforce RTI reporting among all private and public health services. The practicality of such enforcement is doubtful, because it would be difficult to check the accuracy of the reporting, and doing so would mean overburdening a system with little capacity to respond to an increased demand. This being so, sentinel surveillance may be a better alternative for Brazil.

AIDS. A meeting on Mother-Child AIDS in the Americas, sponsored by the World Health Organization (WHO) and held in São Paulo in August 1990, recommended monitoring the epidemic by anonymous HIV testing among pregnant women, drug abusers, STD clinic and family planning clients, and adolescents in selected centers representing each region of the country.[36] Data from periodic seroprevalence studies would track the epidemic and be used to persuade the public to take preventive actions. As a follow-up, the Ministry of Health and the São Paulo State Health Secretariat are preparing collaborative, multicenter studies of HIV infection prevalence in specific groups.

Puerperal Infections. The possibility of national surveillance for postpartum and postabortion infection is remote, because in-hospital assistance is mostly private. In the short run, the only reasonable prospect is to collect data from samples of hospital patients in the various regions, in order to establish an incidence of septic complications after vaginal delivery, cesarean section, and abortion. Care should be taken to include several hospitals at each site, as there are large interhospital differences in the pregnancy outcome (normal delivery, cesarean, abortion) and in the incidence of infection.

BIOMEDICAL CONSEQUENCES OF RTIs FOR GIRLS AND WOMEN

Impact of Infection on Pregnancy Outcome and Child Survival

Available information is limited largely to congenital syphilis, puerperal infection, and, as of more recently, AIDS. In Recife, in the northeast, Silva[37] found 16 percent of serologic tests positive for syphilis in the postpartum period in 1978. Costa and colleagues[38] found a prevalence of 8 percent in 1987 and 6 percent in 1988 among pregnant women receiving antenatal care in the same city, but in a different hospital. Lower prevalence rates are described for Goiania, in the midwest (3 percent), by Viggiano and coworkers in 1983,[39] and for Ribeirão Preto, in the State of São Paulo (2 percent), by Duarte and colleagues in 1987.[40]

In 1986, Huggins[41] reported six cases of congenital syphilis observed at the University Hospital in Recife. The report illustrates the poor quality of antenatal care and the little attention given to STDs, as five of the six mothers of these infected babies had received prenatal care. Cases of congenital syphilis increased in the Federal District from 0.17 per 100,000 inhabitants in 1980 to 1.7 per 100,000 in 1984, a 10-fold increase in a period of five years.[10] Official death information for the country, which is much less reliable, shows death rates from congenital syphilis of 8–12 per 100,000 live births in the period 1979–85.[42]

With respect to AIDS, the national register shows a progressive increase in perinatal infections, which reached 2 percent of all AIDS cases in 1989.[25] The biological interaction between HIV infection and pregnancy is still unclear and is confounded by factors, such as drug use, that are associated with poor perinatal outcome, as well as with HIV infection. A social effect is, however, quite clear. HIV-infected women are isolated and discriminated against; many hospitals simply will not accept them. Some HIV-infected women are, however, able to obtain safe abortions, as the social environment is more favorable to this indication than to other reasons for medical abortion.[43]

Puerperal infection plays an important role in maternal morbidity, and its relevance has increased with the extensive practice of unnecessary cesarean section. Postpartum infection can affect 10–50 percent of all women delivering by cesarean section.[33,34] A large proportion of these infections are not diagnosed by the attending physician, as more than two thirds of infected women show their first symptoms after discharge from the hospital.[33] In a country where cesarean sections represent as many as 50 percent or more of all deliveries,[35] excessive cesarean section is possibly a major factor in RTIs and all their consequences, including maternal mortality.

Maternal mortality in Brazil is high in relation to the economic development of the country. Though the relevant statistics are rather poor,[44] maternal mortality is estimated at over 50 per 100,000 live births in the most developed regions and over 200 per 100,000 in the less-developed ones. Within this somber picture, infection plays a major role, causing one seventh to one half of all maternal deaths, as Table 4 shows.

Impact of RTIs on Contraceptive Use and Safety

According to the international literature, IUD use could be associated with pelvic inflammatory disease (PID), and oral contraceptives with chlamydial cervicitis, while reducing the risk of other PID. The effect of barrier methods is to reduce PID.[53] Not surprisingly, we found no national publications on the possible positive effect of the pill or

Table 4. Percentage of Maternal Deaths Caused by Infection,
as Reported in Several Brazilian Studies

Author	Years	Location	Percentage
Arkader[45]	1965–66	Rio Janeiro	14.2
Neme[46]	1957–70	São Paulo	25.7
Darze[47]	1959–71	Salvador, BA	34.1
Parente[48]	1957–77	Rib. Preto, SP	50.0
Costa[49]	1974–79	Recife, PE	20.6
Magalhães Netto[50]	1973–83	Salvador, BA	27.3
Andrade[51]	1977–86	Juiz Fora, MG	19.7
Cunha[52]	1980–88	Marilia, SP	20.3

barrier methods. This is probably because diaphragms are hardly available and condoms and pills are used largely outside the health system. The present campaign for condom use seems to have been effective, at least among the clients of the one community distribution program that keeps those statistics. If that program's information could be extrapolated to the country, condom use should have a positive effect on reducing the incidence of STDs.[54]

Several studies have looked at infection among IUD users in Brazil. Aleixo and coworkers[55] found a significantly higher prevalence of *Gardnerella vaginalis*-indicative cells and of *Trichomonas* among Pap smears taken from IUD users than among smears from women who used oral contraceptives. Silva and colleagues,[56] studying the causes for removal of IUDs, found that 21 of 440 women (5 percent) who had used the method for up to four years discontinued use because of infection. Ferrari and colleagues[57] found that 1 percent of IUD users had PID. As there is little information on time of exposure, characteristics of the population, and incidence of infection in a comparable population of nonusers, it is difficult to interpret such studies. An evaluation of the clinical performance of the IUD, coordinated by the University of Campinas, showed a very low rate of infection.[58] The authors suggest that the risk could be low if the patient selection and insertion are done correctly.

Impact of Infection on Other Aspects of Women's Health

Cervical Cancer. Cervical cancer is the second leading cause of death by neoplasm among women 15–49 years old in Brazil; in 1985, it represented 2 percent of all deaths among women in this age group.[10] In the least developed regions—such as the north, northeast and center-west—cervical cancer is the leading cause of female death by neoplasm.

An association between some strains of human papilloma virus (HPV) infection and cervical cancer is strongly suspected. One study has been done on the prevalence of infections by HPV 6/11 and 16/18 among women in three hospitals in Recife and São

Paulo. The prevalence of HPV 6/11 was 2 percent in São Paulo and 5 percent in Recife; for HPV 16/18, the figures were 2 percent and 6 percent, respectively.[59]

RTIs and Infertility. A Latin American WHO-sponsored five-center study included one center from Salvador, Brazil. The cumulated experience of these five centers showed that tuboperitoneal factors were present among 44 percent of couples consulting for infertility.[60] A study carried out at the infertility clinic at the State University of Campinas Hospital showed that tuboperitoneal factors were present in 37 percent of such couples.[61]

Other Health Problems. Virtually all Brazilian women experience some kind of RTI, and many spend a large part of their lives with some kind of genital infection. Even when the infection is not life-threatening and does not have serious medical consequences, it may still cause constant discomfort in the form of itching, swelling, irritation, and emotional stress. For many women, these problems are so frequent that they become part of their lives, an additional disadvantage to being a woman; furthermore, health service providers often do not pay any attention to them.

Women's Health Programs and RTIs

PAISM, the women's health program proposed by the government, could make significant contributions to the prevention and reduction of infections if it were implemented. Unfortunately, the present health system, with few exceptions, not only fails to protect women, but may even contribute to RTIs—for instance, through the failure to screen for infection in antenatal and family planning clinics; the high rates of cesarean section, exposing women to greater risk; and the virtual unavailability of safe abortions.

Abusive use of antibiotics by the general public also increases the risk of infection and its consequences. The pharmacy is often consulted before a health service.[62] Antibiotics of all kinds are sold over the counter with no real control, contributing to the development of bacterial resistance and difficulties in future treatment of infections.

Another important factor is poor delivery care. With the loss of the professional midwife, delivery has been left in the hands of inexperienced personnel or very busy obstetricians. There is an excessive use of vaginal examinations, early artificial rupture of membranes, and neglect of aseptic technique. All of these factors increase the rate of intrapartum, neonatal, and postpartum infections. Busy individual physicians, who do not work in teams, have tended to resort excessively to cesarean sections, which represent from 30 percent to over 50 percent of births across regions; some cities have cesarean section rates as high as 70 or 80 percent. The association of cesarean section with puerperal infection is well known in the international literature and is no different in Brazil.[33]

SOCIAL, CULTURAL, AND ECONOMIC CAUSES AND CONSEQUENCES OF RTIs

Patterns of Sexual Behavior and Other Culturally Based Factors

In Brazil, having multiple partners is a culturally accepted sexual behavior for men, but not for women. However, infections acquired outside the home will be transmitted from husband to wife, and to other sexual partners. A study of sexual behaviors that might increase the risk of acquiring STDs was carried out among university students in Campinas. It showed that while 4 percent of female students admitted to having multiple partners, 27 percent of males did so.[63]

The practice of anal sex also increases the risk of RTIs because it favors contamination with bacteria that are normally present in the rectum, but that become pathogens in the reproductive and urinary tract. The same study of university students found that 31 percent of males and 19 percent of females practiced anal sex before becoming aware of the high risk of contamination with HIV brought about by this practice. Nevertheless, as Table 5 shows, the percentages remained essentially the same—31 percent and 17 percent, respectively—after the students were made aware of this risk.

Women's Status and Risk of Acquiring RTIs

Social Status. Women's inferior social status in Brazil has a direct influence on their risk of infection. Generally, they cannot control when and how they have sex with their partners, much less with whom and how many other sexual contacts their partners have. A good example is the limited power of women—even those with higher education—to decide on the use of condoms. The study among university students asked about sexual behaviors before and after becoming aware of the risk of AIDS and the protective effect of the condom. Male university students had a threefold increase in the use of condoms, from 22 percent to 61 percent. In contrast, female students had a smaller increase, from 24 percent to 42 percent.[63] Data among women of lower economic status are not available, but our experience during the last 35 years shows that many women who accept condoms at family planning clinics do not succeed in getting their partners to use them.

Table 5. Percentage of Students Practicing Risk Behavior Before and After Obtaining Knowledge about AIDS

Risk behavior	Male		Female	
	Before	After	Before	After
Nonuse of condoms* (N)	77.8 (270)	39.3 (270)	76.1 (138)	58.0 (138)
Anal sex† (N)	30.5 (275)	30.9 (275)	19.3 (140)	17.1 (140)
Multiple partners (N)	27.3 (275)	16.4 (275)	4 3 (140)	2.1 (140)

* Cochran test (for related samples), significant for both sexes ($p < 0.0001$).
† Cochran test, significant only for males ($p < 0.0001$).
Source: reference 63.

Abortion is another area that reflects the inferior status of women in Brazilian society, and where again they are exposed to risk. A legal abortion is practically unattainable; women with unwanted pregnancies either accept their fate or seek illegal (and generally unsafe) abortions and suffer their consequences: infection or even death. Moreover, even in cases of rape and imminent danger of death, when abortion is legal, a clean and safe interruption of pregnancy is seldom obtained. The usual "machista" cliché that "you never know if the woman encouraged the rape" is used to deny or delay interruption of that pregnancy in health services, as well as on the judiciary level.

In addition, there are indications that women may not seek treatment for infection. They tend to give less attention to their own "minor" health problems than to the problems of their children and other family members. An evaluation of gynecologic disturbances among women consulting for nongynecologic symptoms at the University of Campinas Hospital showed that 10 percent of these women had trichomonas infections. Nevertheless, they did not consider the symptoms of the infection sufficiently bothersome to justify a visit to the doctor.[35]

Economic Status. The lower the social and economic status of women, the higher their exposure to RTIs and the risk of infection after abortion or delivery.

Even illegal abortion varies in levels of safety according to economic power. In Recife, a study of women who underwent induced abortion showed that two fifths of lower-income women in the sample used the dangerous procedure of introducing a sound or probe into the uterus, while only one tenth of middle-income women did so. All lower-income women had the abortion outside a hospital, and about half the middle-income women had theirs in a clinic or hospital. Higher-income women were not included in the study.[64]

A recent study of female students and employees at the State University of Campinas found complications after illegal abortion among 53 percent of women with no more than elementary education, 35 percent of those with some high school education, and 13 percent of women who had reached the university.[65]

Personal, Social, and Economic Consequences of RTIs for Women

RTIs may have social, psychological, and economic consequences as a result of the negative connotations of the diseases, the symptoms of acute or subchronic episodes, or the sequelae that women suffer during the rest of their lives.

Syphilis and, more recently, HIV infection are illnesses with very negative social connotations, which deeply affect the lives of individuals. These include the rejection of behaviors associated with infection and the unreasonable fear of contamination through social contact. Though no studies have been carried out, mass media frequently report communities' strong and boisterous attacks on AIDS patients' homes, families' rejection of infected individuals, and extraordinary efforts taken to hide the true nature of the disease, even in the terminally ill. As these illnesses affect both men and women, the excessive attention given to female prostitutes as contaminating agents seems to be the only gender-related discrimination.

Symptoms of acute episodes or subchronic manifestations of RTIs also affect women's lives and have psychological impact. Repeated episodes of vaginal discharge that has a foul odor or irritates the external genitalia interferes with normal sexual functions. Infected women are often rejected by their sexual partners or hear derogatory remarks, even if the disease was brought home by the male. This is the case with trichomonas or candida infections that usually have few medical consequences. It also happens with condyloma, because the external manifestation can be visually distasteful and can reach dimensions that directly interfere with intercourse.

In addition to encountering her partner's rejection, a woman may be affected by the suspicion that her partner transmitted an infection acquired by sexual contact with other women. Whether true or not, the suspicion will have a negative effect on family life and the woman's psychological well-being. Women with STDs are also at risk of other emotional disturbances. One study found that most patients had a negative emotional reaction after being informed that they had an STD, and sometimes adopted aggressive behavior.[66]

Psychologically and socially, a major consequence of RTIs is tubal infertility, especially among young, childless women. The capacity to conceive is still a condition strongly associated with a woman's worth in the eyes of her male partner. Though this feeling is more prevalent among the less-educated, there have been cases of highly educated professional men who abandoned their infertile wives to start a family with another woman able to bear children. The loss of the capacity to conceive has a great negative impact on self-esteem, and the lack of the husbands' economic support can be disastrous for women culturally prepared only to be housewives and have children.

INTERVENTIONS FOR PREVENTION AND CONTROL OF RTIs

Public Education Programs on STDs and RTIs

The Ministry of Health, in collaboration with some state Secretariats of Health, has developed educational materials on STDs, through joint efforts by the Maternal-Child Health (MCH) and STD/AIDS Divisions. Two booklets have been distributed through PAISM since 1985. One booklet, for clinical staff, is a technical document describing the various STDs, including PID. It provides health staff with basic orientation on procedures for the diagnosis and treatment of each disease, including AIDS. The second booklet is simpler, including a written description of the diseases and advice on what to do if someone suspects he or she has acquired an infection. The information on prevention is less extensive and relatively weak.

The Secretariat of Health, State of São Paulo, has produced and distributed a less-technical and easier-to-read booklet for the general public. This publication has less written information and more illustrations (drawings and photographs) pertaining to each of the diseases. This booklet seems to be much more appropriate to inform the general public. The federal and state governments also have used mass media for campaigns on how to prevent STDs and AIDS. However, these are only sporadic messages transmitted via TV and radio. A number of posters on AIDS and AIDS prevention have been widely distributed and are fixed in health posts, hospitals, post offices, bus and railway stations, and elsewhere.

We are not aware of any evaluation of the impact such educational efforts may have had on sexual behavior, practice of preventive measures, or incidence of STDs and AIDS. The coincidence between the presence of these messages and the slowing in the reporting of new cases of AIDS in the country cannot be considered a cause-and-effect relationship without a careful study of the two phenomena. It may reflect only a greater difficulty in confirming each case, and a consequent delay in reporting, as the number of new cases increases without a parallel reinforcement of staff at the state level.

Involvement of the public education system is still missing. Though there are frequent demands to introduce sex education into primary and secondary school education, there is no effective initiative. Only a few isolated activities are being carried out by some more progressive teachers. With very few exceptions, sex education is missing even at the medical school level.

Interventions for Managing RTIs

Screening and Prevention. There is no specific screening program for RTIs in the country. Cervical cancer prevention programs, based on Pap smears, have long been under way, but are still weak. They are supposed to be integrated with all other health activities addressed to women, including antenatal care, family planning, and consultations for specific illness, but they still function as isolated activities. An evaluation of PAISM in São Paulo State showed that Pap smears had been taken among only one fifth of the women receiving antenatal care during 1987.[67] This is especially significant because São Paulo is one of the states that gives greatest emphasis to cervical cancer prevention.

It is equally distressing that little if any attention is given to information on trichomonas, candida, papilloma virus, and gardnerella picked up by Pap smears. Health personnel have not been instructed on how to manage these cases. Even when a woman is treated, her sexual partner is usually ignored, allowing for rapid reinfection.

Inappropriate management of RTIs can be attributed to three groups of factors: low priority within PAISM, inadequate or no training in RTI management for health personnel, and the high cost of medication. To the best of our knowledge, neither the federal and state government health programs, private institutions, universities, nor hospitals have taken specific steps for the screening of STDs or prevention of infection during contraceptive use. Some state governments are trying to improve screening among clients for different contraceptive methods. The only official contraceptive initiative that is likely to have an influence on RTIs is the promotion of condoms.

Institutional Capacity for Laboratory Identification of RTIs. In-country technical capacity to use more complex techniques (chlamydia or anaerobic culture) are almost nonexistent. Furthermore, few personnel are skilled in simpler bacteriological diagnosis, and the capacity to carry out existing simpler techniques is not fully utilized. Many primary health care clinics have a microscope that is underused, sometimes because of the lack of skilled personnel, lack of initiative, or low priority.

RECOMMENDATIONS FOR PREVENTION AND CONTROL OF RTIs

Recommendations fall into the following categories: health education/motivation, access to services, and research priorities.

Health Education/Motivation

Policymakers and Health Authorities. Policymakers and health managers do not have a clear concept of all the social, economic, and even political consequences of RTIs, nor of the important implications these infections have for several of the more visible issues of maternal and child health. Consequently, efforts should be made to inform policymakers and health managers, to help them understand the relevance of RTIs, so as to obtain the political support that could increase the allocation of resources to this problem. Internationally, WHO and the International Federation of Gynecology and Obstetrics (FIGO), which have played a key role in raising awareness and funds, and in coordinating programs for women's health (human reproduction, perinatal and maternal mortality, and, more recently, AIDS), could also lead the movement to shift attention toward the effects of RTIs on women's health.

Health Providers. The poor attention given to RTIs in health care services is due in part to lack of training and equipment. Nevertheless, a lot depends on motivation. Health workers should understand that activities related to RTIs are critical to achieve better health for women and children, and are second to no other services in terms of their efficiency and relevance. In the same way as a lack of motivation can be an obstacle to any program, the presence of motivation can overcome weaknesses in the system and encourage health providers to become actively involved in demanding more resources for, and more attention to, RTIs.

General Public. Public education campaigns should be continued and expanded. They should improve information, influence behavior toward "safer sex," and stimulate a demand for services. The new awareness that AIDS poses a real threat to everyone offers the possibility of greater acceptance of sex education and new opportunities to permanently include it in the school system and in health professionals' training.

Women's Groups. Raising awareness among women's groups of the importance of RTIs to so many aspects of women's health merits specific attention. The feminist movement, which is particularly strong in Brazil, may play a very important role in prevention, diagnosis, and treatment of RTIs. It can make women aware of their disadvantages regarding RTIs and can put pressure on health authorities and health providers to respond with policies and services. Safe abortion, proper delivery care (avoiding unnecessary cesarean sections), and more concern about STDs should be part of feminist demands at all levels.

Internationally, the alliance of women's groups and WHO, FIGO, other professional organizations, and their national equivalents, will have a decisive influence on the attention RTIs receive in the future. A strong coordinated effort can make the difference between the present neglect and the high priority this problem deserves.

Access to Services

Diagnosis and Treatment. The basic recommendation is to include the prevention, diagnosis, and treatment of RTIs in PAISM and to coordinate and integrate these activities with the AIDS control program. Including RTIs in a package with cervical cancer and contraception would make PAISM more cost-effective. AIDS prevention is only starting in Brazil, and integrating STDs within the national program for AIDS control will be very important.

Improved detection of RTIs and attention to the findings will require changes in priorities within PAISM, improved standards for care, staff training, and qualified supervision. This is all within the health system's grasp, but implementation will depend on the political commitments of health authorities and on the strength of the social pressure groups that demand change. Simpler techniques for both laboratory and clinical diagnosis of RTIs should be developed and evaluated, along with methods to identify groups with a particularly high risk of these diseases.

In the meantime, procedures that are already available or that can easily be made accessible at the primary health level should be better applied. A vaginocervical smear for cytologic diagnosis can identify infections such as *Trichomonas vaginalis*, *Candida albicans*, and papilloma virus. The cost of installing a simple light microscope and of training a nurse to diagnose trichomonas and yeast in a fresh sample of vaginal discharge is minimal. With a little training, it is possible to identify bacterial vaginosis from vaginal mucus samples.

Diagnosis and treatment of RTIs would most appropriately and effectively begin at antenatal care and family planning services. Close to 70 percent of pregnant women receive antenatal care, and addressing RTIs may be one of the most effective interventions to improve pregnancy outcome. The cost-effectiveness of routine HIV testing during pregnancy in low-risk populations does not justify its practice. However, there should be efforts to identify risk factors that, if present, require serodiagnosis of infection. The same criteria should be applied to other STDs.

In terms of family planning, clinical screening of STDs should be included in the provision of all contraceptive methods. While costly laboratory screening for every subject is not feasible, an evaluation of the risk of infection and clinical observation for STDs should be undertaken for every woman who requests a contraceptive method. At this time, when there is general agreement that modern IUDs should be more widely known and used in Brazil to reduce the improper use of other methods (pill, tubal ligation), special care should be taken to assure careful clinical screening before each IUD insertion.

In general, the efforts to screen for STDs should be initiated with priority among sexually active adolescents and young adults, who have a higher risk of STDs and among whom the consequences of RTIs are most destructive.[68] This recommendation implies the need to train health providers and to increase the availability of simple diagnostic techniques and of low-cost treatments.

Safe Abortion. Provision of safe abortion would have an important role in reducing RTIs and their sequelae. The most immediate priority is to seek the means to make abortion effectively available in cases where the law permits it: when a pregnancy results from rape or seriously endangers the woman's health. A medium-term objective should be to change the law in order to expand the conditions under which abortion is legal. The laws in Brazil do not allow for eugenic abortion, though many physicians perform abortion in cases of rubeola in early gestation or of demonstrated severe genetic anomaly. In the case of HIV infection, for example, the mother should be informed that her baby has a 30–40 percent chance of being infected,[69,70,71] and should be given medical, social, and psychological support for her decision as to whether or not to carry out the pregnancy.

Appropriate Birth Care. The most important action to reduce RTIs in relation to birth is to reverse the trend of an ever-increasing cesarean section rate. This is not the place to give details on what can be done; let us say only that priorities include changes in social security rules, the introduction of new routines, the recovery of the profession of midwifery, and public education.

Condom Distribution. The use of condoms should be facilitated by their sale not only in pharmacies, but also in newspaper stands, supermarkets, vending machines, and all kinds of commercial outlets. The present price (approximately US$1.00 per condom) should be reduced by government subsidy, which can be fully justified, as condom distribution could be a very cost-effective mechanism for STD/AIDS prevention.

Research Priorities

Local Demonstration. The role of illegal abortion and cesarean sections in puerperal infections of variable severity, including infections leading to death, should be seriously studied. The effects of these aggressions on women's bodies should be objectively documented, and the extent of their consequences should be clarified with objective data obtained by scientifically sound studies.

Given the potential effect of contraceptives on RTIs, it is important to know the incidence of infections among contraceptive users, and to develop practical and cost-effective means to diagnose STDs among these women. Studies of risk factors for STDs within this population could help identify those at high risk, for whom more expensive laboratory procedures would be justified.

Other topics that are emerging as priority research issues are the association between sexual behavior, RTIs, and tubal infertility; the prevalence of vaginosis; and the possible association between vaginal infections and premature rupture of membranes.

Program Evaluation. There is an urgent need to evaluate alternative approaches to screening and treatment of RTIs wherever sexually active women and men are in contact with health services. The best examples are the evaluation of STD screening for women choosing the IUD and an assessment of the effect of screening on the incidence of infection during IUD use; evaluations of the effectiveness of treatment of clinical infections on pregnancy outcome, and of simple diagnostic techniques to detect them, are other good examples.

Another example is operations research to evaluate strategies to reduce unsafe abortion and its complications, and to lower the unacceptable cesarean section rate.

Social Research. Diagnosis and treatment of RTIs depends as much on availability of services as on women's requesting care. This interaction between women's demand and the existence and quality of service is probably at least as important as the technological advances in RTI screening and treatment. Social research can play an important role in identifying the obstacles to care seeking, such as office hours conflicting with women's work schedules, locations that are difficult to reach, attitude of health providers, and the range of services available. A specific example would be the study of the practical obstacles posed to women seeking legal abortion, and the strategies followed by those who have succeeded in obtaining it.

Behavioral Research. There are several issues that should be the subject of behavioral research: the underlying factors that lead women to accept the symptoms of some RTIs as "normal" and that influence their lack of demand for services; the factors influencing the adoption or not of protective behavior, such as condom use; and interventions addressed to change all of the above.

CONCLUSIONS

In the attention Brazil has given to RTIs during last 20–30 years, the country has followed the rest of the world. The advent of antibiotics created a false sense of assurance, and infections were viewed with complacency, as no longer being a problem. Following this trend, Brazil gave priority to other themes within women's health, such as gynecologic cancer, the new techniques for treatment of infertility (assisted fertilization, microsurgery), contraception, fetal and perinatal medicine, and, more recently, maternal mortality and AIDS.

Present knowledge about these subjects strongly suggests that neglecting infections was a big mistake: in preventing cervical cancer, the control of HPV infection may play a key role; in reducing infertility, avoiding RTIs could be more effective than all the new technology to reverse their effects; in contraception, the opportunity simultaneously to address protection against infection has been missed; in fetal and perinatal health, the treatment of vaginocervical infection may save more babies' lives, by preventing prematurity, than all the very expensive paraphernalia currently used; in reducing maternal mortality, the prevention of infection and its determinants during childbirth could be a major mechanism; in AIDS control, a stronger emphasis on preventing STDs could have been and may still be a key strategy to prevent the spread of HIV to women.

These six themes are legitimate priorities in women's health in which large intellectual and financial investments have already been made. The acceptance of RTIs as a new priority may be easier if presented not so much as a new theme, but as an issue that underlies all of the others, and one that may have a decisive contribution to make toward their solution.

REFERENCES

1. Anuário estatístico do Brasil. Rio de Janeiro: Fundação IBGE, 1988.
2. Constituição do Brasil, 1988. Rio de Janeiro: Bloch, Editores, 1988.
3. Farah CA, Matheus ED, Trabuls LB. Frequência de Haemophilus vaginales em vaginites e seu tratamento com Nimorazol. Folha Médica 1981; 83:441–2.
4. Magalhães M, Andrade M, Véras S. Uretrites não gonococicas masculinas associadas a Chlamydia, Ureaplasma e Trichomonas. Rev Microbiol, 1982; 13:156–60.
5. Passos M, Lopes PVC. Levantamento sorológico para sífilis no Instituto de Ginecologia da UFRJ. Bol Inform União 1983; 8:29.
6. Teramussi LA, Franchini M, Souza AI, Araújo NA. Inquérito epidemio-dermato-laboratorial em uma população de alto risco para DST. Bol Inform União 1983; 8:48.
7. Kruse W, Naud P, Barcellos S et al. A detecção de Chlamydia trachomatis em processos inflamatórios. Rev HCPA & Fac Med Univ Fed Rio Grande do Sul 1985; 5:117–9.

Annex 1. Summary of Brazilain Studies that Present Percentage of Sexually Transmitted Diseases in Selected Populations

Author	Year	Sample population	% diagnosed										
			Gonococcol	Syphilis	Chlamydia	Condyloma	NGU	Candida	Trichom.	Gardnerella/Haemopilus	Chancroid	Ureaplasma	Herpes genit.
Farah[3]	1981	Vaginitis	-	-	-	-	-	-	-	-	-	-	-
Magalhaes[4]	1982	Male-NGU	-	5.10	-	-	-	3.0	-	-	39.0	-	-
Passos[5]	1983	Gynecol.	-	5.18	-	-	-	-	-	-	-	-	-
Teramussi[6]	1983	Prisoners	-	15.5	-	-	-	-	-	-	-	-	-
Kruse[7]	1985	PID	-	-	22.0	-	-	-	-	-	-	-	-
Lira[8]	1985	Vagin./cyst.	-	-	0.5	-	-	9.7	4.4	-	19.2	-	0.1
Paciornik[9]	1985	Prostitute	13.0	77.0	-	6.0*-14.0†	20.0*	80.0*	-	23.0†	-	-	-
Bol.I.Ur.[10]	1985	Women	4.0	5.6	-	3.7	-	23.5	-	8.9	0.2	-	0.4
Bol.I.Ur.[10]	1985	Men and women	-	5.3	-	-	-	-	-	-	-	-	-
Souza[11]	1986	Acute salp.	4.1	-	-	-	-	-	-	-	-	-	-
Bedone[12]	1987	Prostitutes	20.0	19.0	-	6.0	-	-	-	-	5.0	-	-
Belda[13]	1987	Population	-	5.6	-	-	-	-	-	-	-	-	-
Maeda[14]	1987	Vagin./cyst.	-	-	0.3	-	-	-	-	-	-	-	-
Pizzol[15]	1987	Policemen	0.9	0.7	-	1.4	3.6	-	-	-	0.2	-	1.7
Tomioka[6]	1987	Gynecol.	18.2	-	18.2	-	-	-	-	-	-	27.3	-
Oliveira[17]	1988	Skin dis.	-	-	-	0.5	-	-	-	-	-	-	0.2
Belda[18]	1989	Cervicitis	-	-	10.0	-	-	-	-	-	-	-	-
Bol.I.Un.[19]	1989	STD	17.4	11.4	-	14.6	15.8	2.9	2.9	4	14.1	-	2.9
Bol.I.Un.[20]	1990	STD	12.1	9.6	-	5.1	68.0	-	-	-	0.9	-	3.0

* Sample of 102 prostitutes.
† Sample of 70 prostitutes.

8. Lira Neto, JB. Achados colpocitológicos em 1987 casos de vaginites. J Bras Ginec 1985; 95:529–35.
9. Paciornik M. Matrizes. Condições Sanitárias de uma concentração de Barrageiros na Foz de Areia. Bol Inform União 1985; 10:5–6.
10. Ministério da Saúde. Bol Inform União 1985; 10:11–12.
11. Souza AZ, Tomioka ES, Santos NC, et al. Bacterioscopia da secreção cervico-vaginal da salpingite aguda. J Bras Ginec 1986; 96:213–6.
12. Bedone DMB, Pastene L, Franzin MMO, Pinotti JA. Prostituição e saúde. J Bras Ginecol 1987; 97:201–6.
13. Belda W, Santos MFQ Jr, Siqueira LSG. Situação atual de algumas das doenças sexualmente transmissíveis no Brasil. Bol Inform União 1987; 12:3–4.
14. Maeda M, Cavaliere M, Shik LWS, Yamamoto LSU. Chlamydia trachomatis em esfregações cervicais e vaginais: importância do método de Papanicolau no rastreamento em grandes populações. Rev Inst Adolfo Lutz 1987; 47:45–50.
15. Pizzol JL. Estudo das doenças sexualmente transmissíveis em policiais militares no Espirito Santo. An Bras Dermatol 1987; 62:197–200.
16. Tomioka ES. Agentes sexualmente transmissíveis em ginecologia: incidência e importância. J Bras Ginec 1987; 97:183–7.
17. Oliveira Filho J, Nunes EA, Calado ER, Bossa FV, Almeida MCM, Guidoni VGR. Incidência das dermatoviroses no Centro de Saúde Escola da Faculdade de Medicina de Santo Amaro, SP. An Bras Dermatol 1988; 63:353–7.
18. Belda W, Siqueira LSG, Santos MFQ Jr, Muniz W, Siqueira MC, Muniz L. A imunofluorescência direta na pesquisa da Chlamydia trachomatis em cervicite crônica. Bol Inform União 1989; 14:2–3.
19. Ministério da Saúde. Notas Epidemiológicas. Bol Inform União 1989; 14:6.
20. Ministério da Saúde. Notas Epidemiológicas. Bol Inform União 1990; 19(57):5.
21. Vilar MLL, Santos MA, Maciel GMFL, Meireles TEF, Santiago LH, Cabral MEF. Levantamento epidemiológico das DST no Serviço de Dermatologia do Hospital Universitário Prof. Walter Cantílio da Universidade Federal do Ceará. An Bras Dermatol 1988; 63:359–365.
22. Gonçalves AC, Gonçalves NMS. As doenças de transmissão sexual como um problema de saúde pública no Brasil. Rev Hosp Clin Fac Med Univ São Paulo 1987; 42:185–9.
23. Pires MFC, Loureiro ECB, Lopes F et al. Avaliação sobre o atendimento das doenças sexualmente transmissíveis: inquérito realizado em farmácias do bairro de Pinheiros, Município de São Paulo. Bol Inform União 1988; 13:3–4.
24. Piot P, Laga M, Ryder R et al. The global epidemiology of AIDS infection: continuity, heterogeneity and change. J AIDS 1990; 3:403–12.
25. Ministério da Saúde. Notas Epidemiológicas. Bol Epidemiol AIDS 1991 (Março).
26. Andrade ALSS, Martelli CMT, Pinheiro ED, Santana CL, Borges FP, Zicker F. Rastreamento sorológico para doenças infecciosas em banco de sangue como indicador de morbidade populacional. Rev Saúde Publ 1989; 23:20–5.
27. Romão JE Jr, Daher EF, Machado MM, Sabbaga E. Prevalência de anticorpos anti-HIV em pacientes dialisados. Rev Hosp Clin Fac Med São Paulo 1989; 44:80–3.
28. Aoki FH, Lima JN, Pavan MHP, Pedro RJ. HIV infection among prostitutes and transvestites in Brazil. Presented at the Fifth International Conference on AIDS, Montreal, June 4–9, 1989.

29. Giraldes PR, Santos MC, Rivetti PS, Porto AG, Mendes NF. Pesquisa de anticorpos anti-HIV pelo teste Elisa na rotina pré-natal. Rev Bras Med 1989; 46:106–8.

30. Duarte G, Pinhata MMM, Pasti MJ, Takida E, Del Lama J. Problemas práticos na determinação da prevalência e assistência às parturientes com sorologia positiva para HIV. Presented at the Fifth International Conference on AIDS, Montreal, June 4–9, 1989.

31. Amaral E, Passini R Jr, Faúndes A, Milanez H. Infecção pelo HIV e obstetrícia; revisão e reflexão sobre as várias faces de um problema. Femina 1991; 19:104–114.

32. Ministério da Saúde. Bol Epidemiol AIDS 1991; Year III, No. 9, 1990.

33. Albuquerque RM. Antibiótico profilático na operação cesariana. Estudo em pacientes de baixo risco. Tese de Mestrado. 1989, Universidade Estadual de Campinas (UNICAMP).

34. Belfort P, Machado S, Goulart MG, Baptista AM, Guimarães ML. Antibioticoterapia profilática na operação cesariana: validade ou inanidade? J Bras Ginec 1981; 91:475–8.

35. Pinotti JA, Faúndes A, Hardy EE et al. Avaliação da assistência ginecológica no estado de São Paulo. Rev Ginec Obst 1990; 1:7–21.

36. PAHO, WHO, UNFPA. Relatório da Reunião Internacional sobre a AIDS Materno Infantil na Região das Américas. 31 de julho a 3 de agosto de 1990, São Paulo, Brazil.

37. Silva AS. Incidência de sífilis em puérperas, recém-nascidos prematuros e a termo: associação entre sífilis materna e prematuridade, risco de transmissão fetal. 39 f. Dissertação. Mestrado UFPE. Faculdade de Medicina, 1978.

38. Costa EL, Porto AMF, Silva Filho AJ, Santos LC, Pinto MB. Frequência de sífilis em recém-nascidos de gestantes luéticas tratadas com dois esquemas posológicos de penicilina-benzatina. Mimeograph. Instituto Materno-Infantil de Pernambuco (IMIP), 1989.

39. Viggiano MGC, Ximenes YR, Moraes VA et al. A sífilis no ciclo gravídicopuerperal. Rev Bras Ginec Obst 1983; 6:277–82.

40. Duarte G, Cunha SP, Yamada RT, Bailão A, Philbert PMP. Sífilis e gravidez. Ainda um problema. Rev Bras Ginec Obstet 1987; 3:75–8.

41. Huggins DW. Sifilis congênita. Pediat Med 1986; 21:275–80.

42. Ministério da Saúde. Divisão Nacional de Epidemiologia. Estatítica de mortalidade: Brasil, 1979–1985. Brasília, 1982–1988.

43. Pinotti JA, Faúndes A, Zeferino LC. The concept of integral assistance to women's health. Historical development. In: Pinotti JA, Faúndes A, eds. Women and their right to a health policy, Casterton Hall, UK: Parthenon Publishing Group, 1990: 11–20.

44. Siqueira AAF. Como melhorar a informação sobre a mortalidade materna. In: Faúndes A, Cecatti JG, eds. Morte Materna: Uma tragédia evitável, Campinas: Editora UNICAMP, 1991 (in press).

45. Arkader J. Considerações sobre a mortalidade materna no Brasil. Tese Faculdade de Medicina. UFRJ, 1969.

46. Neme B. Mortalidade Materna: Relatório oficial XIX Jornada Brasileira de Obstetrícia e Ginecologia, Rio de Janeiro, 1971.

47. Darzé E, Magalhães Netto JM. Mortalidade materna na maternidade tsylla balbino: Revisão de 13 anos (1959–1971). Matern Inf, 1974; 33:101–6.
48. Parente JV, Martinez AR, Franco JG Jr, Costa OLN, Lima MJM, Meirelles RS. Mortalidade materna no hospital das clínicas da faculdade de medicina de Ribeirão Preto (USP) no período de 1957–1977. Parte II: causas. J Bras Ginec 1979; 88:105–8.
49. Costa CFF, Maia VO, Lomachinsky G. Mortalidade materna na maternidade Prof. Monteiro de Moraes, de 1974 a 1979. Parte II: fatores causais. J Bras Ginec 1981; 91:339–41.
50. Magalhães Netto JM. Mortalidade materna. Femina, 1985; 13:490–8.
51. Andrade ATL, Andrade DN, Faza MC, Cotta MCM, Clarck LH, Araujo DA. Mortalidade materna: estudo de 60 anos. Rev Bras Ginec Obstet 1988; 10(9):205–10.
52. Cunha DC, Salgado Neto J, Halbe HW, Ottoboni WR, Gotardo D. Comitês de Morte Materna. In: Faúndes A, Cecatti, eds. Morte materna: uma tragédia evitável, Campinas: Editora UNICAMP, 1991 (in press).
53. Grimes DA, Cates W, Jr. Family planning and sexually transmitted diseases. In: Holmes KK, Mårdh P-A, Sparling PF et al., eds. Sexually transmitted diseases, second edition, New York: McGraw-Hill, 1990:1087–94.
54. Costa NFP. BEMFAM community distribution statistics. Personal communication, 1990.
55. Aleixo Neto A, Peixoto MLS, Cabral ACV. Estudo Comparativo da incidência de *Gardnerella vaginalis* em usuárias de dispositivos intra-uterinos e anticoncepcionais orais. J Bras Ginec 1987; 97:315–6.
56. Silva PAR, Martelly JU, Gauza JE, Barbosa LCR. Avaliação do DIU: causas de retirada. J Bras Ginec 1987; 97:211–3.
57. Ferrari AN, Lomando SR, Galvão LW, Saldanha C. Análise retrospectiva de quatro anos do dispositivo intra-uterino T de cobre 200 B. J Bras Ginec 1987; 97:95–9.
58. Díaz J, Díaz MM, Pastene L, Asaki R, Faúndes A. Randomized clinical study of the T-Cu 380 A and the Lippes Loop, in Campinas, Brazil. Contracept 1982; 26:221–8.
59. Villa LL, Franco ECF. Epidemiologic correlates of cervical neoplasia and risk of human papilloma virus infection in asymptomatic women in Brazil. J Nat Cancer Inst 1989; 81:332–40.
60. Cates W, Farley TMM, Rowe PJ. Worldwide pattern of infertility: is Africa different? Lancet 1985; 1:596–8.
61. Cunha e Silva M. Estudo descritivo de casais que consultaram no Ambulatório de Esterilidade da FCM/UNICAMP no período de 1972–1980. Tese de Mestrado. Universidade Estadual de Campinas (UNICAMP), 1983.
62. Giovani G. A questão dos remédios no Brasil: produção e consumo. São Paulo: Polis, 1980:148.
63. Díaz M, Goodson P, Faúndes A, Aoki F, Pinto e Silva JL. Risco de contaminação com vírus da AIDS e percepção desse risco entre estudantes da UNICAMP. Accepted for publication in Revista da Faculdade de Ciências Medicas da UNICAMP, 1991.
64. Ramos MEG, Correa SO, Avila MBM. Causas e condições do aborto provocado no Grande Recife. Mimeograph. SOS-Corpo, Recife, 1983.

65. Hardy EE, Department of Obstetrics and Gynecology, School of Medical Sciences, State University of Campinas, SP, Brazil. Personal communication, 1991.
66. Oliveira MHP, Vietta EP, Moriya TM et al. Reações emocionais dos portadores de doenças sexualmente transmissíveis no momento da confirmação do seu diagnóstico. Rev Bras Enfermagem 1987; 40:38–42.
67. Hardy EE, Silva IR, Montanini LAG, Osis MJD, Rodriguez T, Moraes TM. Resultados da área metropolitana e do interior de estado: informações relativas ao pré-natal, parto e revisão pós-parto. In: Avaliação do Programa de Assistência Integral à Saúde da Mulher no Estado de São Paulo, Relatório II, 1988, CEMICAMP. Mimeograph.
68. Ory HW. A review of the association between intrauterine devices and acute pelvic inflammatory disease. J Reprod Med 1978; 20:200–4.
69. Ryder RW, Nsaa W, Hassig SE et al. Perinatal transmission of the human immunodeficiency virus type 1 to infants of seropositive women in Zaire. N Engl J Med 1989; 320:1637–42.
70. Blanche S, Rouziouse C, Moscato MG et al. HIV infection in newborns. French Collaborative Study Group. A prospective study of infants born to women seropositive for human immunodeficiency virus type 1. N Engl J Med 1989; 320:1643.
71. Tovo PA, Martino M. Epidemiology, clinical features and prognostic factors of pediatrics HIV infection—Italian multicentre study. Lancet 1988; 2:1043–6.

REPRODUCTIVE TRACT INFECTIONS IN KENYA: INSIGHTS FOR ACTION FROM RESEARCH

Dr. A. B. N. Maggwa
Research Fellow/Lecturer
Department of Obstetrics and Gynecology
P.O. Box 30288

Dr. E. N. Ngugi
Lecturer
Department of Community Health
P.O. Box 19676

College of Health Sciences
University of Nairobi
Nairobi, Kenya

INTRODUCTION

Reproductive tract infections (RTIs) include not only sexually transmitted diseases (STDs), but also endogenous infections, caused by an overgrowth of organisms normally present in the reproductive tract, and iatrogenic infections, caused by procedures that manipulate the reproductive tract, including induced abortion, delivery, and traditional practices. Although data are inadequate and are drawn primarily from clinic and hospital populations, it appears that RTIs are common and have severe consequences for women in Kenya. Nonetheless, national health planning and policies have given little priority to these diseases. This chapter explores the reasons for this neglect and attempts to offer a range of possible interventions.

FACTORS INFLUENCING DATA AVAILABILITY

Factors affecting the availability of data on RTIs include lack of appreciation of the prevalence and severity of these diseases, restricted health resources, and stigma associated with STDs. In both medical and nonmedical circles, STDs are often looked at as self-inflicted problems that are relevant only to the sufferers. This perception has led to the

Reproductive Tract Infections, Edited by A. Germain *et al.*
Plenum Press, New York, 1992

neglect of RTIs in most national health programs. As evidence of this neglect, only two facilities exist in the country that are designated for the diagnosis and treatment of STDs. In Nairobi, with a population of approximately 2 million people, only one clinic treats STDs free of charge or at a minimal fee.

Kenya, like other developing countries, is financially hard-pressed; it spends only 7 percent of its national budget on health services. RTIs rank very low in health priorities because the mortality associated with them is relatively low and most of their consequences (e.g., infertility and chronic pelvic pain) are invisible and delayed. Although the Ministry of Health has a division dealing with communicable diseases, no attempt was made to set up a national STD control program until 1990, and in 1987, a special national AIDS control program was established without regard to other STDs. The situation is worse for the other kinds of RTIs. Abortion is legally restricted, and women are forced to resort to unsafe procedures that often result in sepsis. Most pregnant women deliver outside of hospitals, also in conditions where infection is likely. No attention at all is given to the problem of overgrowth of endogenous organisms.

Sex is a topic that is considered taboo in most African communities, including Kenya. Therefore, any diseases linked to it are not openly discussed, and this leads to several problems. First, lack of awareness about RTIs is widespread, and unless these conditions cause very significant symptoms, care is not sought. Second, even those who are aware may avoid going to known special STD treatment facilities, choosing instead self-medication or treatment by untrained persons or private practitioners. These treatment approaches do not result in the reporting of cases or partner notification. In addition, inadequate or improper medications obtained this way may result in severe   complications and emergence of resistant organisms. Third, specific beliefs stigmatize people with RTIs, and thus inhibit treatment-seeking behavior and reporting of cases. For example, in some communities, STDs are considered a punishment from God for having been unfaithful to one's spouse.

RISK FACTORS FOR RTIs

The risk factors for RTIs include sexual behavior; transcervical procedures, such as childbirth, abortion, and IUD insertion; and traditional practices.

Sexual Behavior

Adolescent sexuality. In a study of adolescents in a rural community in Kenya, A. B. N. Maggwa[2] found that the mean age at first sexual exposure was 14.9 years for girls and 13.7 for boys. Similar observations have been reported by V. M. Lema,[3] and C. G. H. Obongo,[4] studying adolescent groups in different parts of the country. Maggwa[2] also found that 43 percent of the sexually active girls and 75 percent of the sexually active boys had multiple sex partners. All three studies documented that knowledge about sexuality- and fertility-related issues is very low among adolescents.[2,3,4] Thus, in Kenya, exposure to STDs is common and prolonged, and the consequences have proved to be severe—early age at first sexual intercourse and multiple sex partners have been shown to be significant risk factors for human immunodeficiency virus (HIV) infection among women attending family planning clinics in Nairobi.[5]

Commercial Sex. A large number of women earn or supplement their meager incomes by selling sex. This practice has been necessitated by a shortage of income-generating jobs and the ever-increasing cost of living. The problem is compounded by the high dropout rate of school girls, due to pregnancy. A. Ferguson[6] found that between 8,340 and 10,400 Kenyan schoolgirls drop out of school each year for this reason. Most of these girls never return to school after delivery. Maggwa,[7] working in a rural community, found that fewer than 5 percent of the girls who became pregnant while in school ever went back to complete their education after delivery. These girls may be rejected by their immediate families and the community. With the added pressure of bringing up an unplanned child, they frequently resort to selling sex. Other factors that lead women to commercial sex include divorce and widowhood, which are on the increase in Kenya. As long as these factors exist, commercial sex will thrive and increase.

Once these women are in the trade, they have multiple daily sexual exposures. In one study in Nairobi,[8] it was found that these women serve an average of four male clients per day (range, 1–10). In contrast, married women in Kenya usually have only one sexual partner, and an average of two lifetime sexual partners.[5] However, it is important to note that married women still get infected; most probably this is the result of their spouses' sexual behavior outside the marital institution. Extramarital sexual affairs are common in Kenya, and society does not condemn men for engaging in them.

In addition to female commercial sex workers (CSWs), the daily newspapers have carried stories about men in one of the coastal towns who admit to practicing anal sex with other men as a means of earning an income. Although most of the customers are tourists visiting Kenya, some are Kenyans of African origin.

Homosexuality. The role that homosexuality plays in spreading HIV infection in Kenya remains to be studied. Most Africans would like to believe that homosexuality does not exist in their communities. Although the extent to which homosexuality is practiced in Kenya is not documented, there is evidence that sexual activities that increase the risk of STD and HIV transmission, such as anal intercourse, are practiced.

Transcervical Procedures

Some studies have shown a variety of vaginal flora in Kenyan women. W. L. Kirumbi,[9] working at Kenyatta National Hospital (KNH), found that 26 percent of antenatal women had *Staphylococcus aures*, 24 percent had *Escherichia coli*, 40 percent had *peptostreptococcus*, and 29 percent had *Candida albicans* organisms isolated from their genital tract. G. W. Ingari,[10] working at the same hospital, reported that 9 percent of antenatal women had asymptomatic bacteriuria. A study of women with incomplete abortion at KNH found that 82 percent of them had at least one bacterial organism isolated from either the genital tract or the products of conception.[11] These findings, though limited to selected populations, have some implications for transcervical procedures in Kenya.

The majority of women in Kenya live in rural areas, where health services are not easily available. Several studies show that although the majority of these women receive modern antenatal care at least once during each pregnancy; over 80 percent of them do not deliver in a modern health care facility.[12,13] The majority deliver in places where it may be impossible to achieve asepsis, and are attended by traditional midwives, who may know very little about aseptic techniques.

Abortion is common in Kenya and accounts for up to 60 percent of admissions to most gynecology wards. A high proportion of abortions are the result of unwanted pregnancies,[14] and many of the incomplete abortions seen are likely to have been induced. Lema and colleagues[15] found that 11–16 percent of incomplete abortions seen in eight district hospitals were probably induced. In a study at KNH, it was found that 63 percent of the incomplete abortions were induced.[14] In the studies above, 49 percent and 26 percent, respectively, of induced abortions had been carried out by nonmedical personnel. The risk of introducing exogenous organisms or disseminating organisms normally resident in the vaginal tract into the upper genital tract is likely to be extremely high in the setting of these procedures.

Women using IUDs have been shown to have an increased risk of developing pelvic inflammatory disease (PID): the odds ratio of 4.8 suggests they are 4.8 times as likely as others to develop the disorder. The risk of infection is highest in the period immediately following insertion. This raises the possibility that the infection is introduced into the upper genital tract during insertion.

Traditional Practices

Both male and female circumcision appear to be common practices in Kenya, but their extent and impact have never been studied. These procedures are carried out in places where sterility cannot be guaranteed. The risk of iatrogenic infection may therefore be substantial. Many cases of genital tract infections, some fatal, have been reported in local newspapers.

In some Kenyan communities, certain rituals may increase the risk of infection with HIV. These include wife inheritance, where the younger brother inherits his late brother's wife or the younger sister is given to the husband of her late sister. In each of these situations, the person concerned is expected to have sex with the new partner regardless of the former spouse's cause of death.

Among the Masaai, it is an accepted practice for age-mates to share wives. One needs only to place a spear in front of the house of an age-mate, and this is enough to inform the age-mate that someone is having sex with his wife. The age-mate, in turn, seeks the wife of another age-mate with whom to have sexual relations. This type of tradition may exacerbate the spread of STDs in the community. It is important to note that the women do not have the same rights. Furthermore, there may be similar practices in other tribes, but these are not as freely discussed and therefore go unnoticed.

MAGNITUDE OF THE PROBLEM

As mentioned earlier, data on the prevalence of RTIs in Kenya are scanty. Most deal with the prevalence of STDs in selected populations. The available data are summarized here by the populations studied.

Pregnant Women

Antenatal clinics provide an important opportunity for STD screening during pregnancy, but no policy exists for routine screening. Special studies[1,16–19] show differing

Table 1. Prevalence of STDs among Pregnant Women,
Various Study Populations (Percentage and Percentage Positive % +VE)

STD	Rural (N=68)[16]	Urban (N=1,013)[18]	Urban (N=15,649)[1]	Urban (N=200)[17]	Urban (N=402)[19]
Syphilis	9	NS	1	NS	NS
Gonorrhea	10	7	NS	5	1
Chlamydia trachomatis	6	21	NS	NS	16
Mycoplasma hominis	19	NS	NS	NS	19
Trichomonas vaginalis	2	NS	NS	8	NS
Candida albicans	2	NS	NS	NS	NS
Herpes simplex virus (HSV)	NS	NS	NS	NS	NS

Note: NS = not studied.

prevalence rates for various STDs (Table 1). The prevalence of gonorrhea ranges from 1 percent to 10 percent, with the highest prevalences reported in rural women. Chlamydia infection ranges from 6 percent to 21 percent. All women attending antenatal clinics are supposed to be routinely screened for syphilis. However, because of operational problems, this does not happen. The data available show prevalence rates ranging from 1 percent to 9 percent.

Women Presenting with Abortion Complications

Two Kenyan studies have looked at the prevalence of sepsis among women presenting with incomplete abortion (Table 2). In these studies, sepsis was defined as the presence of any of the following clinical signs: fever, purulent vaginal discharge, adnexal tenderness, peritonitis, or evidence of pelvic abscess. In one study, sepsis occurred in 43 percent of all cases and in 87 percent of women who had had induced abortions.[14] The second study found sepsis in 9 percent of all abortion cases and in 38 percent of women who had had induced abortions.[15] The study that reported lower rates of sepsis involved women from rural communities, while the second study involved an urban population, which has access to more hygienic facilities for the induction of abortion. The reasons for this discrepancy are not clear.

Table 2. Prevalence Complications of Abortion, by Type
of Abortion, Two Study Populations (% +VE)

Complication	Induced		Not induced		Total	
	Rural (N=115)	Urban (N=230)	Rural (N=962)	Urban (N=380)	Rural (N=1,077)	Urban (N=610)
Sepsis	38	87	4	18	9	43
Genital injury	17	2	0	1	3	1
Hemorrhagic shock	13	NS	7	NS	8	NS
Anemia	18	NS	9	NS	10	NS
Other	4	NS	1	NS	1	NS
None	9	11	90	81	69	56

Note: NS = not studied.
Sources: references 14 (urban data) and 15 (rural data).

Family Planning Clients

Family planning services provide another opportunity for women to be screened for STDs and other RTIs. In Kenya, the prevalence of family planning use is about 27 percent of eligible women.[20] If this opportunity were fully utilized to screen women for RTIs, over one quarter of sexually active women would be covered. However, among women attending these clinics, only the relatively few who present with complaints undergo screening for RTIs.

T. N. Mulandi,[16] working in a rural community, found the following levels of STDs among asymptomatic women attending four family planning clinics: gonorrhea, 8 percent; syphilis, 3 percent; and chlamydia, 5 percent. In another study,[21] involving women attending two urban family planning clinics, prevalence rates were 2 percent for syphilis, 4 percent for gonorrhea, and 5 percent for HIV. The prevalence of chlamydia in women attending another urban family planning clinic was 5 percent.[22] None of the women studied had symptoms. Although these studies are few, they suggest that women attending family planning clinics are an important reservoir of untreated infection.

Groups at High Risk

CSWs, truck drivers, and adolescents generally have a higher risk of RTIs than the women discussed above. Studies of these groups are summarized in Table 3.

Table 3. Prevalence of STDs among Various High-risk Groups (% +VE)

STD	CSWs (N=193)[23]	CSWs (N=NS)[24]	Truck drivers (N=600)[25]	Students (N=205)[26]
Gonorrhea	30	NS	32	33
Syphilis	33	NS	5	NS
Chlamydia trachomatis	11	NS	NS	NS
Haemophilus ducreyi	5	NS	NS	NS
HSV	3	NS	NS	NS
HIV	NS	66	26	NS

Note: NS = not studied.

CSWs. In a study involving 193 CSWs seen over a six-month period at the special treatment clinic in Nairobi, L. DeCosta and colleagues[23] found that 30 percent had gonorrhea, 33 percent had syphilis, 11 percent had *Chlamydia trachomatis*, 5 percent had *Haemophilus ducreyi*, and 3 percent had herpes simplex virus (HSV). These prevalence rates are much higher than those reported for pregnant women and family planning clients. In another study, F. A. Plummer and coworkers[24] found that 66 percent of low-income CSWs were HIV-positive. This high prevalence rate reflects not only a danger to the CSWs themselves, but also a potential source of infection for the male clients of the workers.

Truck Drivers. Mombasa is a coastal town that serves as an entry port for goods from abroad for several African countries. The goods are picked up by trucks that have to travel across Kenya. The drivers of these trucks spend most of their time on the road and may have several sexual partners along the route. They therefore constitute a group that can spread diseases in several places over very short periods of time. In one study, 26 percent of truck drivers were found to be infected with HIV, 5 percent with syphilis, and 32 percent with gonorrhea.[25] This is the only study that has ever screened the male population for such diseases. The prevalence of these infections in low-risk men is not known.

Adolescents. As mentioned earlier, adolescents initiate sexual activity at very early ages, and know little about sexuality-related issues, including STDs. Several studies have shown that STDs are common among Kenyan youth. E. A. Orwenyo,[17] working at KNH, found that 23 percent of antenatal women aged 15–19 years were infected with *Neisseria gonorrhoeae*, *Chlamydia trachomatis*, or HSV. Mulandi[16] observed similarly high infection rates among adolescents in maternal-child health/family planning clinics, where 41 percent of the women aged 15–24 years had STDs. One study by the Department of Community Health at the University of Nairobi[26] found that 33 percent of 205 primary school children aged 13–15 years were infected with *Neisseria gonorrhoeae*. All the cases in these studies were asymptomatic.

Extent of HIV Infection and Relationship with RTIs

In May 1990, it was estimated that 200,000 Kenyans were HIV-infected and 9,139 had AIDS. The ratio of females to males infected is approximately 1:1, and the majority of infected persons are in the economically productive and childbearing years (18–40 years).[27] However, no national serosurvey has been done to date. Special studies indicate that 24–88 percent of CSWs[24] are infected. Blood donors had a seroprevalence of 0.5–1.0 percent in 1986 and 2–4 percent in 1990.[27] These blood donors are apparently healthy individuals who do not get paid for their service, and who represent the general population. J. K. G. Mati and colleagues,[21] working at two family planning clinics serving women considered to be at low risk of acquiring HIV infection, have found the HIV prevalence to be 5 percent.

Studies done in Kenya have documented associations between HIV infection and other STDs, particularly genital ulcer diseases and *Chlamydia trachomatis* infection.[1,10] Furthermore, one of these studies demonstrated that male-to-female transmission of HIV was highly efficient in the presence of genital ulcers, on the order of 10–40 percent, as evidenced by monthly follow-up for six months.[28] Thus, the problem of HIV infection is a major one in Kenya, and as the available data show, it is inextricably interrelated with the other STDs.

THE IMPACT OF RTIs

The impact of these infections must be assessed for individuals, families, and society at large in terms of mortality, morbidity, and socioeconomic consequences.

Pregnancy Outcome

The consequences of RTIs include a variety of adverse effects on both pregnant women and their newborns, as described below.

Antenatal Infections. A study done at KNH found that pyrexia occurred in the antenatal period in 6 percent of the 4,276 women who delivered in a 12-month period.[29] In this study, urinary tract infections (UTIs) and genital tract infections (GTIs) accounted for 18 percent of all cases of pyrexia, while malaria and upper respiratory infections accounted for 19 percent. The rest of the women had pyrexia of unknown origin. Among the women with clinical evidence of UTIs and GTIs, the most common bacterial agent isolated was *Escherichia coli* (37 percent), followed by *Klebsiella* (24 percent) and *Staphylococcus albus* (18 percent). However, the significance of these isolates is not clear, as they were isolated from the lower genital tract.

Postpartum Infections. Plummer and colleagues[18] found that 20 percent of 1,013 women delivering in one institution had signs of postpartum infections within seven days of delivery. They found that the risk of developing postpartum infection if a woman had *Neisseria gonorrhoeae* was 4.4 times greater than that for uninfected women (p value, 0.0001). The risk among women who had chlamydia was 1.7 times greater (p value, 0.02). Given the high prevalence rates of these infections during pregnancy (1–10 percent for gonorrhea and 6–21 for chlamydia), the potential for postpartum infection due to these organisms in Kenya is very high. Of all the cases of postpartum infection, 83 percent were positive for *Neisseria gonorrhoeae*. As further evidence for the role of these organisms in postpartum infection in Kenya, M. Termmerman and coworkers[30] found that 11 of 35 women with postpartum endometritis had *Neisseria gonorrhoeae* isolated from the upper genital tract, compared with two of 30 controls; for chlamydia, the figures were six out of 30 and two out of 29, respectively. Although limited to only two possible causative agents, these studies demonstrate the major role that RTIs play in the etiology of postpartum infections in Kenya.

Maternal Mortality. Maternal mortality in Kenya is estimated at 6–7 deaths per 1,000 live births. Most of the data are institution-based and may not present the true picture in the community. The causes of maternal mortality in studies done at KNH and Pumwani Maternity Hospital, where over 10,000 deliveries take place annually, are shown in Table 4.[31,32] Puerperal sepsis and postabortal sepsis accounted for 43 percent of all the maternal deaths at KNH, while puerperal sepsis alone accounted for 19 percent of deaths at Pumwani. This makes RTIs the single most important cause of maternal mortality at these institutions.

Neonatal Infections. Although few studies have been done, neonatal infections appear to be common, with prevalence rates of 10–40 percent. Most of the studies in Kenya have been concerned with ophthalmia neonatorum. G. N. Riara[19] found that of the 315 infants in his study, 9 percent had *Chlamydia trachomatis* organisms isolated from both the eyes and the throat, while 0.3 percent (only one case) had gonorrhea organisms isolated from the eyes and none from the throat. The risks of a mother's transmitting these organisms to her infants were 55 percent and 33 percent, respectively, if the mother was positive at the time of delivery. The implications of these findings were not established, as the children were not followed up for a long enough period. Similar transmission rates have been reported by L. Fransen and colleagues.[33]

Preterm Delivery, Premature Rupture of Membranes (PROM), and Low Birth Weight (LBW). One study in Nairobi, involving a total of 5,293 births over a three-month period, found that 24 percent of the women had preterm deliveries, 2 percent had PROM, 8 percent had LBW babies (infants weighing under 2,000 g); and the perinatal mortality rate (PMR) was 36.6 per 1,000 live births.[34] The role of RTIs in these various outcomes of pregnancy was not studied.

In a retrospective study of women who had delivered at KNH between 1970 and 1979, F. O. Nana[1] found that women who had syphilis and were not treated in the antenatal period had a poorer pregnancy outcome than those who received treatment. The PMR was 391 per 1,000 live births among the untreated group, compared with the overall PMR of 171 per 1,000 live births. These women also had a high prevalence of LBW infants (46 percent). Riara[19] found that women with preterm deliveries and PROM had higher prevalences of chlamydia—23 percent and 30 percent, respectively, compared with the overall prevalence of 16 percent in his study population. Similar observations were reported by C. N. Mbwiria[35] in a study of women delivering at the Pumwani Maternity Hospital.

Complications of Abortion. As reported earlier, postabortal sepsis is a very common problem, and this may lead to death, acute pelvic infections, chronic pelvic infections, and infertility. At KNH, it was found that peritonitis occurred in 8 percent of women who had induced abortions, and pelvic abscesses occurred in 4 percent of a similar group of women.[14] If not adequately treated, these conditions can be fatal or lead to chronic illnesses.

In Kenya, mortality due to abortions is high; the abortion-related mortality rate ranges from one to six per 1,000 abortions reported.[14,15,36] The major cause of death is hemorrhage; sepsis is the next most common cause. In his series, J. N. Fomulu[36] reported that 83 percent of deaths were due to sepsis.

PID

The prevalence of PID in Kenya is not known. At KNH, PID accounts for 30 percent of the cases admitted to the gynecology ward,[37] an estimated 1,860 women each year.

Table 4. Causes of Maternal Mortality, KNH (1972–77)
Pumwani Maternity Hospital (1975–84) (% +VE)

Cause	KNH (N=99)[31]	Pumwani (N=150)[32]
Postabortal sepsis	22	NS
Puerperal sepsis	21	19
Hemorrhage	15	13
Ruptured uterus	6	14
Ectopic pregnancy	5	NS
Anesthesia	5	6
Renal disease/failure	4	NS
Perforated uterus	3	NS
Malignant disease	3	NS
Tuberculosis	3	NS
PET/eclampsia	3	21
Pulmonary embolism	3	5
Hemolytic anemia	3	NS
Cardiac disease	2	7
Hyperemesis	1	NS
Unknown	NS	7
Other	NS	7

Note: NS = not studied.

In one study of women presenting with acute PID complicated by pelvic abscess, a variety of organisms were cultured from the pus obtained at laparotomy. *Escherichia coli* and *Peptococcus* were the most commonly isolated organisms.[37] These organisms were similar to the organisms isolated from the lower genital tract of women with no clinical signs or symptoms. This finding suggests that organisms found in the lower genital tract of women may become pathogenic when they find their way into the upper genital tract.

S. H. Abdulla,[38] working at KNH, found that women using IUDs had an increased risk of developing PID (odds ratio, 4.8); this risk was related to the time since insertion, being highest in the first two weeks following insertion. The same study showed that among long-term users of IUDs, there was a tendency to develop PID-related symptoms around the time of menstruation. These findings tend to suggest that improper insertion techniques and the hanging threads play roles in introducing infection to the upper genital tract.

Gonococcal infection is common among women in Kenya and is thought to be the single most important cause of PID.[39]

Infertility

The prevalence of infertility in Kenya is not known. However, it is estimated at 3 percent countrywide, and 75 percent of consultations in the gynecology clinics in Nairobi and the Coast Province are due to infertility problems. A study of 105 infertile couples at KNH found that 6 percent of the females and 37 percent of the males had a history of STDs, while 13 percent of the females had a history of PID.[40] In the same study, 61 percent of the infertile females had postinfection tubal abnormalities or pelvic adhesions. For the males, clinical evidence of past prostate gland infections and obstruction of the vas deferens were present in 38 percent of the cases. These findings suggest that RTIs play an important role in infertility in Kenya.

Abnormal Cervical Cytology

Cancer of the cervix has been shown to be associated with the human papilloma virus infection, which is sexually transmissible.[41] The prevalence of abnormal cervical cytology is, therefore, yet another reflection of the impact of RTIs on women's health. In one rural area of Kenya, the prevalence of abnormal cytology is about 21–25 per 1,000 women.[42-46] In urban women, the reported prevalence is 19–20 per 1,000.[45] From the available data, one sees that this problem is prevalent in Kenya. Furthermore, many women are seen with cervical cancer in medical institutions; for example, nearly 300 new cases are diagnosed at KNH every year. Women with cervical cancer usually present in the late stages of the disease, which are not amenable to treatment. Most of the cases seen at KNH present in stage 3 and above; only 7 percent are seen with stage 1 of the disease.[41,46]

Family Planning Implications

RTIs play a major role in the acceptance and continuation of use of family planning. Although the family planning programs in Kenya began in 1966, only 27 percent of eligible women were using modern contraception in 1989, despite the fact that more than 80 percent knew of at least one method of contraception and where to obtain the method.[20] Several important barriers to contraceptive use exist. Studies in both urban and rural areas show that poor pregnancy outcome is associated with low contraceptive use and shorter subsequent birth interval. This finding reflects the desire of the woman or couple to replace the wasted pregnancy.[47,48] RTIs contribute significantly to poor pregnancy outcome and indirectly influence contraceptive acceptability.

Another problem is that women who do not know that they have infections when they initiate family planning use may blame the contraceptive for complications resulting from the infections. This not only increases discontinuation rates, but also can influence acceptance. Finally, certain contraceptives may increase the risk of acquiring RTIs (e.g., chlamydia and gonorrhea).[19] This will also tend to discourage women from using those particular methods.

Socioeconomic Impact

The socioeconomic impact of RTIs has not been studied in Kenya. However, on the basis of the authors' knowledge about Kenyan society and the cost of management of these conditions, our assessment is that they have a major impact.

Several impacts on health services have been mentioned. We estimate that more than 75 percent of consultant gynecologists' time is spent on managing cases of infertility. This is a serious problem since consultants are scarce in Kenya. Substantial hospital resources are used to treat women who suffer complications of induced abortions. V. P. Aggarwal and J. K. G. Mati[14] found that these women stay, on average, three days, compared with 1.5 days for women who have spontaneous abortions. Serious consequences of infections demand specialized care and equipment that is expensive and scarce, and that requires special training of staff. For example, women with infertility require specialized X rays, laparoscopy, and special laboratory investigations, the cost of which is enormous. Women who present with cancer of the cervix in the late stages require costly radiotherapy, which most cannot afford. The total cost of such services and equipment is usually many times what would be required to prevent these conditions.

In addition to the impact on health resources, there are substantial social impacts. RTIs afflict primarily the most useful members of society, in particular women aged 15–49 years, who are the major contributors to economic development, as well as the childbearers and household managers. RTIs can be debilitating, reducing work days and productivity. Although death is an uncommon event following RTIs, when it occurs, the family of the person will be deprived of that person's contribution to the well-being of the other family members. Chronic morbidity is common, and this will affect the family resources, as there will be the tendency to spend more on health at the expense of other requirements. RTIs are stigmatizing for women and often lead to infertility, a problem that is frowned upon in most African communities. The affected individual is often made to feel rejected, and this rejection may lead to a variety of psychological and psychiatric conditions, with disastrous results.

CONTROL PROGRAMS

The Kenyan government's national AIDS control program has four main committees: epidemiology; information, education, and communication; clinical management; and laboratory and diagnosis.[50] The program policy is that everybody should know about HIV, including how it is transmitted and how it is not. It is assumed that, after exposure to information, individuals will protect themselves and others. However, not all the intended audiences have access to the different communication media used. A national survey found that of 7,595 people studied, 58 percent said they had learned of AIDS from the radio, 56 percent from public meetings, 42 percent from newspapers, 22 percent from posters, and only 7 percent from television. The same study found that only 13 percent of 3,193 respondents knew that the condom protects against HIV infection.[50] The level of awareness was higher among men than among women; this finding implies that women were less exposed to information. The conclusion of this study was that while radio, print media, and public meetings should continue to be used, other modes of communication media need to be explored, including such traditional modes as music, drama, and folklore.

The government initiative was initially addressed only to HIV. Kenya's Ministry of Health has now produced a national STD control program (a two-year plan for 1990–91),[49] as well as national guidelines for control of STDs.[52] The program includes epidemiology and surveillance, early detection and management of STDs, standardization of management and partner notification, setting up of a laboratory infrastructure, professional training, and research. The program will not be a vertical one, but decentralized and integrated with other programs based on the district focus and primary health care principals. The program shall have close interaction with the national AIDS control program, the maternal-child health/family planning program, and others found appropriate.

The question the majority of policymakers and health workers ask is, can people, particularly those who participate in the commercial sex industry, change their behavior? With tenacity and stamina, a targeted strategy can work, as shown by E. N. Ngugi and F. A. Plummer.[53] Their study was designed to assess the impact of STD and AIDS health education among four groups of women working in the sex trade in different parts of the country. The women were educated and counseled to become partners in upgrading the status of their reproductive health by reducing their number of sexual partners as far as possible, using condoms with every partner, examining clients for symptoms of STDs, and refusing sexual contact with any infected man. Peers were trained to support others.

The women reduced their average number of clients from 8.6 to 3.5. Frequency of condom use increased from 6 percent to 71 percent. In two of these sites, clinical presentation of STDs decreased by 14 percent and 21 percent; reports were not available from the other two sites.[53] At one site, 5 percent of the women opted to leave the trade. The key point here is that such programs are possible and within available resources to a certain extent. The inputs include in-service STD training of a multidisciplinary team, provision of condoms, education and counseling of the study population, and training of peer educators and counselors.

It is government policy and a legal requirement that all communicable diseases, including STDs, be controlled.[51] However, as mentioned earlier, there are currently only two facilities designated for the treatment of STDs in the country. In order for the policy to be implemented, an estimated US$10 million is needed for the initial two-year period.

Currently, youth are not given any special focus in STD control efforts. Although they should be educated and counseled on how to prevent infections and to protect others from getting infected, this does not often happen. The reasons for this are numerous, including lack of time due to overcrowding, negative attitudes of health care workers, and lack of drugs in public health institutions.

POSSIBLE CONSTRAINTS TO CONTROL OF RTIs IN KENYA

Available Facilities

Kenya, with a population of nearly 24 million people and a growth rate of 3.4 percent, has 1,963 health facilities of various types (Table 5). The majority of these are located in urban centers and as such are not accessible to the nearly 80 percent of the population who live in rural areas. A survey by the World Bank in 1984 found that fewer than 50 percent of these institutions were providing good-quality services. Laboratory diagnostic facilities exist only in a few of the hospitals, which account for only 9 percent of the total health facilities in Kenya.

Personnel Available

The institutions mentioned above are staffed by a variety of personnel, as shown in Table 6. Apart from the doctors, the rest of the cadres are not adequately trained to diagnose and treat RTIs; yet, they manage 90 percent of the health facilities. This problem, together with a lack of adequate diagnostic equipment, will make any institution-based intervention programs fairly difficult to implement.

Utilization of Health Facilities

Antenatal Care Clinics. The majority of women receive antenatal care at least once during pregnancy (Table 7). Visits for such care would thus provide a good opportunity for screening these women, but several constraints need to be addressed. The majority of

Table 5. Available Health Facilities

Type of institution	Government/ private	Church	Total
Hospital	139	42	181
Health center	375	81	456
Dispensary	1,054	272	1,326
Total	1,568	395	1,963

Source: reference 51.

Table 6. Available Personnel

Cadre	Total	No. per 100,000 population
Doctors	3,336	14
Registered nurses	10,752	45
Enrolled nurses	14,352	60
Clinical officers	2,472	10
Public health officers	528	2
Public health technicians	2,232	9

Source: reference 51.

women seek care late: only about 20 percent do so before 20 weeks' gestation, and about 30 percent after 30 weeks'. Such timing influences the number of visits during which women can be screened and treated adequately. Thus, if antenatal services sites are to be used as catchment areas, there is need for rapid tests and simple treatments. The importance of diagnosis and treatment needs to be emphasized to health providers also. Two studies have found that only 37–46 percent of women receiving antenatal care get their blood taken for syphilis tests, and of these, nearly half do not get their results; yet, this is one of the routinely recommended investigations during antenatal care in Kenya. Reasons for this kind of situation need to be investigated.[13,20,34,54]

Table 7. Distribution of Pregnant Women by Number of Visits
for Antenatal Care, Various Study Populations (%)

Number of visits	Mombasa[54] (N=300)	Nairobi[34] (N=5,293)	Machakos (rural)[13] (N=835)	Demographic and Health Survey[20] (N=7,150)
None	7	4	12	20
At least one	93	96	88	80

Table 8. Distribution of Deliveries,
by Type of Attendant, Two Study Populations (%)

Attendant	Demographic and Health Survey[20]	Machakos (rural)[13]
Doctor/trained nurse/midwife	50	24
Relative/friend/self	33	15
Traditional birth attendant	14	61
Not stated	3	0

Labor and Delivery. Most of the women in Kenya live in rural areas, where modern health facilities do not exist. Many of them deliver outside the medical facilities, attended by untrained personnel (Table 8). Studies have shown that 50–75 percent of births take place outside the hospital environment. Thus, interventions during delivery will be difficult unless they are made simple enough for untrained birth attendents to administer. In order for intervention programs to influence RTIs at this stage, there is need to enlist the assistance of the birth attendants or to train the mother during antenatal care.[13,20]

Child Welfare Services. In Kenya, these are both preventive and curative services. The 1989 Demographic and Health Survey found that 61 percent of children aged 12–23 months had both clinical and documentary evidence of having utilized preventive and promotive health services. These services, however, were utilized primarily for curative care.[20]

Family Planning Services. These have also been suggested as possible catchment areas for prevention and management of RTIs. In 1989, 28 percent of married women aged 14–49 years were using contraception. However, only 18 percent were using methods that require clinic visits. Of the women using clinic-based methods, 71 percent utilized government facilities; 18 percent, nongovernmental facilities (e.g., church-based or the Family Planning Association of Kenya); and the rest, the private sector. Family planning clinics are not equipped with facilities for diagnosing RTIs. Furthermore, they are staffed by nurses, whose current training does not enable them to make proper diagnosis and provide the required management.

CONCLUSIONS AND RECOMMENDATIONS

During this era of HIV infection, African women are particularly threatened. Because women are the caretakers of the children and spouse, the family unit often suffers levels of disintegration when women get infected. Child survival programs are likely to be adversely affected. Women in most African countries have little or no say in sexual relationships, and yet they suffer more severe consequences from RTIs than men do. They therefore deserve more attention. However, the control of RTIs should be the responsibility of both men and women, and not merely of women, who, according to some societies, are the more available target.

This review has shown that, while RTIs appear to be a very serious problem in Kenya, there are still major gaps in the available data. There are no data on the general population, and some issues (especially the social and economic impact) have simply never been studied. In summary, the major features of RTIs in Kenya are as follows:

1. Data are almost entirely lacking on the extent of RTIs and their sequelae in the general population. Nonetheless, the data available through institution-based studies, indicate there is a serious problem with RTIs and their sequelae in Kenya.
2. Health facilities and personnel trained in the diagnosis and treatment of RTIs are very few. Furthermore, even the available services are not adequately utilized.
3. Most cases of RTIs are found through routine screening. This may reflect women's lack of awareness of the symptoms of RTIs. An ongoing study supports this hypothesis by showing that while over 90 percent of women attending two family planning clinics could name at least one STD, the majority were not aware of any symptoms or signs.[55]

What Can Be Done at Maternal-Child Health/Family Planning Clinics

Maternal-child health/family planning clinics can make four important contributions with reference to RTIs:

1. Screening of women and provision of treatment for RTIs
2. Treating infants as soon as contact is made
3. Educating women about means of prevention of RTIs and about signs and symptoms so that they may recognize RTIs early and seek treatment
4. Changing the attitudes of men toward these clinics so that they can be encouraged to utilize them

Proposed Interventions

1. Family health education aimed at better reproductive health should start early in life—in primary school—and special efforts should be undertaken to reach out-of-school youth. The role of peer group education needs to be emphasized in order to overcome sociocultural barriers. Education initiatives need to utilize focused educational methodology targeted to different population groups. In addition to addressing "high-risk" groups (e.g., CSWs, truck drivers, adolescents), a special effort has to be made to address the general population. This can be done through antenatal and maternal-child health/family planning clinics, and informal groupings (e.g., sports clubs, business clubs, unions, church groups). This would increase coverage to include men.

2. Health personnel and institutions urgently need investment so that they can diagnose, treat, and follow up on RTIs. This should be done within existing health services, as opposed to being a vertical program.

3. Programs should promote safe, effective, and acceptable methods of contraception, to reduce both infection and unwanted or unplanned pregnancies. These efforts should include information on methods that protect against most STDs, including AIDS, especially

the condom. Special emphasis is needed on female-controlled methods that will protect women from both infection and unwanted or unplanned pregnancies. The female condom currently under development is expensive and cumbersome; there is a need to do better than this. For those women who want more children, there is a need for methods that will protect them against infection with no contraceptive effects.

4. Research on culturally acceptable and affordable intervention measures is urgently required. The research should cover the following: perception of RTIs and the treatment-seeking behaviors associated with them in the community; sexual behavior in different communities; and communication media about issues like sex that may be considered taboo in certain communities.

5. Research is also necessary to determine the extent of the problem of RTIs and their complications. This should include population surveillance, which can be done using the same sample populations used in other national estimates; and studies to determine both the medical and the socioeconomic implications of RTIs at the individual, family, community, and national levels.

6. Research on simple, effective, and affordable diagnostic techniques and treatment modalities that can be used at the primary health care level is needed.

7. The impact of RTIs on pregnancy outcome is not clearly understood and needs to be studied.

8. The current and potential roles of nonmedical personnel and institutions in the control of RTIs and their sequelae needs urgent review.

9. The cost-effectiveness of interventions at various levels of health care facilities needs study.

10. Implementation of strategies that have proven successful should be undertaken without further delay in order to bring down the prevalence of RTIs.

11. In order for any of the above activities to take place, there is need for financial support to assist the already strained resources available to the Ministry of Health. There has been increasing political will and awareness in relation to AIDS and selected STDs. However, there is little awareness of the other causes of RTIs. Owing to the lack of information even among scientists and medical personnel, political awareness and will to assist is bound to be lacking. The two-year national STD control program was estimated to cost US$10 million—which does not include a research component or control of other causes of RTIs and their sequelae—RTI programs will require much more. Donor agencies and other international institutions should play a role in strengthening institutions and provision of funds for research on appropriate techniques.

REFERENCES

1. Nana FO. Syphilis in pregnancy at Kenyatta National Hospital. Thesis. University of Nairobi, 1981.
2. Maggwa ABN. Knowledge, attitude and practice survey on adolescent fertility and sexuality among adolescents in rural set up in Kenya. Thesis. University of Nairobi, 1987.
3. Lema VM. Adolescent fertility and sexuality among secondary school girls in a cosmopolitan city, Nairobi, Kenya. Thesis. University of Nairobi, 1987.
4. Obongo CGH. Adolescent sexuality and contraceptive practices in a rural community in Kenya. Thesis, University of Nairobi, 1989.

5. Hunter D, Maggwa ABN, Mati JKG et al. Risk factors for HIV among women attending family planning clinics in Nairobi, Kenya. In: Proceedings of the Sixth International Conference on AIDS, San Francisco, June 20–24, 1990.
6. Ferguson A. School drop out rates in Kenya, Nairobi: Ministry of Health and GTZ, 1988.
7. Maggwa ABN. Parents' knowledge, attitudes and practices toward adolescent fertility and sexuality in Kenya. Unpublished data.
8. Ngugi E, Plummer FA et al. Prevention of HIV transmission in Africa: the effectiveness of condom promotion and health education among high risk prostitutes. Lancet 1988; 2:887–90
9. Kirumbi WL. Microflora in women with a McDonald stitch at Kenyatta National Hospital. Thesis. University of Nairobi, 1989.
10. Ingari GW. Asymptomatic bacteriuria in pregnancy at Kenyatta National Hospital. Thesis. University of Nairobi, 1987.
11. Kibwana. Isolation of bacterial flora from genital tract and products of conception in incomplete abortion at Kenyatta National Hospital. Thesis. University of Nairobi, 1990.
12. World Health Organization offset publication No. 18, Geneva, 1975.
13. Maggwa ABN. The role of traditional birth attendants in reproductive health care. In: National Center for Research in Reproduction and Population Council. Proceedings of seminar on Norplant® and family planning in a rural set up, New York, 1989.
14. Aggarwal VP, Mati JKG. Epidemiology of induced abortion in Nairobi, Kenya. J Obstet Gynaecol East Cent Afr 1982; 1:54.
15. Lema VM, Kamau RK et al. Epidemiology of abortion in eight district hospitals in Kenya. Report for Population Council, New York.
16. Mulandi TN. Prevalence of sexually transmitted diseases in women living in a rural set up in Kenya. Thesis. University of Nairobi, 1985.
17. Orwenyo EA. Cervical infections with N. gonorrhea, C. trichomatis and H. simplex during pregnancy at Kenyatta National Hospital. Thesis. University of Nairobi, 1984.
18. Plummer FA et al. Postpartum upper genital tract infections in Nairobi: epidemiology, etiology and risk factors. J Infect Dis 1987; 156:92–8.
19. Riara GN. Pregnancy outcome in women with STDs (mycoplasma, N. gonorrhea, and chlamydia trachomatis). Thesis. University of Nairobi, 1987.
20. National Council for Population and Development. Kenya Demographic Health Survey 1989, Nairobi, 1989.
21. Mati JKG, Maggwa ABN, Hunter D. The relationship between oral contraception and HIV infection. In: Proceedings of the Sixth International Conference on AIDS, San Francisco, June 20–24, 1990.
22. Ger JO. Chlamydia infection among family planning clients at Kenyatta National Hospital. Thesis. University of Nairobi, 1986.
23. De'Costa L, Plummer F et al. Sexually transmitted diseases among Nairobi prostitutes. In: Proceedings of the Third African Regional Conference on Sexually Transmitted Diseases, March 1983, Nairobi, Kenya, Basel: African Union against Venereal Diseases and Treponematosis, and Ciba Geigy, 1983.

24. Plummer FA, Simosen JN, Ngugi EN et al. Incidence of HIV and related diseases in a cohort of prostitutes in Nairobi. In: Proceedings of the Sixth International Conference on AIDS, San Francisco, June 20–24, 1990.
25. Omari MA, Mutere JJ et al. Sexual behavior of long distance truck drivers and their contribution to the spread of sexually transmitted diseases in East Africa. In: Proceedings of the Sixth International Conference on AIDS, San Francisco, June 20–24, 1990.
26. Department of Community Medicine, University of Nairobi, Kenya.
27. National AIDS Control Program, Ministry of Health. Internal reports. Nairobi, 1990.
28. Pierre P, De'Costa L, Plummer FA et al. Incidence of seroconversion in women with genital ulcers, Nairobi, Kenya. In: Proceedings of the Sixth International Conference on AIDS, San Francisco, June 20–24, 1990.
29. Badia WA. The outcome of pregnancy in patients admitted with pyrexia at Kenyatta National Hospital. Thesis. University of Nairobi, 1980.
30. Temmerman M et al. Microbial aetiology and diagnostic criteria of postpartum endometritis in Nairobi, Kenya. Genitourin Med 1988; 64:172–95.
31. Makokha A. Maternal mortality at Kenyatta National Hospital. East Afr Med J 1980; 57:151.
32. Ngoka WM. Maternal mortality at Pumwani Maternity Hospital, Nairobi, Kenya. East Afr Med J 1987; 64:277.
33. Fransen L, Piot P, Nsanze H et al. Aetiology and management of opthalamia neonatorum in Nairobi, Kenya. In: Proceedings of the Third African Regional Conference on Sexually Transmitted Diseases, March 1983, Nairobi, Kenya, Basel: African Union against Venereal Diseases and Treponematosis, and Ciba Geigy, 1983.
34. Mati JKG, Aggarwal VP, Lucas S et al. The Nairobi birth survey: the study design, the population and outline results. J Obstet Gynaecol East Cent Afr 1982; 1:132.
35. Mbwiria CN. The relationship between prematurity and STDs. Thesis. University of Nairobi, 1989.
36. Fomulu JN. Aetiology of postabortal sepsis at Kenyatta National Hospital. Thesis. University of Nairobi, 1982.
37. Chebroit SC. Pelvic abscesses in the female genital tract. Thesis. University of Nairobi, 1985.
38. Abdulla SH. The risk of pelvic inflammatory disease in women using IUDs at Kenyatta National Hospital. J Obstet Gynaecol East Cent Afr 1982; 1:156.
39. Carty MJ, Nzioki JM, Verhagen AR. The role of the gonococcus in acute PID. East Afr Med J 1972; 49:376.
40. Mati JKG, Sinei SKA, Oyieke JB et al. Clinical aspects of infertility in Kenya: a comprehensive evaluation of the couple. Unpublished.
41. Rogo OK. Human papilloma virus and human immunodeficiency virus infection in relation to cancer of the cervix. Dissertation. Umea University.
42. Ndavi M. Cervical cytology in rural Kenya. Thesis. University of Nairobi, 1986.
43. Kitavi JM. Cervical cytology in rural Kenya. Thesis. University of Nairobi, 1984.
44. Mati JKG, Mbugua S, Maggwa ABN. Control of cancer of the cervix: further experience with screening for premalignant lesion in an African environment. Unpublished, 1990.

45. Kirima J. Cervical cytology at Kenyatta National Hospital. Thesis. University of Nairobi, 1980.
46. Ojwang SB. Cancer of the cervix at Kenyatta National Hospital. East Afr Med J 1978; 55:194.
47. Kamau RK. Birth intervals in women delivering at Kenyatta National Hospital. Thesis. University of Nairobi, 1986.
48. Maggwa ABN. Determinants of birth intervals in women living in a rural set up in Kenya. Thesis. University of Nairobi, 1987.
49. National AIDS Control Program, Ministry of Health. Internal reports, Nairobi, 1988.
50. Ngugi EN, Plummer FA. Health outreach and control of AIDS. J AIDS 1:566–77.
51. National STD Control Program, Ministry of Health, A two year plan for 1990–1991. Nairobi, 1990.
52. Ministry of Health. National guidelines for the control of STDs, Nairobi, 1990.
53. Ngugi EN, Njeru EK. Dynamism of focussed AIDS/STD education/counseling: a cohort study of women with high frequency partner change. Presented at the 30th Scientific Meeting and General Assembly of the Association of Physicians of East and Central Africa, 1990.
54. Kibwana S. Antenatal care in a provincial hospital, Mombasa, Kenya. Thesis. University of Nairobi, 1991.
55. Mati JKG. The relationship between contraceptive use and HIV infection, ongoing study. Personnel communication.

REPRODUCTIVE TRACT INFECTIONS IN NIGERIA: CHALLENGES FOR A FRAGILE HEALTH INFRASTRUCTURE

Dr. Adeyemi O. Adekunle
Senior Lecturer in Obstetrics and Gynecology

Professor Oladapo A. Ladipo
Professor of Obstetrics and Gynecology

Department of Obstetrics and Gynecology
College of Medicine
University of Ibadan
University College Hospital
Ibadan, Nigeria

INTRODUCTION

Reproductive tract infections (RTIs) are frequent and troublesome disorders during the reproductive life of women. In many developed countries, accurate annual data on RTIs are available; in Nigeria, however, most information on RTIs emanate from hospital-based studies that often are not representative of the true incidence of RTIs at the community level.

Despite the absence of accurate national data, it is clear that RTIs constitute great socioeconomic and medical problems among both urban and rural dwellers. Regrettably, the low status of women and their roles in a male-dominated culture make them vulnerable to RTIs. Women are powerless to prevent or control exposure to these risks. They suffer agonizing pelvic pain due to chronic pelvic infection, as well as more serious consequences. Compromise of their reproductive potential is often a regretted major sequelae. Pelvic inflammatory disease (PID) probably accounts for more than half of all cases of infertility seen in Nigerian clinics; the most common causative organisms are *Neisseria gonorrhoeae* and *Chlamydia trachomatis*.

The observed high incidence of RTIs in Nigeria is due to inadequately trained health manpower, scarcity of functional laboratories, inadequate financial resources to support any comprehensive screening and treatment programs, and probably the sexual behavioral patterns in some of the population. The causative organisms are varied and can be adequately treated. However, many women in Nigeria do not have access to medical care.

The few medical personnel and laboratory facilities are concentrated in urban areas and thus exclude the rural community, where the majority of the population live. This problem is compounded by low utilization of limited facilities because of financial constraints and increased patronage of traditional healers.

SEXUALLY TRANSMITTED DISEASES (STDs)

At present, it is impossible to determine the incidence of STDs in Nigeria, as there are no specific mandates or government policies dictating the reporting of these cases. For instance, at Ibadan, which is the largest city in Nigeria, with a population of about 2 million, there is only one recognized STD clinic, based at University College Hospital (UCH). About 1,500 new cases are seen annually, with no significant difference between males and females (Table 1).

Table 1. Distribution of STD Cases Seen at the Special Treatment Clinic, UCH, by Patients' Sex, 1988 and 1989

	1988				1989			
	Male		Female		Male		Female	
STD	N	%	N	%	N	%	N	%
NSU, nongonococcal urethritis, PGU	239	42.1	7	1.2	335	38.9	—	—
Bacterial vaginitis	—	—	141	24.9	—	—	134	18.9
Candidiasis	10	1.8	175	30.9	—	—	254	35.8
Trichomonal infection	6	1.1	95	16.8	8	0.9	103	14.5
Gonococcal infection	170	29.9	99	17.5	346	40.3	153	21.6
Herpes genitalis	47	8.3	1	0.2	44	5.1	5	0.7
Tinea cruris	28	4.9	13	2.0	35	4.1	30	5.2
Genital warts	19	3.3	24	4.2	14	1.6	20	2.8
Lymphogranuloma venereum	25	4.4	3	0.5	42	4.8	5	0.7
Treponemal disease	2	0.3	5	0.8	9	1.0	1	0.1
Chancroid	22	3.8	2	0.3	27	3.1	4	0.5
Total	568	99.9	565	99.3	860	99.8	709	100.8

Source: Courtesy of Dr. F. A. B. Adeyemi-Doro, UCH, Ibadan, personal communication.

The overcrowded government hospitals are busy treating life-threatening and endemic diseases; hence, the management of STDs has been left to private physicians, pharmacists, and herbalists.[1] This makes it difficult, if not almost impossible, to gather reliable statistics, as record keeping is poor among these practitioners. In general, however, it appears that the incidence of STDs is on the increase because of a more liberal attitude toward sex, in particular among teenagers. Socioeconomic and cultural attitudes toward sex constitute important factors in the epidemiology of STDs, particularly in areas where polygamy is widely practiced. For example, a man infected with an STD may seek treatment, but may not be able to afford the cost of treatment for all his wives. Some men even believe that their wives can be cured by their seminal fluid, which they believe contains antibacterial agents. In addition, some communities preferentially allow young men to indulge in promiscuous sexual activities with sexually active women and prostitutes, while young, unmarried females are expected to remain chaste. Older men may indulge in extramarital relations; and in some cultures, a urethral discharge is regarded as evidence of sexual potency or adolescence, while in others, sexual exposure to a virgin is believed to provide a cure for a resistant urethritis.

Gonococcal Infection

The true incidence of gonorrhea is unknown. Various workers have reported different rates over the years, from a low rate of 3.4 percent to a high incidence of 600 per 1,000 (Table 2).

Most males who become infected with gonorrhea develop symptoms such as painful micturition, while urethral strictures and epididymo-orchitis are common sequelae. Chronic epididymitis was the etiologic factor in 32 percent of infertile males (N=510) treated at the UCH between 1972 and 1979.[9] Among women, the infection is usually asymptomatic, and complications are more common, including ascending infections that result in chronic ill health and reproductive failure.[10,11]

While it is widely known that gonorrhea is difficult to control because of its rapid incubation and the large reservoir of asymptomatic women,[12] socioeconomic and cultural attitudes toward sex compound the problem. The improved survival of the gonococcus in humid conditions may be a factor in the increasing observed cases of prepubertal gonorrhea, which was once believed to be rare. Among 578 patients presenting at an STD clinic in Ibadan, 131 (20 percent) had postpubertal gonorrhea, while 27 (4 percent) had prepubertal gonorrhea.[13] Some of the latter cases may be related to child sex abuse, which is rarely reported. In-depth studies are lacking completely.

This unfortunate picture of gonorrhea infection in Nigeria is compounded by the emergence in West Africa in 1976 of penicillin-resistant strains of *Neisseria gonorrhoeae* (PPNG). In Nigeria, among cases diagnosed with gonococcal infection, the prevalence of PPNG has been documented as ranging from 44 percent in Zaria[14,15] to 74 percent in Ilorin[16] and 80 percent in Ibadan.[17,18]

Nongonococcal Urethritis

It has been suggested that causes of urethritis other than gonorrhea may be of equal if not greater importance in Nigerians. These include herpes simplex virus, *Gardnerella*

Table 2. Reported Gonorrhea Incidence and Prevalence in Nigeria, Various Studies

Author	Study population	Infection rate
Osoba (1972)[1]	Ibadan:* Asymptomatic women Prostitutes Female hospital patients	5.0% 15.8% 17.0%
Wilcox (1946)[2]	Nigeria troops (wartime)†	600 per 1,000
World Health Organization Expert Committee on Gonococcal Infection (1963)[3]	Lagos: Adult population*	490.8 per 1,000
Romanowski (1952)[4]	Sokoto survey†	97 per 1,000
Osoba, Onifade (1973)[5]	Ibadan: Asymptomatic pregnant women*	3.4%
Rotimi, Somorin (1980)[6]	Lagos: Males and females (N=276)*	19.2%
Bello (1982)[7]	Zaria: Asymptomatic males and females*	5.5%
Bello, Elegbe, Dada (1983)[8]	Zaria: Males and females (N=910)*	28.1%

* Incidence.
† Prevalence.

vaginalis, Ureaplasma urealyticum, and Staphylococcus saprophyticus.[19] The few reports available in Nigeria (Table 3) document the prevalence of nongonococcal urethritis (NGU) as varying from 26 percent to 61 percent among men seen at an STD clinic. Again, these data are hospital-based, and it is probable that private physicians and herbalists treat more patients with NGU than with gonorrhea. In a study of 442 males with urethral discharge in the UCH, 271 (61 percent) had gonococcal urethritis, and mycoplasma isolation was found in the genital secretions of 24–60 percent of the subjects.[1]

It is also noted in a study that 35 percent of women attending the family planning clinic and 10 percent of those attending the antenatal clinic at Ibadan had seroepidemiological evidence of chlamydial genital infection.[20] In another study, of 1,485 IUD acceptors in Ibadan, approximately 7 percent tested positive for chlamydia.[59] In general, however, there is very little information on chlamydia and NGU in Nigeria, as the technology for culture or immunofluorescent is not available.

Trichomonal Infection

Trichomonas vaginalis is one of the most common causes of vaginal discharge among

Table 3. Reported NGU Prevalence among Men
Seen at an STD Clinic in Nigeria, Various Studies

Author	Study population	Prevalence (%)
Osoba (1972)[1]	Ibadan: Males with urethral discharge (N=442)	61
Rotimi, Somorin (1980)[6]	Lagos: Males (N=276)	59
Sogbetun, Alausa, Osoba (1977)[13]	Ibadan: Males (N=578)	26

Nigerian women, and it sometimes coexists with *Candida albicans.* Several reports have indicated that the prevalence of trichomonal infection in Nigeria varies from 3 percent to 27 percent (Table 4). Overall, 10 of the 842 men (1 percent) and 87 of the 414 females (16 percent) diagnosed at the STD clinic, UCH, had trichomonal infections.[22]

Table 4. Reported Trichomonal Infection Prevalence in Nigeria, Various Studies

Author	Study population	Infection rate (%)
Rotimi, Somorin (1980)[6]	Clinic patients (N=276)	11
Osoba, Onifade, Alausa (1973)[21]	Ibadan: Pregnant women Clinic patients complaining of vaginal discharge Asymptomatic women Infertile women	21 15 27 21
Abioye-Huteyi, Osoba (1978)[22]	Ibadan: Male STD clinic patients (N=842)	1
Aimakhu (1974)[23]	Ibadan: Clinic patients with vaginal discharge	22
Ogunbanjo, Osoba (1987)[24]	STD clinic patients (females)	20
Acholonu (1984)[25]	Imo State	10
Konje et al. (1990)[26]	Female family planning clinic patients (N=2,224)	3

Candidiasis

Candidiasis causes troublesome vaginal discharge and is usually associated with intense vulvitis. The prevalence among Nigerian women ranges from 2 percent in family planning clinics to 33 percent among pregnant women in Ibadan (Table 5).

Among patients attending an STD clinic at Ibadan, a prevalence of 4 percent was reported,[13] while a higher prevalence—9 percent—was found in Zaria.[8] It is well recognized that candidiasis can be sexually transmitted, causing lesions in both sexes. Nine (2 percent) of 442 males investigated for urethritis at Ibadan were found to have urethral candidiasis.[1] However, the role of genital candidiasis in reproductive failure is still undetermined.

Genital Herpes

The incidence of this disease is not known, as most patients with mild genital herpetic lesions probably self-medicate or seek treatment from pharmaceutical outlets. Serological studies at Ibadan showed that 13 percent of young women presenting at UCH had experienced infection with the genital herpes virus type 2.[27,28] A much lower prevalence—1 percent—was reported in Zaria.

Human Papilloma Virus (HPV)

HPV infections have strong epidemiological links with the genesis of cancer of the cervix. In Nigeria, as in other parts of Africa, cancer of the cervix is the most common female malignancy, with a relative cancer frequency ratio of 20 percent. Although no HPV studies have been done on cervical cancer in Nigeria, there is clinical evidence that genital warts are detected among patients attending STD clinics (Table 1). Male partners who are promiscuous tend to transfer the infection to their spouses, and vice versa. Early detection of HPV and appropriate therapy could reduce the incidence of invasive lesions.

Table 5. Reported Vaginal Candidiasis Prevalence in Nigeria, Various Studies

Author	Study population	Infection rate (%)
Osoba (1972)[1]	Ibadan: Males (N=442, of whom nine had urethral candidiasis)	2
Bello, Elegbe, Dada (1983)[8]	Zaria: STD patients	9
Onifade, Osoba (1975)[11]	Ibadan: Pregnant women	33
Sogbetun, Alausa, Osoba (1975)[13]	Ibadan: STD clinic patients	4
Osoba, Onifade, Alausa (1975)[21]	Ibadan: Asymptomatic women	12
Konje et al. (1990)[26]	Ibadan: Family planning clinic clients (N=2,224)	2

Bacterial Vaginosis

Various types of vaginitis have been described, but the most controversial has been that associated with *Gardnerella vaginalis*. The occurrence of *Gardnerella vaginalis* in Lagos prenatal clinic patients is 30 percent among pregnant women and 51 percent among nonpregnant women.[29] At Ibadan, 43 percent of 312 patients presenting with vaginal discharge were infected with *Gardnerella vaginalis*.[30] In a recent study among 2,224 adult women attending a family planning clinic in Ibadan, *Gardnerella vaginalis* occurred in 25 percent of those presenting with discharge and in 9 percent of asymptomatic controls.[26]

Syphilis

The overall picture of syphilis in Nigeria is still unclear, as there are no reliable statistics on its prevalence. The clinical impression, however, based on the diminishing number of patients presenting with symptoms and signs of *Treponema pallidum* infection at urban hospitals and the increasing rarity of cardiovascular syphilis and neurosyphilis,[31] is that the incidence has fallen. Some believe that this apparent decline may be related to the increasing and often indiscriminate use of penicillin and other antibiotics. Furthermore, it is generally believed that yaws has been successfully eradicated in Nigeria. However, 5–6 percent of blood donors and antenatal clinic patients studied had reactive serological tests for syphilis, while 3 percent of 15,399 hospital patients were reactive.[32,34] In Lagos, 95 (10 percent) of 930 antenatal clinic patients had positive serological tests for syphilis.[6] The reported prevalence of syphilis ranges from 1.2 percent in Zaria[34] and 1.4 percent in Lagos[6] to 2.5 percent in Ibadan.[13]

Tropical Venereal Diseases

The so-called tropical venereal diseases comprise lymphogranuloma venereum (LGV), granuloma inguinale, and chancroid. Their incidence is unknown, as they are frequently unrecognized and therefore unreported by most practitioners. Yet, these diseases are said to be prevalent in tropical areas of West and East Africa.[35,36] LGV and chancroid are well-known causes of genital ulcerations among Nigerians. These conditions, when ignored, produce tissue destruction of the external genitalia and perineum. However, the conditions respond readily to antibiotic therapy if diagnosed early. As early as 1937, 11 cases of LGV complicated by rectal stricture were reported among northern Nigerians,[37] while in 1963, 26 cases were found in southern Nigerian women.[35] The few reports that have appeared since then are mainly hospital-based. These include a prevalence rate of 3 percent at Ibadan[13] and a prevalence of 5 percent at Zaria. In a seroepidemiological study of LGV involving 5,006 individuals from various population groups and social classes in two large cities in Nigeria, the seroactivity rates ranged from 5 percent to 18 percent.[33]

Chancroid, too, is not uncommon in Nigeria, though it appears to be less frequent than in Central and East Africa. For instance, 27 (3 percent) of the 860 males and 4 (0.5 percent) of the 709 females seen at the STD clinic at UCH in 1989 had chancroid diagnoses. At Ilorin, it was observed that 19 percent of all genital sores were caused by chancroid.[38]

POSTABORTAL SEPSIS

The incidence of abortion in Nigeria is unknown, although evidence on the morbidity and mortality associated with abortion indicates that it is a serious public health problem. Septic abortion is one of the most commonly treated conditions in obstetrics and gynecology services.[39] The majority of cases follow clandestine illegal abortions, although sepsis can also follow spontaneous abortions or premature spontaneous rupture of membranes, especially in communities where medical services are inaccessible or inadequate.[39-42]

In a 10-year review in Ibadan,[43] there were 400 cases of septic abortion out of 2,700 hospitalized cases of abortion, giving an incidence of 15 percent. The largest proportion (34 percent) occurred in the age group 21–25 years. Of these, 26 percent were among young primigravidae. At the UCH, 7 percent of all maternal deaths over a 10-year period (1960–69) resulted from complications of abortion.[44]

In a review of maternal deaths at Benin City (1973–85), abortion was one of the three major causes of death, accounting for 37 (22 percent) of 165 deaths.[45] Induced abortion was responsible for 34 (92 percent) of these deaths. The usual victims were sexually active teenagers who had no ready access to contraceptive services. Similar findings have been reported by other workers.[46,47]

In a more recent review from Ibadan, it was observed that 119 women with septic abortions were admitted to UCH between 1981 and 1985; of these, 82 percent had had induced abortions.[48] Single girls between the ages of 12 and 20 were the largest group (37 percent). The duration of hospital stay varied from one day to 300 days; *Escherichia coli* was the most causative organism. Findings from the same hospital revealed that among 420 women admitted after induced abortion between 1980 and 1989, 86 percent had sepsis, and septicemia accounted for three of the six maternal deaths.[49]

The role of sepsis is becoming increasingly significant as illegal abortion continues to thrive among quacks, charlatans, and traditional healers. When abortion is complicated by sepsis, particularly *Clostridium welchii* or tetanus infections, the morbidity and mortality rates are phenomenal.[50] In a review of maternal death at Benin City,[45] tetanus infections were factors in seven deaths, six of which resulted from postabortal sepsis. Most tetanus complications arise from the unsanitary methods of illegal abortion.

POSTOPERATIVE SEPSIS

The majority of cases of maternal morbidity and mortality from operative deliveries are due to severe hemorrhage and postoperative septicemia. Most of the septic cases occur partly because many patients and their relatives waste valuable time consulting oracles, native doctors, or prayer houses when difficulties arise and report to the hospital rather late, and partly because health care facilities are not available.

Analysis of a report on maternal deaths from Port Harcourt showed that one of the main causes of death was bacterial infection following operative delivery.[51] Most of these deaths occurred in primigravidae. It was also reported that most deaths that occurred 24 hours after the woman's arrival at the hospital were mainly the result of infection.

Incidence of infection following abdominal deliveries is high. In Port Harcourt, bacterial infection contributed to death both in those who had had and in those who had not had antenatal care (33 percent and 35 percent, respectively).

The major cause of deaths associated with emergency cesarean section at Enugu was postoperative sepsis, contributing to 29 percent of the 17 maternal deaths.[52] In a similar review of maternal deaths following cesarean section at Ile-Ife, sepsis was a common cause of death.[53] This includes wound sepsis (6 percent), genital sepsis (2 percent), and urinary tract infection (0.4 percent). This experience is similar to those from other centers in Nigeria[54,55] and is in sharp contrast to those from developed countries. In a review from UCH, it was reported that postcesarean section wound was associated with pelvic sepsis involving the pelvic organ, which affected subsequent fertility.[56]

Among factors that contribute to the morbidity and mortality associated with abdominal deliveries in Nigeria are prolonged labor, preexisting genital sepsis, ruptured uterus, and antepartum hemorrhage. However, improving the standard of hygiene of the hospital, adoption of proper aseptic techniques at surgery, gentle handling of tissues, and prompt treatment of sepsis would go a long way to reduce the incidence of deaths from infection.

INFECTION ASSOCIATED WITH CONTRACEPTIVE USE

With the high incidence of STDs in Nigeria, the potential increase in the incidence of PID among contraceptive users has been a major concern among providers and policymakers. Several studies from outside Nigeria have suggested an association between PID and the use of IUDs.[57,58] Current information suggests that PID among IUD users is most likely caused by bacterial contamination of the endometrial cavity at the time of IUD insertion.

Studies on the association of RTIs and IUD use are scarce in Nigeria, although the IUD is currently the most popular method among contraceptive acceptors. Recently, a randomized clinical trial of 1,485 women in Nigeria evaluated the effectiveness of 200 mg doxycycline (vs. placebo) given orally at the time of IUD insertion in reducing the incidence of PID during the first three months of IUD use.[59] It was observed that the rate of PID in the doxycycline-treated group (1.7 percent) was, in fact, higher than that in the placebo-treated group (1.3 percent), and the rate of unscheduled IUD-related visits to the clinic was not significantly lower among the doxycycline-treated group. It would appear that the population studied was at a lower risk for IUD-related PID than was previously thought. These rates are lower than expected in view of the general opinion that RTIs are widespread in Nigeria. This is the only case-control IUD-PID study in Nigeria; hence, other centers should be encouraged to replicate this study.

A review of cases of pelvic abscess at the University of Nigeria Teaching Hospital, Enugu, revealed that 23 percent of patients were IUD users, as were 18 percent of patients with pelvic sepsis, previously reported from the same institution in 1975.[60,61]

Other contraceptive methods available in Nigeria have not been implicated in the pathogenesis of PID. In fact, they appear to be of advantage in this regard. Barrier methods may prevent cervical infection by PID-causing pathogens, but information is lacking on this in Nigeria.

CONSEQUENCES OF RTIs

RTIs can lead to male and female infertility. In the Nigerian culture, there is a high premium on fertility, particularly as a demonstration of consummation of the marriage and as one expression of the couple's social role. Information on the prevalence of infertility at the community level is scanty. However, two studies, in Oyo and Kwara states, indicate that there are pockets of high levels of infertility.[62,63] The overall prevalence rate in Kwara was 30 percent—9 percent for primary infertility and 21 percent for secondary infertility. The higher incidence of secondary infertility suggests a postconception factor, which in this environment is due to RTIs—either an STD, postpartum or postabortal sepsis, or, occasionally, pelvic tuberculosis. Primary infertility is rare after the age of 30 years. In about two thirds of infertile females, tubal disease as a sequelae of PID is the major cause of infertility.

The incidence of ectopic pregnancy is also higher in patients who have had pelvic infection. A follow-up study of such patients indicates poor reproductive performance[64]— while 40 percent subsequently conceive, 37 percent remain infertile, and 14 percent have recurrent ectopic pregnancy.

Other sequelae of RTIs include chronic pelvic pain, congestive dysmenorrhea, menstrual disorders, increased risk of fetal wastage, funiculitis, urethritis, epididymo-orchitis, and sometimes filariasis, which can lead to hydrocele and lymphovaricocele. Between 40 percent and 50 percent of males in infertile union have abnormal spermograms. In the majority of these cases, gonadal atrophy and previous genital tract infection are the major causes of compromised reproduction; hence, results of chemotherapy are generally poor.

SOCIOECONOMIC AND CULTURAL VARIABLES THAT AFFECT PREGNANCY AND THE SEVERITY OF RTIs

Although there are studies that have identified socioeconomic and cultural factors that affect the health of women in Nigeria, very few have specifically highlighted the impact of these factors on RTIs. Some traditional practices are beneficial, some are harmful, and others have no effect at all.[65]

Widely Dispersed Population

The majority of Nigerians are rural dwellers living in widely dispersed villages that are distant from health centers. Poor transport is also responsible for underutilization of health facilities, while the nomadic life-style of the Fulanis makes follow-up of RTIs in this community difficult. Rural/urban migration by people seeking gainful employment has created a severe strain on limited urban infrastructures and led to overcrowding, poor housing conditions, inadequate water supply and waste disposal, and other social problems that enhance RTIs.

Cultural Practices

In Nigeria, marriage patterns vary from one region to another. However, of relevance to the subject of RTIs is the practice of purdah (the system of secluding women) by Muslims, who believe that this reduces promiscuity among their wives and young girls. In polygamous settings, however, a woman runs the risk of contracting RTIs, especially if her husband has extramarital sexual relationships with an infected individual. Women in purdah sometimes seek extramarital affairs out of sexual frustration, with the potential risk of infecting not only the husband but other wives. While the men in such circumstances often seek medical care, the subordinate and secluded status of the women makes access to health care difficult for them, especially when medical units are staffed by male doctors. Thus, women are generally denied the opportunity to discuss their reproductive health problems, and the potential risk of reinfection is real.

Clitoridectomy, which is still practiced among some Nigerian tribes, has short- and long-term sequelae, including RTIs, subsequent PID and infertility, and failure to consummate marriage due to genital scarification. It is estimated that 50 percent of Nigerian females undergo clitoridectomy[66] for a variety of reasons, including religious sacrifice, attenuation of sexual desire, and initiation rites.

The "Gishiri cut" is a traditional operation practiced among the Hausa in northern Nigeria[67] in which the vagina is cut, usually by old women using unhygienic razor blades. It is used to treat various gynecologic and obstetric conditions, including prolonged labor. RTIs, vesicovaginal fistula, and fatal hemorrhage are common complications. Some of these result in extreme social stigma and personal discomfort. The traditional Hausa custom of child marriage and early sexual initiation often results in pregnancy at a time when the young girl has not achieved the necessary physical growth. The consequence is prolonged obstructed labor and its life-threatening sequelae, among which are RTIs.

Jehovah's Witnesses refuse blood transfusions; hence, uncorrected anemia among this group would increase susceptibility to postpartum infection, in particular RTIs. Recently, the emergence of new churches has created concern because their practices are different from those of orthodox churches that have established hospitals run by medical personnel. Many women use valuable time consulting oracles and prayer houses, and resort to health clinics or hospitals only when all else has failed. These new practices have emerged as community culture, probably influenced by the depressed economy, rather than by Islamic or Christian practice.

To a large extent, Nigerians depend on traditional systems of health care for a variety of reasons, despite the potential risks. For example, traditional birth attendants are known to be responsible for about 70 percent of all deliveries.[68,69] They have acquired practical skills over the years, but they practice in unhygienic circumstances that may increase the patient's risk of acquiring RTIs. Such infections are often treated with traditional methods that may not have therapeutic effects and may be harmful (e.g., insertion of caustic herbs into the birth canal).

Economic and Social Pressures

In recent times, because of economic depression and limited job opportunities, women have been under profound social pressure to enter occupations in which they are vulnerable to forced sex and its consequences. For example, several incidents of sexual molestation in the course of street hawking have been reported.[70-72] Noncommercial prostitution is very common, usually for material or financial gain. For example, married women and females in institutions of higher learning accept food or money from older men with whom they establish casual sexual relations. They are often pressured into this because of the prohibitive cost of living.

Various studies suggest that levels of premarital sexual activity are high. In a study of motivation for birth control,[73] almost one third of women respondents indicated they began practicing contraception because they were unmarried or in school. More recently, it was reported that premarital sexual behavior has become more common over time, as Nigerian society has undergone marked social change, and that this behavior appears to be more common among women from nontraditional backgrounds.[74] Reports from Ibadan have indicated that a substantial proportion of unmarried adolescents are sexually active (38–91 percent); the highest percentage is among nonstudents.[75] This liberal attitude to sex exposes the adolescent to STDs. It is noteworthy that this change in behavior is multifactorial; it may be partly due to the abolition of traditional and religious norms that regulated sexual behavior, the relaxation of parental control, and the influence of pornography and the media, which frequently portray women and sexuality.

Taboos against Discussion Related to the Reproductive Tract

In most African societies, discussion related to the reproductive tract is a taboo. Most women know that the reproductive organs are the part of their body responsible for procreation, and while they realize that the genital area must be kept clean (which must occasion minimal contact), they also know they are not supposed to look at it or touch it.[76] Additionally, young girls having their first babies are expected to be shy and modest; thus, the Hausa custom of "kunya" prevents a girl during her first pregnancy from discussing her pregnancy or its outcome with anyone.[77]

STDs as a Gender Issue

In periods of economic depression and political oppression, cultural forms of aggression projected on vulnerable groups abound in society, for they provide catharsis and diversion from frustrating economic and political realities.[78] Among these are sexual harassment and abuse perpetuated especially on young girls and women, which seems to be on the increase in Nigeria. These practices not only inflict mental torture on the victims, but also may create residual effects, sometimes manifested as reproductive tract pathologies, especially STDs. Some members of the society, for example, believe that urethritis can be cured by sexual intercourse with a virgin.

The cultural pattern in most communities in Nigeria is such that women occupy a subordinate position, and this may have a profound effect on their health. Most women of reproductive age are poor, malnourished, overworked, powerless, and pregnant or lactating most of the time. In most communities, they must obtain permission from their husbands to seek medical assistance. Therefore, the acceptance or not of modern medical care depends upon the husband, who is not likely to appreciate the physical discomfort and personal embarrassment caused by RTIs.

The women generally are expected to provide sexual pleasure on request and to produce as many children as possible, preferably males. The woman is blamed, therefore, for infertility, reproductive failure, and so on. The issue of women's social status has been ignored, largely because of religious and cultural barriers, and partly because of the low literacy level. This aspect requires in-depth social science studies and documentation. For example, sex roles also influence the power relationship within the couple, making it very difficult, often impossible, for females to determine when, with whom, and under what conditions they have sexual relations. More often than not, for example, women are unable to ascertain from a partner whether he has multiple sexual relationships or any signs of genital infection, unable to restrain their partners from having multiple relations, and unable to persuade their partners to use condoms or to obtain appropriate treatment for genital infection. Even when there is obvious genital infection, the male expects his wife to play her sexual role.

The complex dynamics of fertility preferences and attitudes about, as well as access to, modern contraception are largely affected by women's social status. This, in turn, affects their exposure to infection. In general, a woman's social and economic status is highly dependent on her fertility; hence, many Nigerian women value pregnancy more than their state of health and may engage in risky sexual relationships. Despite intensive public education on the protective value of condoms and spermicides in reducing the risk of genital infection, many women still are not able to insist that men use these barrier methods.

INTERVENTIONS FOR PREVENTION AND CONTROL OF RTIs

Symptomatic or asymptomatic vaginal discharge with or without PID represents a major medical and public health problem in Nigeria. This is evident from the World Health Organization multicenter study on worldwide patterns of infertility, in which the UCH participated.[79] Nigerians, like other African couples in that study, were more likely than those from elsewhere to have secondary infertility, a history of STDs or pregnancy complications, and infertility diagnosis suggestive of previous genital infection (e.g., bilateral tubal occlusion or pelvic adhesions). Although the available data base in Nigeria is limited to hospital records, the general consensus among clinicians is that STDs are on the increase in the general population, resulting in more cases of acute or chronic PID, ectopic pregnancy, infertility, and chronic pelvic pain.

Policy Issues

From the point of view of the woman, the priorities are as follows:

1. Control PID associated with STDs.
2. Prevent lower genital tract infections from ascending to the upper genital tract.
3. Limit the frequency and severity of long-term sequelae.
4. Strengthen the status of women through education and legislation that can also positively change the attitudes and sexual behavior of men.

In public health terms, this means that greater attention must be focused on prevention, diagnosis, and treatment strategies that combine complementary behavioral and biomedical approaches if any significant decline in rates of STDs is to be achieved. Prevention of exposure to chlamydial, gonococcal, herpes, and human immunodeficiency virus (HIV) infection depends primarily on the following interventions to change sexual behaviors:

1. Postpone age at first sexual contact.
2. Encourage one-to-one relationships.
3. Discourage sexual relationships with high-risk individuals.
4. Encourage abstention from intercourse during treatment of STDs.
5. Discourage coital and pericoital practices such as douching, using traditional medications, and engaging in intercourse during menstruation.

With specific reference to AIDS, Nigeria is regarded as a low-risk country. For example, out of 118,330 individuals screened to date, 516 were seropositive, while 84 cases were confirmed AIDS patients, according to the Western blot test.[80] Nigeria therefore has an opportunity to prevent widespread AIDS through a variety of interventions used for preventing other STDs.

Women with little social or economic power have the highest risk of HIV infection. Lack of access to basic resources, like condoms and STD treatment, and inadequate information on safer sex options compound their risks. Cultural constraints on sexual behavior and poverty often mean that women are unable to change their behavior, even if they are well informed. There is a need to sensitize various interest groups who collectively will have a long-term positive effect on attitudes and sexual behavior. Among the organizations and institutions that can help achieve behavioral change are the Multidimensional Approach to Fertility Management (MUDAFEM) program, which uses peer group counselors at tertiary institutions; the Society of Women for Prevention of AIDS in Nigeria; and the federal government, which can express its political and financial commitment through the national population program and through family life education in primary and secondary schools. Women can also mobilize and develop innovative strategies to change gender power relationships such that women and men will have equal status in terms of their roles.

Fertility Regulation

Contraceptive practice represents an important means of both primary and secondary prevention of RTIs. Some contraceptives help to reduce STD-related infertility. With regard to STD control, condoms and some spermicides protect against infection; oral contraceptives are also associated with reduced risk of PID. Efforts to enhance the safety of contraceptives (the IUD in particular) and to provide quality reproductive health services to women would encourage them to recognize family planning services as supportive of their needs.

Furthermore, family planning services reach women in the general population who would not otherwise have access to RTI information and services. Increasing demand for contraceptives requires a policy decision to make services available through both fixed and social marketing networks for selected contraceptive methods. Such services should run concurrently with intensive information, education, and communication (IEC) programs that are aimed at the high-risk groups (i.e., youths, commercial sex workers and men who patronize them, communities where multiple sexual relationships are condoned by social norms and religion or for economic reasons).

It is necessary to screen for STDs among clients requesting IUDs in order to reduce the risk of PID. Furthermore, contraception should be promoted in order to reduce the currently high risk of unwanted pregnancy. This effort will certainly reduce the risk of genital sepsis associated with induced abortion. Safe abortion procedures within the family planning setup are desirable, but will require changes in current restrictive law.

Primary Health Care

In Nigeria, only about 30 percent of the population are served by modern health facilities. In the past five years, primary health care (PHC) has been the focus of government health policy. In this effort, community mobilization and participation is a prerequisite; hence, an ideal opportunity exists for integrating STD information and relevant services into the PHC program. The village health system provides the foundation at the community level from which other tiers of service provision are built up to secondary and tertiary levels. The Village Development Committee consists of responsible individuals within the community whose role is to ensure community support and supervision of voluntary health workers. The committee also assists with information dissemination. Under the PHC strategy, women at the grass-roots level can be taught to recognize their own and their partners' RTI symptoms early in the course of infection, to use health care services, and to ensure compliance with specific therapy. Furthermore, since some genital infections are asymptomatic (e.g., gonococcal infection), women should be advised to have periodic medical examination if they are at high risk.

Facilities for Diagnosis and Treatment of STDs

Currently, the facilities for the diagnosis and treatment of STDs in Nigeria are abysmal, and the true incidence of all forms of STDs is unknown. However, some diagnostic and therapeutic interventions can be established at family planning, antenatal, and gynecology clinics, while specialized clinics can be strengthened for referral purposes. Adequate financial and material resources are required; thus, it is imperative that the government be politically committed to this strategy.

In most parts of Nigeria, diagnosis is based on clinical observation. Development of more adequate facilities for management of STDs and sound backup research are recognized as essential components for an STD control program.[80,81] Priority should be given to effective diagnosis of *Trichomonas vaginalis*, gonorrhea, and *Chlamydia trachomatis*. An STD clinic should be planned as an integral part of the outpatient department. Patients attending these clinics often do so with some reluctance; hence, such clinics are discreetly located, but should be adequately sign-posted.

The provision of good diagnostic and treatment services also implies training of various cadres of staff, in particular microbiologists and laboratory technicians, with a focus on STDs. Regional training seminars should be sponsored by the government to ensure that all health workers are familiar with contemporary views on the management of RTIs. Ideally, each local government should have both physical and manpower needs to provide STD management, or a functional STD clinic should be established in every major town as an initial step to control STDs. Such clinics would serve not only as reference centers for their environments, but also as training centers for all grades of medical personnel. Daily collection of data would provide information for health authorities that would enable future planning and control strategies to be developed.

With reference to AIDS control, the federal government of Nigeria has established an AIDS task force, funded by both the government and the World Health Organization, to ensure continued surveillance and public enlightenment. This is a positive effort to address the menacing subject of STDs. Finally, because of the epidemiological link of STDs with cervical cancer, it is imperative that the STD program include screening programs for cervical cancer. IEC programs should emphasize the potential risks of cervical cancer among high-risk women and wives of men who have STDs.

Research on Sexual Behavior and on Health Provider Behavior

An appropriately designed research project on sexual behavior is a sine qua non for effective secondary and tertiary prevention initiatives. It would also benefit primary prevention by helping identify means to decrease the prevalence of infection in the partner pool. There is a need to investigate the factors leading to sex with multiple partners or high-risk partners, young age at first intercourse, and sex during symptoms and therapy for STDs. Appropriate interventions to change these behaviors are essential.

Research is also needed on health providers' knowledge about both the behavioral and the medical aspects of RTIs, their sequelae, and their management. Simple research is needed to identify ways to ensure that health providers do not introduce infection, and ways that providers can encourage compliance with drug therapy, partner notification, and abstention from intercourse during infection and therapy. Interventions to promote these behaviors should be designed and tested. For example, a critical appraisal of counseling and partner notification approaches should be made. Equally important in a resource-poor country like Nigeria is evaluation of integrated programs (e.g., family planning plus STD control) vs. general education programs in terms of cost-effectiveness and cultural acceptability; further assessment of the cost-effectiveness of prophylactic use of antibiotics following IUD insertion by women who are at high risk is essential for a policy decision.

CONCLUSION

RTIs are a major socioeconomic and medical problem with myriad complications that have physical and psychological effects. Principal among the complications is the potential risk of reproductive failure, which is tragic in a society that places a high premium on childbearing and parenthood. Although both financial and institutional capacity for diagnosis and management are limited, the government should move quickly to set up a committee or use existing committees for AIDS surveillance to specifically integrate the above strategies within the PHC initiative. The IEC program is an effective conduit for information dissemination to the masses. While advocating for improved diagnostic and treatment strategies, women's organizations could help generate support for appropriate programs designed to identify RTIs and their consequences. Finally, resources should be available for continued research and surveillance if the level of RTIs is to decline significantly.

ACKNOWLEDGMENTS

This is to express gratitude to Mrs. Ronke Akinleye, Mrs. Margaret Adewunmi, and Mr. Samuel Onuoha for their secretarial assistance.

REFERENCES

1. Osoba AO. Epidemiology of urethritis in Ibadan. Br J Vener Dis 1972; 48:116–20.
2. Wilcox RR. Venereal disease in British West Africa. Br J Vener Dis 1946; 22:63–68.
3. World Health Organization Expert Committee on Gonococcal Infection. WHO study on world trends of early syphilis and gonorrhea during 1950–1960, WHO Technical Report 1963 (WHO publication no. 262, Geneva).
4. Romanowski V. A venereal disease survey in Sokoto town. W Afr J Med 1952; 1:166–70.
5. Osoba AO, Onifade A. Venereal disease among pregnant women in Ibadan, Nigeria. W Afr J Med 1973; 1:39–41.
6. Rotimi VO, Somorin AO. Sexually transmitted diseases in clinic patients in Lagos. Br J Vener Dis 1980; 56:54–6.
7. Bello CSS. Population screening for gonorrhoea in northern Nigeria. W Afr J Med 1983; 2:49–52.
8. Bello CSS, Elegbe OY, Dada JD. Sexually transmitted diseases in northern Nigeria. Br J Vener Dis 1983; 59:202–5.
9. Awojobi OA, Nkposong EO, Lawani J. Aetiologic factors of male infertility in Ibadan, Nigeria. Afr J Med Sci 1972; 12:91–4.
10. Osoba AO, Alausa KO. Gonococcal urethral stricture and watering-can perineum. Br J Vener Dis 1976; 52:387–92.
11. Onifade A, Osoba AO. Venereal diseases among women complaining of infertility. W Afr J Med 1975; 23:284–6.
12. Alausa KO, Sogbetun AO, Montifiore D. Effect of drying of Neisseria gonorrhoeae in relation to non-venereal infection in children. Nig J Paediatr 1977; 4:14–8.
13. Sogbetun AO, Alausa KO, Osoba AO. Sexually transmitted diseases in Ibadan, Nigeria. Br J Vener Dis 1977; 53:155–60.
14. Bello CS. Penicillinase producing Neisseria gonorrhoeae: report of first isolates from northern Nigeria. W Afr J Med 1982; 1:39–41.
15. Joshi RM, Lawande RV. Sensitivity pattern and beta-lactamase screening of Neisseria gonorrhoeae strains isolated in Zaria, northern Nigeria. Trop Geogr Med 1985; 37:74–6.
16. Odugbemi T. Sensitivity pattern of Neisseria gonorrhoeae in Nigeria and the significance of PPNG. Presented at the National Seminar on STD, Kano, Nigeria, September 19–22, 1984.
17. Osoba AO, Ogunbanjo BO. Penicillinase producing Neisseria gonorrhoeae in Nigeria. E Afr J 1983; 60:694–8.
18. Osoba AO, Montifiore DG, Sogbetun AO et al. Sensitivity pattern of Neisseria gonorrhoeae to penicillin and screening for beta-lactamase production in Ibadan, Nigeria. Br J Vener Dis 1977; 53:304–7.

19. Ogunbanjo BO. Sexually transmitted diseases in Nigeria. W Afr J Med 1989; 8:42–9.
20. Darogar S, Forsey T, Osoba AO, Dines RJ, Adelusi B, Crocker GO. Chlamydia genital infection in Ibadan, Nigeria: sero-epidemiological survey. Br J Vener Dis 1982; 58:366–9.
21. Osoba AO, Onifade A, Alausa KO. Genital tract infection and reproductive failure in developing countries. Nig J Med 1975; 5:401–6.
22. Abioye-Kuteyi EA, Osoba AO. Trichomoniasis in Nigeria: epidemiology and control. Unpublished data, 1977.
23. Aimakhu VE. Trichomonas vaginalis treated with a single dose of Trinidazole: full report. Int J Gynecol Obstet 1974; 12:84–7.
24. Ogunbanjo BO, Osoba AO. Trichomonal vaginitis in Nigerian women. Trop Geogr Med 1984; 36:67–70.
25. Acholonu WAD. Trichomoniasis in Imo State, Nigeria: a first report. Afr J STD 1984; 1:27–8.
26. Konje JC, Otolorin EO, Ogunniyi JO, Obisesan KA, Ladipo OA. The prevalence of Gardnerella vaginalis, Trichomonas vaginalis and Candida albicans in the cytology clinic at Ibadan, Nigeria. Afr J Med Sci 1991; 20:29–34.
27. Adelusi B, Osunkoya BO, Fabiyi A. Antibodies to herpes type 2 virus in carcinoma of the cervix in Ibadan, Nigeria. Am J Obstet Gynecol 1975; 123:758–61.
28. Adelusi B, Osunkoya BO, Fabiyi A. Sero epidemiology of herpes type 2 virus and carcinoma of the cervix in Ibadan. Afr J Med Sci 1977; 7:394–6.
29. Abudu OO, Odugbemi TO. Gardnerella vaginalis vaginitis in pregnancy. W Afr J Med 1985; 4:5–8.
30. Rotowa NA. Gardnerella vaginalis vaginitis in Ibadan. Dissertation, Nigeria Medical College, 1982.
31. Rampen F. Venereal syphilis in tropical Africa. Br J Vener Dis 1978; 54:356–64.
32. Osoba AO. Serological tests for syphilis among hospital patients in Ibadan. In: Proceedings of first medical research seminar, Lagos: West African Council for Medical Research, 1972.
33. Osoba AO. The control of gonococcal and other sexually transmitted diseases in developing countries with particular reference to Nigeria. W J Med Sci 1979; 2:127–33.
34. Adeoba A. Interpretation of positive serological tests for syphilis in pregnancy. Br J Vener Dis 1967; 43:249–51.
35. Lawson JB. Lymphogranuloma venereum in Nigerian women. W Afr J Med 1963; 12:89–94.
36. Lomhott G, Nsibarrbi J. Venereal diseases. Uganda Med J 1972; 1:109–13.
37. Ellis M. Benign tubular structive of the rectum in the African. Trans R Soc Trop Med Hig 1973; 30:515–20.
38. Onile BA, Odugbemi TO. Unpublished data.
39. Ladipo OA. Preventing and managing complications of induced abortion in third world countries. Int J Gynecol Obstet 1973 (Suppl); 3:21–8.
40. Akinla O. Abortion, maternity and other problems in Nigeria. Nig J Med 1971; 7:465–7.
41. Botu M. Septic abortion and septic shock. S Afr Med J 1975; 47:432–8.
42. Santamariva BG, Smith SA. Septic abortion and septic shock. Clin Obstet Gynecol 1970; 13:291–304.

43. Ojo AO. Septic abortion in Ibadan: a ten year review of cases. W Afr Med J 1978:51–3.
44. Ojo AO, Savage VY. A ten-year review of maternal mortality rates in the University College Hospital, Ibadan, Nigeria. Am J Obstet Gynecol 1974; 118:517–22.
45. Unuigbe JA, Oronsanye AU, Orhue AAE. Preventable factors in abortion related maternal mortality in Africa: focus on abortion deaths in Benin City, Nigeria. Trop J Obstet Gynecol 1988; 1(Special Edition):36–9.
46. Omu AE, Oronsanye AU, Faal MKS, Asuquo EJ. Adolescent induced abortion in Benin City, Nigeria. Int J Obstet Gynecol 1981; 19:495–9.
47. Oronsanye AU, Ogbeide O, Unuigbe E. Pregnancy among school girls in Nigeria. Int J Obstet Gynecol 1982; 20:409–12.
48. Konje JC. Septic abortion in Ibadan. Dissertation, Nigerian Postgraduate Medical College, 1986.
49. Adewole IF. University College Hospital, Ibadan, Nigeria. Personal communication, 1991.
50. Adadevoh BK, Akinla O, Post-abortion and post-partum tetanus. J Obstet Gynecol Br Commonwealth 1970; 77:1019–23.
51. Briggs ND. Maternal death in the booked and unbooked patients: the University of Port Harcourt Teaching Hospital experience. Trop J Obstet Gynecol 1988; 1(Special Edition):26–9.
52. Megafu U. Maternal mortality from emergency caesarean section in booked hospital patients at the University of Nigerian Teaching Hospital, Enugu, Nigeria. Trop J Obstet Gynecol 1988; 1(Special Edition):29–31.
53. Okonofua FE, Makinde ON, Ayangbacle SO. Yearly trends in caesarean section and caesarean maternity at Ile-Ife, Nigeria. Trop J Obstet Gynecol 1988; 1(Special Edition):31–5.
54. Adeleye JA. Primary elective cesarean section in Ibadan. Int Surg 1977; 62:97–9.
55. Oronsanye AU, Diejomah FME, Omene JA. A review of caesarean section at the University of Benin Teaching Hospital, Benin City, Nigeria (1973–1976). In: Ojo OA, Ainakhu VE, Akula O, Emmanuel LA, Chukudebelu WO, Brodena Ekstrands-Tryckeri AB, eds. Obstetrics and gynaecology in developing countries: proceedings of an international conference by Society for Gynecology and Obstetrics of Nigeria. Ibadan, Nigeria, 1977. Lund, 1980, 1977:402–9.
56. Ibeziako PA. Effect of post-caesarean section sepsis in subsequent fertility. W Afr J Med 1986; 5:35–9.
57. Grimes BA. IUCDs and pelvic infection. Am J Gynecol Health 1989; 111:23–6.
58. Senakaye P, Kramer DG. Contraception and the etiology of pelvic inflammatory disease: new perspectives. Am J Obstet Gynecol 1980; 138:852–60.
59. Ladipo OA, Farr G, Otolorin EO et al. Prevention of IUCD related pelvic infection: the efficacy of prophylactic doxycycline at IUCD insertion. Adv Contracept 1991; 7:43–54.
60. Okehilanu MG. Pelvic abscess at University of Nigeria Teaching Hospital, Enugu. Long commentary for fellowship examination, West African College of Surgeons, 1989.
61. Chukudebelu WO. Acute pelvic infection. W Afr J Med 1975; 23:284–6.
62. Nylander PPS, Ladipo OA. Infertility status in rural Nigeria. World Health Organization Community Survey, 1979. Unpublished.

63. Adetoro OO, Ebonmoyi EW. The prevalence of infertility in a rural Nigerian community. Afr J Med Sci 1991.

64. Akingba JB, Eneli AC. A review of 100 cases of ruptured ectopic pregnancies in Lagos, Nigeria. Nig J Med 1975; 5:241–6.

65. Odebiyi AI. Socio-cultural factors affecting health care delivery in Nigeria. J Trop Med Hyg 1977; 80:249–54.

66. Hosken FP. The Hosken report: genital and sexual mutilation of females. Women in Nigeria News 1979 (second enlarged edition).

67. Harrison KA. The influence of maternal age and child-bearing with special reference to primigravidae age 15 years and under. Br J Obstet Gynecol 1985; 92 (Supplement 5):23–31.

68. Ekabem II, Ebigbola JA, Ugyn AA. The role of traditional birth attendants in southeastern Nigeria, Ile-Ife: Ile-Ife Institute of Population and Manpower Studies, 1975.

69. Maclean U. Traditional healers and their female clients: an aspect of Nigerian sickness behaviour. J Health Soc Behav 1969; 10:172–86.

70. Stanching H, Kisekka MN. Sexual behaviour in Sub-Saharan Africa: a review of annotated bibliography. Project report submitted to British Overseas Development Administration, 1989.

71. Kisekka MN, Ahmadu Bello University, Zaria, Nigeria. Personal communication, 1990.

72. Obot I. Sexual abuse of children in Calabar, Cross River State, Nigeria. In: Child labour in Africa, Chuka Printing Company, 1986.

73. Ware H. Motivation for the use of birth control: evidence from West Africa. Demography 1976; 13:479–93.

74. Feyisitan B, Pebley AR. Pre-marital sexuality in urban Nigeria. Stud Fam Plann 1989; 20:343–54.

75. Nichols D, Ladipo OA, Patmen JM, Otolorin EO. Sexual behavior, contraceptive pill practice and reproductive health among Nigerian adolescents. Stud Fam Plann 1986; 17:100–6.

76. Koso TO. The circumcision of women: a strategy of eradication, London: Zed Books, 1987.

77. Trevitt J. Attitudes and customs in childbirth among Hausa women, Zaria City. Savannah 1973; 2:223.

78. Kisekka MN. Aspects of childhood and adolescent health needs in Nigeria. Presented at the UNICEF seminar on Maternal and Child Health in Nigeria, Ile-Ife, February 26–28, 1990.

79. Cates W, Farley TMM, Rowe PJ. Worldwide patterns of infertility: is Africa different? Lancet 1985; 2:596–8.

80. Federal Ministry of Health, Lagos. Unpublished data.

81. Rotimi VO, Somorin AO, Itafiz S. Suggestion for the facilities required for the management of sexually transmitted diseases in developing countries. Nig J Med 1982; 12:61–9.

REPRODUCTIVE TRACT INFECTIONS IN INDIA: THE NEED FOR COMPREHENSIVE REPRODUCTIVE HEALTH POLICY AND PROGRAMS

Dr. Usha K. Luthra
Indian Council of Medical Research
Institute of Cytology and
Preventive Oncology

Dr. Suman Mehta
Indian Council of Medical Research

Dr. N. C. Bhargava
Regional STD Centre
Safdarjung Hospital
New Delhi 110029, India

Dr. Prema Ramachandran
Indian Council of Medical Research

Mr. N. S. Murthy
Dr. A. Sehgal
Institute of Cytology and
Preventive Oncology

Dr. B. N. Saxena
Indian Council of Medical Research

Indian Council of Medical Research
Ansari Nagar
New Delhi 110029, India

Institute of Cytology and
Preventive Oncology
Maulana Azad Medical College
New Delhi 110002, India

INTRODUCTION

Worldwide, the subject of human reproduction is shifting from a mainly "demographic issue" to a broader women's health and development issue that is viewed as a key determinant of both individual well-being and societal prosperity. A general consensus now exists that reproductive health not only should include the ability to regulate fertility, but must also ensure optimal conditions for safely fulfilling the biological role of reproduction, namely, bearing and raising healthy children. Sound reproductive health policy and programs also must help both women and men to handle their sexuality with responsibility and dignity. These programs would enable women and men to cope with problems such as reproductive ill health—by preventing and treating sexually transmitted diseases (STDs) and other reproductive tract infections (RTIs)—as well as providing infertility and safe abortion services. Though many diseases place a heavy burden of morbidity and mortality on both men and women in developing countries, women are more often seriously affected because of synergistic effects of infection, malnutrition, and reproduction.

Reproductive Tract Infections, Edited by A. Germain *et al.*
Plenum Press, New York, 1992

The situation needs to be examined in India, a country with a very large absolute number of women in need of reproductive health care: approximately 133 million Indian women are in the reproductive age group, and they have 26 million births and 3–4 million induced abortions annually.[19,21] The demographic trends in India are important indicators of women's health status. The ratio found in the 1981 census,[21] 933 females per 1,000 males, reflects the higher mortality risk experienced by female children and women during the reproductive ages. The higher mortality for such women is largely preventable through use of appropriate health technologies, and development-oriented interventions and strategies, which emphasize a holistic approach to reproductive health care in national programs. The average Indian woman has about eight pregnancies and live births; typically, four or five of her infants survive. She is estimated to spend 80 percent of her reproductive years pregnant or lactating.[19] Thus, reproductive morbidity, including RTIs, exercises an adverse influence on her productive role in the society and a baneful effect on her health profile.

HEALTH SERVICE INFRASTRUCTURE

The population of India is increasing by more than 15 million every year and is approximately 845 million at present. Only 23 percent of the people reside in urban areas. To meet the health needs of the community, an extensive health infrastructure provides a comprehensive package of basic health care to the population residing even in the remote areas (Figure 1). There are about 130,000 subcenters (SCs), 20,000 primary health centers (PHCs), and nearly 2,000 community health centers (CHCs) functioning in the country. An SC staffed by two health workers, one male and one female, is expected to serve a population of 5,000 (3,000 in tribal areas and difficult terrain), and a PHC (with six subcenters in its jurisdiction) is supposed to serve a population of 30,000. The Indian Council of Medical Research (ICMR) carried out an evaluation of the family planning and maternal-child health (MCH) service components of the primary health care system during 1987–89. The results of this evaluation, conducted in 398 PHCs, indicated that the quality of care rendered was below prescribed norms.[27] In addition to the health providers functioning at PHCs and CHCs, a large work force is available at the grass-roots level to assist the community in utilizing health services — e.g., 500,000 traditional birth attendants and 400,000 community health guides.[22] The proportion of women attended by trained personnel during delivery has increased steadily in recent years.

While the present financial investments are below the national needs, they are not unimpressive. The national government's outlay for health and family welfare during the period 1980–85 represented 4 percent of the national "plan outlay," which includes the entire national budget, exclusive of spending on permanent infrastructure. Within the health and family welfare segment, the family welfare component (including family planning and MCH), which deals largely with reproductive health issues, more than doubled from the period 1975–80 to a value of about half the total health and family welfare budget during the period 1980–85. These nationally sponsored services are augmented greatly by nongovernmental organizations. By virtue of their flexibility in approach and the dedication of their workers, they have been successfully delivering primary health care in many locations, such as rural areas of Aurangabad, Pune, Ahmedabad, and Rajasthan.

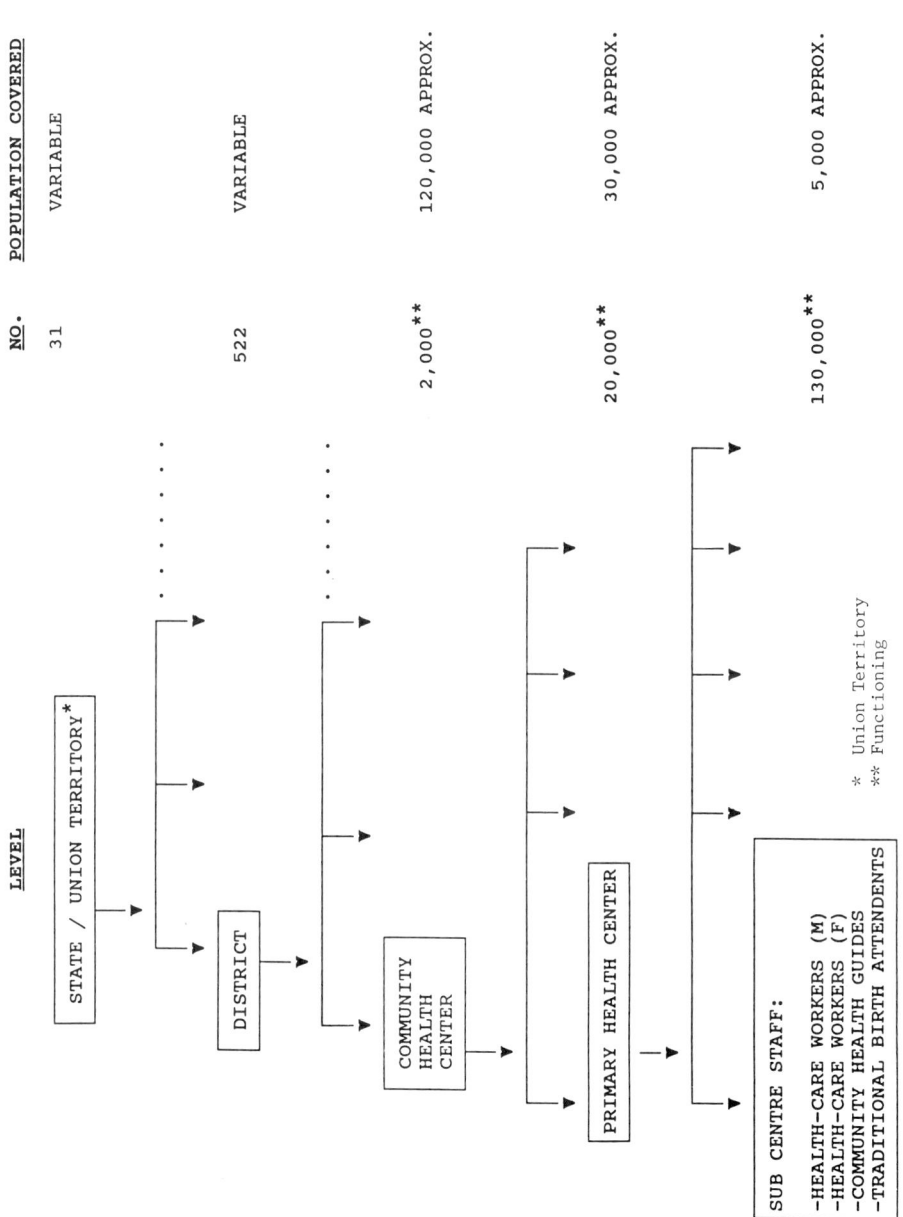

Figure 1. Health Service Infrastructure

MAGNITUDE OF THE RTI PROBLEM

RTIs, especially among females, are recognized by researchers and health professionals to be an important health problem in India, as evidenced by the large number of studies carried out in the country over recent years. However, the majority of these studies are limited to urban populations and to small sample sizes. In spite of these inadequacies, they provide useful information on the pattern, magnitude, and types of infection prevailing in different locations; they also supplement the data available from official sources.

At present, health services for women are mainly limited to care during pregnancy and childbirth, and contraception. Little, if any, attention has been given to the reproductive health needs of nonpregnant women and adolescents. Sociocultural barriers and taboos associated with diseases even remotely connected with reproduction and sexuality are major hindrances to seeking help when needed. Most Indian women are reluctant to talk to or be examined by male doctors, especially for gynecologic or sexual disorders. Nurses and paramedical workers are not trained to deal with gynecologic diseases, and the availability of female doctors in rural areas is very limited. Consequently, gynecologic care has remained limited to urban areas.

It is therefore not surprising that regional or national related to infection of the reproductive tract, one of the most common types of morbidity, are not available. The fact that the subject cuts across many disciplines and the multifactorial etiology of RTIs make them a challenging problem. Furthermore, the magnitude of the problem is expected to grow in the near future, because of urbanization and changes in sexual behavior of the younger population.

TYPES AND PREVALENCE OF INFECTIONS

Infections of the lower reproductive tract are common in Indian women of reproductive age, as is evident from numerous studies undertaken over the years and referred to in various sections of this paper. Such infections can be classified on the basis of clinical findings alone, such as the site and manifestation of infection; on the basis of the etiological agent; on the basis of microbiological or serological examinations; or on the basis of both clinical and laboratory findings.

Little information is available about the incidence or prevalence of gonorrhea in the population, largely because a substantial number of cases presumably go undiscovered. The prevalence of gonococcal infection was observed to be 2 percent in 271 women attending the gynecology clinic of a large hospital in Chandigarh.[20] Strains resistant to penicillin and other commonly employed antimicrobial agents have been reported from India,[10,13,45] as they have throughout southeast Asia.[46]

Prevalences of *Chlamydia trachomatis* ranging from 20 percent to 30 percent have been reported among men attending STD clinics in India.[12,44] Cervicitis with mucopurulent discharge is the most common manifestation of chlamydial infection in females. About 40 percent of all women with gonorrhea have concomitant infection with chlamydia; and the infection rate for both gonorrhea and chlamydia is highest in young sexually active women.[9,44] Ascending chlamydial infection can result in acute or chronic endometritis and salpingitis. Studies conducted in Delhi over a period of three years in 300 women suffering from acute or chronic pelvic inflammatory disease (PID) have shown the prevalence of *Chlamydia trachomatis* to be 6 percent in acute, and 29 percent in chronic, PID cases.[9]

Among 200 infertile women, the prevalence was observed to be 17 percent in primary infertility cases and 6 percent in secondary infertility cases.[9] Logically, many centers in India have reported a higher prevalence of chlamydial infection among contraceptive users (1–15 percent) and STD clinic attenders (15–30 percent) than among controls.[6,9,46]

In a study of risk factors related to cervical carcinogenesis, a cohort of 1,107 dysplasia cases and 1,077 controls matched by age and parity were tested for herpes simplex virus type 2 (HSV-2) antibodies, using indirect hemagglutination inhibition techniques. Very high proportions of cases (39 percent) and controls (42 percent) were positive for HSV-2, indicating that the virus is a common infection among women.[24] The roles of human papilloma virus (HPV) and HSV-2 in carcinogenesis have been studied and are referred to in later sections of this paper.

Other types of specific RTIs in women or men that have been studied in India include trichomoniasis, syphilis, and other causes of genital ulcers; mycoplasma infections; genital warts; and HPV infections.[7,17,18,23,30,40,42,43] It is recognized that some STDs—hepatitis B, syphilis, HPV, and human immunodeficiency virus (HIV) infection—may have no genital manifestations at all, but can give rise to systemic infection with grave manifestations. Some of these infections are further discussed below.

In addition to studies of specific sexually transmitted infections, some extensive observations have been made in Indian women concerning nonspecific genital inflammation or infection. The reported prevalence of excessive white discharge among women is quite high: approximately 50 percent of women complain of the problem.[12,20,35] However, not all women with white discharge suffer from lower reproductive tract infections. In a small group of rural women from Haryana State, 49 percent were considered to have vaginal discharge of bacterial etiology.[1] The presence of infection was significantly associated with substandard personal hygiene, low socioeconomic status, and husband's occupation: women married to service people had the lowest rate of infection, whereas women married to unskilled laborers had a significantly higher rate. Among women with abnormal vaginal discharge who do not have infection with candida or trichomonas, *Gardnerella vaginalis* found in over 90 percent of cases, whereas in matched controls, *Gardnerella vaginalis* was found in fewer than 10 percent of cases.[4,11]

Various studies conducted in India have shown that *Gardnerella vaginalis* has been isolated from 11–71 percent of women with abnormal vaginal discharge and from 3–16 percent of controls. Quantitative estimates indicate that the organisms were present in higher numbers in vaginitis cases than in controls. These observations are consistent with the possibility that bacterial vaginosis accounts for a proportion of cases of abnormal vaginal discharge. It has also been observed that 30 percent of IUD users had vaginitis; of these, 76 percent yielded cultures with *Gardnerella vaginalis*, with heavier colonization than was found in cultures of nonusers.[41,44]

In summary, a few clinical and microbiological studies have identified the presence of specific and nonspecific RTIs or infection-related syndromes in India. The distribution and extent of these conditions have been assessed in several surveys, as discussed below.

FACILITIES OFFERING STD SERVICES

There are more than 350 STD government clinics providing diagnostic and therapeutic services in India. In addition to these clinics, the medical colleges (about 130 in number) have combined STD and skin clinics. The majority of STD clinics are located in

metropolitan cities or at the district level, except in the states of Tamil Nadu and
Himachal Pradesh, where such services extend to the subdistrict level. Official statistics
point to an increasing trend in the number of cases seen at STD clinics (Table 1).[14] This
increase could be due to changes in sexual behavior, but also to many other reasons, such
as the opening of more facilities; better diagnostic skills; increased awareness of STD among
the population, especially those residing in the cities; or better reporting. Detailed data
pertaining to these diseases and the sociodemographic characteristics of individuals with
STD are lacking.

Table 1. Number of Reported Cases Seen in STD Clinics, 1981–87

Year	Number
1981	557,994
1982	457,414
1983	479,599
1984	919,085
1985	1,226,858
1986	1,275,822
1987	1,302,610

Source: reference 14.

The data in Table 1 are of limited value because the majority of patients suffering from
STDs do not come for treatment to STD clinics or other government-run facilities, such
as hospitals or PHCs. Patients usually seek treatment from general medical practitioners or
pharmacists, who do not report cases to their state governments because STDs are not
considered notifiable diseases. Even cases treated at the government hospitals are often not
documented properly. No large surveys at the national level have been conducted to define
the magnitude of the problem. However, surveys that have been conducted among selected
populations, such as commercial sex workers (CSWs) and pregnant women, indicate very
high prevalence rates of many STDs, particularly in urban settings.

STD PREVALENCE AMONG CSWs AND PREGNANT WOMEN

A large proportion of CSWs (82 percent), from a total of 200 attending a municipal clinic for various ailments, were observed to be suffering from STDs.[46] In addition to the ill health that the CSWs suffer, they pose a potential risk to their clients, who in turn place their other sexual partners at risk.

Antenatal populations are particularly suitable for surveillance of syphilis and other STDs. It has been observed that the rates of seropositivity for *Treponema pallidum* vary from place to place and from year to year. Among 9,380 pregnant women attending antenatal clinics at two hospitals in Delhi, the overall seropositivity rate was 1 percent in 1988.[15] However, review of available reports (published and unpublished) over a period of two decades (1968–88)[5] suggests that the prevalence of syphilis seropositivity in pregnant women elsewhere ranged from 7 percent to as high as 23 percent, as determined by Venereal Disease Research Laboratory (VDRL) testing (Table 2). These rates are as high as any that have been observed around the world. The observed differences could be due to different diagnostic procedures among centers and changes in lab methods, in addition to real changes in rates of syphilis over time.

SYPHILIS SURVEILLANCE OF BLOOD DONORS

Surveillance of syphilis seropositivity among blood donors, like surveillance of antenatal patients' rates, has traditionally been used to assess the extent, distribution, and trends in syphilis in the population. Table 3 shows that, in contrast to the apparent increase in number of reported STD cases seen in STD clinics in India (Table 1), the prevalence of positive VDRL tests among blood donors tested at the Institute for STD in Madras fell by nearly two thirds from 1978 through 1989 (except for a transient increase in 1987).[5] It is not certain if this reflects a true decline in rates of syphilis or simply a shift in the populations donating blood.

Table 2. Prevalence of Reactive Serologic Tests for Syphilis (VDRL) in Pregnant Women

City	Rate %
Bangalore	9
Bombay	7
Delhi	12
Madras	8
Madurai	12
Nagpur	23

Source: reference 5.

COMMUNITY-BASED RTI STUDIES

Perceptions about what constitutes morbidity are important in measuring the extent of a specific morbidity. Women are relatively unlikely to report to health care clinics if they perceive a condition to be normal, if the condition is associated with shame or guilt, or if they do not perceive any symptoms. For example, in a population-based study of gynecologic and sexual diseases in 650 women residing in two villages, 92 percent of

Table 3. Trends in Prevalence of Reactive VDRL Tests
among Blood Donors, 1978–89

Year	Number of donors tested	Total reactive		Reactive ≥ 8 dilutions	
		Number	%	Number	%
1978	8,131	923	11.4	353	4.3
1979	10,047	739	7.4	242	2.4
1983	9,726	626	6.4	205	2.1
1984	8,568	466	5.4	155	1.8
1987	9,612	813	8.4	229	2.4
1988	7,148	460	6.4	121	1.7
1989	9,860	383	3.9	121	1.2

Source: reference 5.

women were found on examination to have a gynecologic problem, but only 55 percent reported having a problem. The average number of diseases per woman was observed to be 3.6; RTIs contributed to half of this morbidity (Table 4).[2] Noteworthy features included the presence of reactive syphilis serology in 11 percent; microscopic evidence of trichomoniasis in 14 percent; clinical evidence of PID in 24 percent; and very high prevalence rates of nonspecific abnormalities, such as cervical erosion (46 percent), cervicitis (49 percent), and bacterial vaginitis (62 percent). However, sensitive tests for gonorrhea and chlamydia infection were not employed.

Table 4. Prevalence of Gynecologic and Sexually Transmitted Disease

Diagnosis	Number of women	% (N=650)
Primary amenorrhea	7	1.1
With mullerian duct aplasia	4	0.6
Without mullerian duct aplasia	3	0.5
Secondary amenorrhea	22	4.7
Functional uterine hemorrhage	6	1.3
Oligomenorrhea/hypomenorrhea	105	22.4
Polymenorrhea	4	0.9
Menorrhagia	71	15.2
Dysmenorrhea	269	57.5
Irregular periods	60	12.8
Primary sterility	20	3.1
Secondary sterility	24	3.7
Frigidity	57	12.3
Dyspareunia	43	9.3
Vaginismus	47	10.2
Senile vaginitis	20	11.0
Trichomonas vaginitis	78	14.0
Candida vaginitis	190	34.1
Bacterial vaginitis	347	62.2
Vaginitis of unknown origin	23	4.1
Cervical erosion	255	45.7
Cervicitis	272	48.7
Endocervicitis	67	12.0
PID	157	24.2
Ovarian cyst	6	0.9
Cystic ovary	5	2.3
Cervical dysplasia	7	1.1
Cervical metaplasia	8	1.2
Cervical polyp	10	1.5
Syphilis	68	10.5
Leucorrhea	22	3.4
Leukoplakia of vulva	4	0.6
Gonorrhea*	2	0.3
Cystocele	3	0.5
Vulvitis	2	0.3
Fibroid uterus	1	0.2
Other gynecologic disease	52	8.0

*The diagnosis of gonorrhea was based upon gram stain, not culture of endocervical specimens.
Source: reference 2.

Another community-based study was carried out in the field practice area (Alipur rural block) of the Institute of Cytology and Preventive Oncology (ICPO), situated near Delhi. In this study of 1,705 women, the feasibility of using paramedical staff to collect cervical smears in PHCs was evaluated (Table 5). It was noted that on direct questioning, 77 percent of women had gynecologic complaints; white vaginal discharge, lower abdominal pain, and backache made up the majority of these complaints. The distribution of symptoms was similar for those under 35 years of age and those 35 or older (Table 5). As shown in

Table 5. Percentage Distribution of Women Screened at Alipur Rural Block PHCs, according to Clinical Symptoms

Symptoms	Age of woman				Total symptoms	
	< 35 years		≥ 35 years			
	Number	%	Number	%	Number	%
White discharge	287	27.6	156	23.5	443	26.0
Contact bleeding	–	–	2	0.3	2	0.1
Irregular vaginal bleeding	13	1.2	9	1.4	22	1.3
Menstrual irregularity/ menstrual disorders	64	6.1	46	6.9	110	6.5
Lower abdominal pain	57	5.5	43	6.5	100	5.9
White discharge, menstrual irregularity, and pain in lower abdomen	73	7.0	46	6.9	119	7.0
White discharge and pain in lower abdomen	33	3.2	33	5.0	66	3.9
White discharge and menstrual irregularity	41	3.9	42	6.3	83	4.9
Backache	87	8.3	72	10.8	159	9.3
White discharge and backache	120	11.5	59	8.9	179	10.5
Menstrual irregularity and backache	11	1.1	5	0.8	16	0.9
Pain in lower abdomen and backache	7	0.7	4	0.6	11	0.6
No complaint	248	23.8	147	22.1	395	23.2
Total symptoms	1,076	134.9	699	135.0	1,705	100.1

Source: reference 29.

Table 6, a cytological diagnosis was possible in only 1,328 women, because some women did not agree to a smear or inadequate material was collected. While 28 percent of smears were normal, 62 percent were observed to be inflammatory (nonspecific type), according to World Health Organization (WHO) morphological criteria,[29] which are based on the presence of altered epithelial cell morphology, with or without the presence of increased numbers of inflammatory cells. An expert group discussed the problem of this high

Table 6. Percentage Distribution of Women Screened at Alipur Rural
Block, according to Cytological Diagnosis

Diagnosis	Number	%
Normal	371	27.9
Nonspecific inflammation	825	62.1
Vaginal trichomoniasis	93	7.0
Candida	5	0.4
Condyloma	9	0.7
Metaplasia	18	1.4
Atypical	1	0.08
Mild dysplasia	2	0.13
Moderate dysplasia	2	0.13
Dysplastic cells (grading not possible)	1	0.08
Malignant cells	1	0.08
Total	1,328	100.00

Source: reference 29.

proportion of nonspecific inflammatory smears at the Transfer of Technology Programme for Cervical Cancer, held in Delhi in 1986. The role of antibiotics in this situation was questioned, and data obtained at ICPO revealed that only 15 percent of the smears respond to such therapy. It is interesting that although the number of rural women tested is small, the prevalence of moderate dysplasia or malignancy in this rural setting was three out of 1,328 (0.2 percent), lower than that found in the urban setting described below.

HOSPITAL-BASED RTI STUDIES

The preliminary data from another ongoing hospital-based study indicated a very high proportion of lower genital tract pathology (72 percent), including pathology consistent with increased risk for cervical cancer (e.g., bleeding erosions, suspicious-looking cervix, unhealthy cervix)[20] (Table 7). Cervicitis, including hypertrophied cervix, was diagnosed in 21 percent of cases. This proportion was significantly less than that found in a community-based survey, reflecting differing diagnostic criteria, or perhaps better access to prior therapy for cervicitis among the hospital population. Several large hospital-based cytological studies of the frequency and type of RTIs reveal a varying picture. The largest study, in terms of sample size, entailed cytological screening of 117,411 women attending gynecology clinics of seven hospitals in Delhi (Table 8). The results showed that only about 26 percent of smears were normal; the remainder were diagnosed with inflammation (72.3 percent), dysplasia of various grades (1.6 percent), and malignancies (0.1 percent).[38]

In another study, cytological monitoring of cervical smears was carried out in a total of 8,307 women attending the gynecology outpatient clinic of Queen Mary Hospital,

Table 7. Distribution of Women Enrolled at Six Hospitals
in Delhi, according to Clinical Diagnosis

Diagnosis	Number*	% (N=21,599)
Vaginitis	523	2.4
Normal cervix	6,019	27.9
Cervical erosion	10,642	49.3
Cervical erosion that bleeds on touch	1,901	8.8
Hypertrophy of cervix	2,227	10.3
Cervical polyp	315	1.5
Cervicitis	2,333	10.8
Unhealthy cervix	1,194	5.5
Suspicion of cancer of the cervix	124	0.6
Cancer of the cervix	17	0.1
Prolapsed uterus	527	2.4
Dysfunctional uterine bleeding	113	0.5
Fibroid	188	0.8

* Some women had multiple diagnoses.
Source: reference 28.

Table 8. Percentage Distribution of Women Screened at
Initial Smear Examination, according to Cytological Diagnosis

Diagnosis	Number	%
Normal	30,397	25.9
Inflammation	84,889	72.3
Mild dysplasia	1,253	1.1
Moderate dysplasia	495	0.4
Severe dysplasia	162	0.1
Malignancy	215	0.1
Total	117,411*	99.9

*A total of 120,411 women were screened; adequate smears were available from 117,411 women.
Source: reference 38.

Lucknow, from 1971 to 1990. Cervical dysplasia was found in 5 percent of cases, and malignant smears in 1 percent. Trichomonas infection was the most prevalent STD (4 percent) detected by cytology, and its prevalence was highest in the youngest women, below 20 years of age. The association between contraceptive use and cervical dysplasia was explored in 3,374 women using different types of IUDs and hormonal contraceptives. No Lippes Loop users or copper IUD users developed cervical neoplasia or severe dysplasia, confirming the previous observations of the investigators.[36,37]

Similar findings have also been reported from a multicenter study where the rate of initial dysplasia among 804 acceptors of copper IUDs (1971–72) was observed to be 4 percent; women who continued IUD use were followed up prospectively. During the period of IUD use, 28 women developed dysplasia. At the end of 48 months of follow-up, all cases of dysplasia observed either initially or during follow-up periods had regressed to normal status.[33]

PATTERNS OF SEXUAL BEHAVIOR AND
OTHER SOCIOCULTURAL CORRELATES OF RTIs

There is little information available on sexual, behavioral, and sociocultural practices and patterns in India, and their correlation with the frequency and severity of RTIs. Such studies would be beneficial for the design of effective intervention strategies for the prevention and control of RTIs. Early marriage and childbearing and frequent births or abortions may increase the risk of infection. At present, nearly 80–85 percent of all births take place at home in rural areas. A large majority of these births are attended by untrained personnel, who are not necessarily using aseptic techniques. The situation with regard to abortions is several times worse, with services underutilized, even when available, because of sociocultural factors.[26] Practices such as abstinence during menstruation, religious ceremonies, and the postpartum period, together with improved patterns of service utilization, may reduce the risk of infections. Sociocultural norms, concerned with age at first intercourse and total number of sexual partners, are reportedly associated with cervical dysplasias and cervical cancer. The extent to which these sociocultural norms are adhered to, and trends in childbirth and abortion practices, can influence the prevalence of RTIs in the future.

In a prospective study of factors influencing the progression of dysplasia, 75 of 1,107 dysplasia cases and four out of 1,077 controls progressed to carcinoma in situ (CIS). The overall rate of progression to CIS in cases was 16 percent at the end of 108 months (follow-up used survival analysis). Early age at consummation of marriage and initially higher grade of dysplasia were identified as factors enhancing the risk of progression to CIS. The associations between progression and other factors—including religion, literacy status, parity, presence of cervical erosion, and HSV-2 positivity—were not statistically significant.[38] More recent data indicate that sexual promiscuity of the male partner is an important risk factor for cervical neoplasia. The husband's having had premarital sex was associated with a relative risk of 2.6 that the woman would develop moderate or severe cervical dysplasia; the relative risk was even higher (4.8) when the husband had extramarital sex. Sex with another partner before and after marriage increased the risk sevenfold.[28]

PROJECTIONS OF STD PREVALENCE

On the basis of observations from various studies conducted, it is apparent that reproductive tract morbidity related to STDs in India is quite substantial. For example, assuming that every tenth person among the sexually active population in the country is suffering from an STD, it could be estimated that as many as 20–30 million people are suffering from STDs. These numbers may grow in the years to come unless large-scale control programs are implemented efficiently and effectively.[5] Since estimates for specific diseases and syndromes are not available on a representative basis, it is not possible to make projections for each disease.

RECOMMENDATIONS FOR IMPROVING NATIONAL RTI SURVEILLANCE

It is clear that a system needs to be instituted for collecting RTI data from a representative population in the country. To ensure that the system remains viable, it should be integrated with the current data sources on health. A mechanism needs to be established whereby a grid of hospitals can network from different regions and pool their data at a central resource center. This center can be responsible for disseminating reports periodically. Since it is essential that the data gathered be of good quality, a uniform methodology for data collection and diagnosis also needs to be developed. Needless to say, a community-based component in addition to the hospital-based one is required, so that a complete picture emerges.

Establishment of a functioning network of hospitals for RTI surveillance is a challenging task, since within each hospital, collaboration among different departments, such as microbiology, ob-gyn, STD clinic, and community medicine, is necessary. However, under the aegis of the ICMR, a preliminary base already exists. The ICMR is supporting a network of centers to focus its research programs in the area of human reproduction, specifically contraception and MCH, and cancer and HIV surveillance, among others. These centers, mostly located in medical colleges, have experience in carrying out hospital- and community-based research programs. With minimal strengthening, these existing networks of collaborating institutions can provide an efficient data base for surveillance of RTIs. To provide data of good quality, the following steps would be required:

1. Retraining research staff in diagnosis of RTIs by visual examination of the cervix, examination of wet vaginal smears, and, where indicated, collection of material for laboratory testing.
2. Strengthening clinical facilities with microscopes, reagents, and other essential supplies.
3. Strengthening laboratories to carry out serology and cytomorphology work.

IMPACT OF RTIs ON CONTRACEPTIVE USE AND SAFETY

The strategy of the National Family Welfare Programme (NFWP) is to offer a variety of fertility control methods to eligible couples, to ensure as far as possible that all couples are able to find a method that meets their particular need. Currently, the NFWP offers sterilization, IUDs, oral contraceptives, and barrier methods. However, because of organizational and operational considerations, the program has depended heavily on sterilization. Some 80 percent of couples effectively rely on sterilization, and the rest on nonpermanent methods, such as IUDs, oral contraceptives, or barriers. Realizing that a sound family planning strategy should advocate emphasis on younger women, the program is making efforts to promote the use nonpermanent methods. In this context, RTIs gain importance.

With the use of nonpermanent contraceptive methods, the relative protective or risk-increasing effects of each method are particularly important. Data on contraceptive use are not routinely collected in India. Contraceptive prevalence is calculated by the family planning program as the proportion of eligible women protected by different methods, based not on the actual number of women accepting specific methods, but on the "distribution of methods" records maintained by health functionaries at different levels. "Equivalent sterilization" is computed by equating one couple protected by sterilization to the distribution of 72 condoms, 13 pill packets, or three IUD insertions per year (because only about one third of IUD acceptors continue with the method for one year or longer). Thus, in a PHC, distribution of 1,300 cycles of pills or 7,200 condoms, and insertion of 300 IUDs, is equated to 100 couples protected by each method for that year.

There are no mechanisms to gather data on long-term safety of contraceptives in the country, though women are screened prior to acceptance of a method. For example, paramedical staff conduct a preliminary screening, utilizing a simple checklist for potential acceptors of oral contraceptives. A supply of up to three months can be given to a woman with the advice that she should be examined by the medical officer. The examination includes complete systemic examination, and includes visual examination of the cervix, but not examination of wet vaginal smears or collection of cervical cytology. IUDs are inserted by female paramedical staff, as well as by medical officers, and visual examination of the vagina and cervix is performed prior to IUD insertion. Data are not available from the family planning service statistics on the extent to which specific contraceptives are not provided because of infection of the vagina or cervix.

The ICMR, through several research institutions, including the network of Human Reproductive Research Centres (HRRCs) located at medical colleges and the ICPO, is supporting operations research activities to improve the quality of care related to contraception and MCH within existing health services. A pilot study is evaluating the feasibility of training and utilizing auxiliary nurse-midwives, village health guides, Anganwadi workers (non-health personnel who are concerned with nutritional supplements for preschool children throughout India), and medical officers of PHCs in the detection of precancerous and cancerous lesions of the cervix by means of Pap smear in high-risk women. A system is being established for referral to secondary and tertiary levels of care for women requiring treatment for cancerous and precancerous lesions.[32] In a multicenter study in progress at 33 PHCs through the network of HRRCs, screening of women for breast and cervical cancer has been integrated with MCH services. Comprehensive training modules have been used to orient all categories of health workers in early detection and management of precancerous and cancerous lesions, and related aspects of antenatal, intrapartum, postnatal, and family planning care.

The outcome of these programs will be assessed on the basis of process indicators of performance and coverage, such as numbers screened, numbers referred, types of services provided, and quality of care rendered. These programs have been initiated recently; it will be some time before results will become available to guide replication on a wider extent.

IMPACT OF RTIs ON PREGNANCY AND CHILD SURVIVAL

No data are yet available on the impact of RTIs on pregnancy and child survival. A multicenter study has been initiated jointly by the ICMR and the United States Agency for International Development (USAID) at four centers in Varanasi, Lucknow, Pune, and Trivandrum. The first phase of the study aims to determine the prevalence of RTIs during pregnancy, and to document associations with adverse obstetric outcomes, including fetal growth retardation and low birth weight, in a sample of 800 women. Urine, blood, and vaginal discharge samples are collected at enrollment and at 34 weeks of pregnancy, for study of various infections, including syphilis, gonorrhea, and infections with *Mycoplasma hominis*, *Ureaplasma urealyticum*, *Trichomonas vaginalis*, and group B streptococcus. The laboratories have been appropriately strengthened with trained manpower and necessary equipment, and patient enrollment is in progress. The results from this study are expected to be available after 2–3 years to assess the need for intervention strategies.

RTIs AND CERVICAL CARCINOGENESIS

Cervical cancer is the most common cancer among Indian women. Data on cancer incidence for different regions are available from the National Cancer Registry Programme (NCRP) of the ICMR. The incidence of cervical cancer reported by the NCRP ranged from about 18 to 44 per 100,000 women for the period 1982–87. From NCRP data, it has been estimated that the number of cases of cervical cancer in India will increase from 92,000 in 1986 to 140,000 by the year 2000,[39] and that 61,000 women died of cervical cancer in India during 1990. Direct information on consequences such as proportion of female deaths due to cancer of the cervix, social stigmatization, and reduction in work capacity is not available.

The ICPO studies are aimed at elucidating the role of HPV, HSV-2, and other preventable possible cofactors for cervical carcinogenesis. Out of 63 cases of cervical cancer subjected to cervical cytology, colposcopy, and colposcopic-directed biopsy, 43 were found to have lesions that, by one or more parameters, suggest HPV infection.[31] A relative risk of 5.9 (with a 95 percent confidence interval of 2.5–14.1) has been found for the association of HPV 16 and 18 with progression of dysplasia to CIS or cervical cancer in Indian women.[17] In a community-based study conducted in Alipur Block, Southern Blot analysis showed a very high proportion of women (31 percent) to be harboring HPV 16.[29] To elucidate the role of HSV-2 in carcinogenesis, 167 cervical smears diagnosed as normal, dysplastic, and CIS were examined for the presence of HSV-2 antigen. Antigen was found in significantly higher proportions of cases of cervical dysplasia and CIS than in normal smears.[24]

In another study conducted at ICPO (1979–88), 1,107 dysplasia cases and 1,058 controls were followed up at periodic intervals.[28] Observations included the following:

1. The majority of the cases of CIS were preceded by various grades of dysplasia.
2. The progression from dysplasia to CIS took an average of 36–48 months. The interval was not affected by age or other risk factors for cervical cancer.
3. The protection afforded by a negative Pap smear was over 95 percent for an average follow-up of three years.
4. The average ages at detection of dysplasia, CIS, and invasive cancer 34.4, 38.6, and 47.8 years, respectively.

While many risk factors for dysplasia are related to behavioral or cultural factors, such as age at marriage and number of sexual partners, we believe that other cervical and vaginal infections and cervical erosions are strong biological risk factors; a prospective study that lasted for 11 years supports this hypothesis.[35] It was estimated that cervical erosions increase the risk of cervical dysplasia threefold, and the risk of infections, such as HPV and HSV infections, as well as vaginal infections, 13-fold. Further, the risk increases 60-fold when both cervical erosion and infection are present among women over the age of 35 years. Keeping in mind the high prevalence of cervical erosions and vaginal infections among Indian women, it is estimated that control of these two factors may lead to a reduction of more than 70 percent in the incidence of cervical cancer.[28]

HIV INFECTION AND ITS RELATIONSHIP TO RTIs

Realizing the potential threat posed by HIV infection and the urgent need to find out how the infection had affected India, the AIDS Task Force of the ICMR recommended initiation of serosurveillance for HIV infection among asymptomatic persons belonging to high-risk groups. The results of screening 102 female CSWs in February 1986, in a port city of Tamil Nadu, showed that 10 were HIV-seropositive.[25] The Task Force further recommended that national serosurveillance and clinical surveillance for HIV infection be initiated to obtain information on prevalence and major mode of transmission of HIV infection.

The national surveillance was established as a collaborative effort of the ICMR, the Directorate General of Health Services, and state health authorities. A network of five reference centers and 43 surveillance centers was established in six months within the existing health infrastructure, entailing a minimum of essential additional inputs. Surveillance was undertaken in three phases. The first two phases included screening of high-risk groups, and the third phase expanded coverage to blood donors and mother-infant dyads.

There was a steep rise in screening activities during the beginning of the third phase, among high-risk groups, and among blood donors and pregnant women. The overall seropositivity rate continued to be low (3.8 per 1,000), but an increase in the seropositivity rate among blood donors and men and women with multiple partners was obvious (Table 9).[25]

During 1990, the ICMR's National Institute of Cholera and Enteric Diseases, Calcutta, in collaboration with the Regional Medical College, Imphal, and state health authorities, carried out screening of intravenous drug users near the Golden Triangle, in northeast India. Preliminary results from the survey indicate that over half the drug addicts screened were seropositive. Efforts are under way to strengthen and expand facilities for HIV screening, for counseling, and for care of seropositive individuals in this region.

Studies undertaken in Vellore and Bombay have demonstrated a rather steep increase in the HIV seropositivity rate in the last five years among CSWs and men with multiple sex partners. By 1990, some 25–30 percent of all CSWs screened by these centers were seropositive. A similar increase in the seropositivity rate has been seen among men attending STD clinics in Vellore and Bombay. In 1990, nearly 10 percent of men attending these clinics were seropositive. Seropositivity rates among low-risk groups, such as pregnant women, and men and women attending hospitals for medical or surgical ailments in these cities, ranged between one per 1,000 and five per 1,000.

Though the AIDS surveillance is an ongoing priority, there are no large-scale programs that are exploring an association between HIV and RTIs. Under the National Medium Term Plan for AIDS Prevention and Control, blood donor screening and diagnostic testing have been strengthened. The program is being channeled through various levels of hospitals and clinics (teaching hospitals; district hospitals; and other hospitals, clinics, and AIDS units) and therefore envisages strong linkages with STD clinics.

THE VALIDITY OF EXISTING PERSPECTIVES ON RTIs

An interesting perspective on the nature of RTIs in women has evolved over the past few years in India. On the one hand, cytological surveys, clinical examinations, and rural population-based surveys have suggested that the prevalences of cervicitis and vaginal discharge are extremely high (up to 80 percent or more for cervical disease), and that these conditions may not be due to conventional STD pathogens. From this perspective, it appears that nonspecific cervicitis and vaginal discharge could be of preeminent importance in the etiology of cervical cancer (perhaps as a cofactor with HPV), as well as in other types of RTI morbidity in women, perhaps even as risk factors for transmission of HIV.

However, we recognize two limitations in these perspectives. There have been two levels of "nonspecificity" in development of the perspective that nonspecific cervicitis and vaginal discharge are a widespread problem in India. Both the clinical criteria used to define these conditions and the microbiological criteria used to infer the absence of conventional "specific" pathogens have been nonspecific or lacking.

First, the criteria used to define the presence of inflammation have themselves been nonspecific (e.g., WHO cytological criteria for nonspecific inflammation actually are based upon epithelial cell cytological and nuclear changes, with or without the presence of increased inflammatory cells; the presence of inflammation is inferred). Similarly, when visual inspection of the cervix shows cervical ectopy, the term "erosion" has been used, although neither colposcopic nor histologic evidence of epithelial discontinuity and inflammation has been documented to establish the presence of an abnormal state, as opposed to a normal physiological state of cervical ectopy. Similarly, the finding of abnormal vaginal discharge is not necessarily defined by microscopic or other criteria. Second, in these studies, laboratory tests for conventional sexually transmitted and cervical pathogens, such a *Chlamydia trachomatis*, *Neisseria gonorrhoeae*, and *Trachomatis vaginalis*, have not always been employed.

Along with the perspective that nonspecific genital inflammation is common in Indian women, it is widely held that STDs such as syphilis, chancroid, gonorrhea, and chlamydial infection may be quite uncommon, especially in rural areas. However, this perspective is not based upon recent surveys using modern laboratory technology. In fact, the high prevalence of reactive VDRL serologies in pregnant women (Table 2), the existence of a large commercial sex industry in larger cities, and the rapid increase in HIV seroprevalence in CSWs all suggest that this perspective must be critically reexamined. There is an urgent need for coordinated clinical and laboratory surveys of RTIs in women in rural and urban settings in India to assess the true prevalence of STDs and the possible relationship of conventional STDs to nonspecific lower genital inflammation, as well as to HIV infection.

INTERVENTIONS FOR RTI PREVENTION AND CONTROL: PLAN OF ACTION

Insights into the magnitude of RTIs have been provided, based on limited primary data from India and considerable secondary information now available from other sources. The evidence indicates that RTIs are an important health problem in the country. While mechanisms to ensure continuing availability of national-level data are needed, the real need is to develop appropriate intervention strategies for the prevention and control of RTIs. Services have remained limited to treatment of a few STDs and are inaccessible, as there are few urban-based clinics and hospitals offering such services, and socially unacceptable to the community. These efforts cannot pay dividends unless a holistic and comprehensive approach is identified and implemented. This will involve viewing reproductive health in a broader perspective, reaching beyond maternity care and family planning services, to include care for gynecologic and sexual problems, safe abortion services, and reproductive health education. Such endeavors must focus on populations at risk, and not just those with disease who seek care. It will also require shifting the emphasis from a *curative* approach to a *prevention and control* approach. Concentrating on specific groups, such as young adults and those at risk (e.g., subpopulations with multiple sexual partners and their partners), can enhance the cost-effectiveness of the approach. It is important that research and development efforts strive to identify ways to integrate the necessary components relating to RTIs with ongoing health and social welfare programs, instead of evolving new vertical programs.

Table 9. Trends in HIV Seropositivity Rates in Selected Groups

Group	October 1985– April 1986	May 1986– October 1986	November 1986– April 1987	May 1987– October 1987	November 1987– April 1988	May 1988– October 1988
MALES WITH MULTIPLE PARTNERS						
Number tested	1,072	3,000	852	7,212	7,105	5,967
Number positive	0	1	2	17	53	53
Rate per 1,000	0	0.3	2.3	2.4	7.5	8.9
Cumulative rate per 1,000	0	0.2	0.7	1.6	2.8	5.0
FEMALES WITH MULTIPLE PARTNERS						
Number tested	306	680	2,863	7,491	3,375	3,752
Number positive	0	3	4	7	14	20
Rate per 1,000	0	4.4	1.4	0.9	4.1	5.3
Cumulative rate per 1,000	0	3.3	1.8	1.2	1.9	2.5
BLOOD DONORS						
Number tested	872	2,184	2,340	5,137	4,413	12,795
Number positive	0	0	0	1	3	37
Rate per 1,000	0	0	0	0.2	0.7	2.9
Cumulative rate per 1,000	0	0	0	0.1	0.3	1.5

Source: reference 25.

The elements and modalities for such an action are outlined in Figure 2.

Prevention. The main group targeted for prevention should be adolescents and young men and women. The major components include enhancing knowledge regarding sexuality, reproductive processes, safer sexual practices (including use of barrier methods, such as condoms), and sexual hygiene. These actions must be undertaken at both the individual and the community levels through involvement of health and welfare sectors. Many approaches should be tested so that those most suitable to meet local needs emerge.

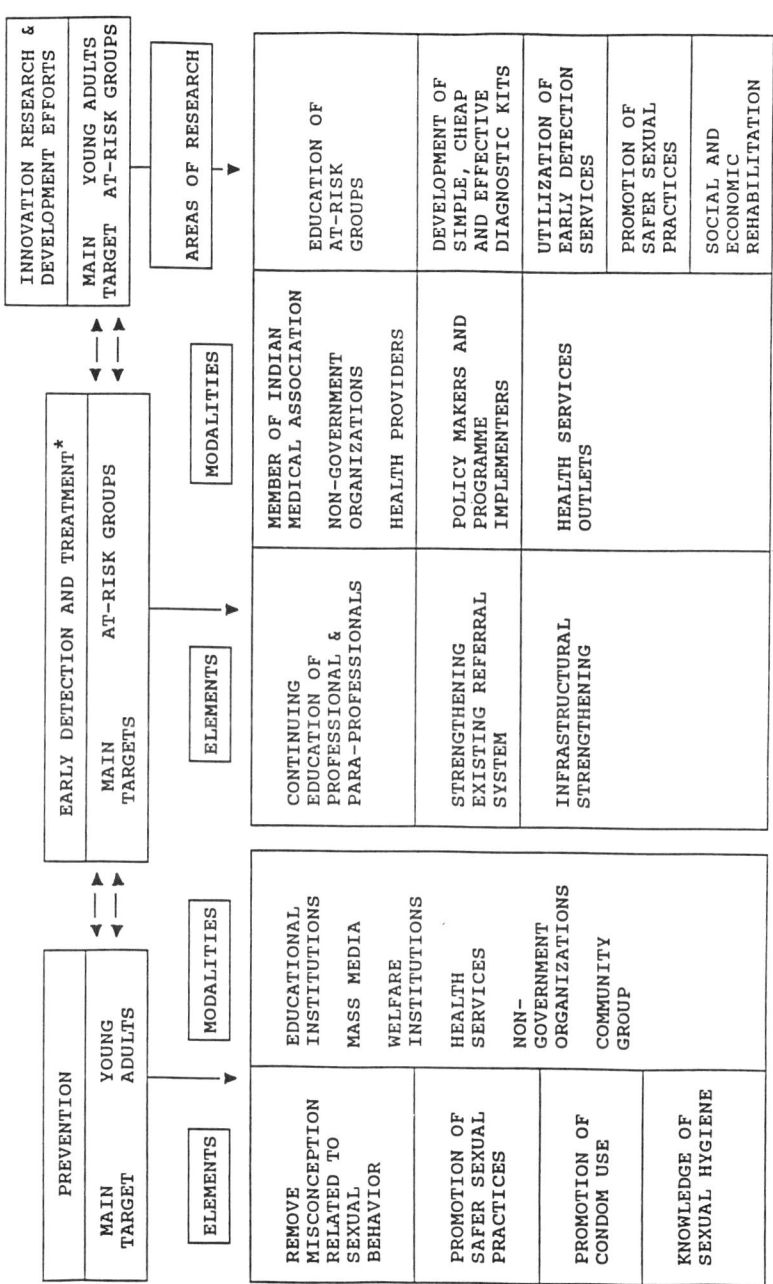

* Early detection and curative treatment of communicable sexually transmitted diseases equals primary prevention of these diseases.

Figure 2. Integrated RTI Prevention and Control: Plan of Action

Early Detection and Treatment. A special interest in India has been the evaluation of so-called downstage screening for early detection of invasive cancers by visual inspection of the cervix before symptoms of cervical cancer develop. Observations of cervical erosions that bleed on touch, growths or an unhealthy cervix (defined as a hypertrophied, elongated cervix with irregular contour and abnormal discharge) provide the basis for diagnosis. As reported, prospective evaluation of a cohort of women with cervical dysplasia has shown that 33 (52 percent) of 63 incidence cases of CIS or cervical cancer were detected at the time of diagnosis by visual inspection of the cervix. Most recently, in a study of 45,000 women attending gynecology clinics, it was found that women with a history of contact bleeding with intercourse had an eightfold increased prevalence of cervical cancer; among 5,135 women (11 percent of the total) with bleeding, erosions, suspicious-looking cervix, or a growth, 149 had cervical CIS or cancer (63 percent of the total cancers).[28,34]

A pilot program has been undertaken that demonstrates that paramedical personnel (medical social workers and auxiliary nurse-midwives) can be trained to do speculum exams and to differentiate between normal and abnormal cervices. Downstage screening, by symptoms and signs, could identify a substantial proportion of presented cervical disorders in India, allowing referral to central facilities that offer colposcopy and cytological screening.[32]

To achieve the objective of early diagnosis of other RTIs, as well as cervical cancer, continuing education of health professionals and paraprofessionals should include risk assessment and specific clinical training in the use of appropriate algorithms for RTI management. The training of health providers must go hand in hand with some strengthening of the current service infrastructure. For example, if vaginal smears are to be examined at the PHC level, provision of a microscope, reagents, and necessary drugs for treatment have to be ensured. Furthermore, financial and operational constraints preclude delivery of all services at the primary or secondary level. An effective system for triage and referral of cases is therefore essential. In concept, a referral system exists whereby men and women requiring special investigation or treatment are referred from SCs or PHCs to district hospitals (secondary level of care) and teaching hospitals or apex institutions (tertiary level). However, in actual practice, the referral system is not optimally functioning for most components of health care, including MCH and oncology.

As mentioned above, the ICMR has a network of collaborating centers in many fields. One such network involves 33 HRRCs, which are located in the medical colleges, but have developed linkages with primary and secondary levels of health services through various research programs. This could be one model for integrating prevention and management of RTIs within the MCH component, and for linking the health and nonhealth sectors. Similar mechanisms can be explored and evaluated.

Innovative Research and Development Efforts. While most of the activities mentioned above will involve operations research from the beginning, innovative research projects can be initiated in several other areas, such as the following:

1. Sociobehavioral research to identify the underlying reasons for RTIs among the at-risk population, to understand the feelings and stigma associated with these diseases, including values attached to commercial sex, sexual promiscuity, and so on. The research findings will be useful in the preparation of training materials for providers and educational materials aimed at encouraging behavioral change within the community.

2. Development of simple, cheap, and effective diagnostic kits. Current diagnostic methods are expensive and are not appropriate for field conditions prevailing in India. The need for diagnostic kits is a global one, and efforts to devise appropriate technologies are being made in both developed and developing countries. Needless to say, such technologies will be useful in India for undertaking large-scale screening programs in field conditions, and for early detection of infections.
3. Evaluation of strategies for rehabilitation, of means to increase utilization of primary health care services, and of efforts to encourage adoption of safer sexual behavior and practices.

Mechanisms for Implementation

A multisectoral approach should be utilized to establish strong linkages between the health, education, and welfare sectors. The mechanisms and their interlinkages are outlined in Figure 3. The existing networks of collaborating centers of the ICMR could be the main operational channel for various programs. It is proposed that while the current focus on utilizing skin and STD clinics should be kept, family planning, gynecology, and antenatal clinics should be made additional service delivery outlets. Further, for a preventive and control strategy to be effective, health providers will have to play a more active role and

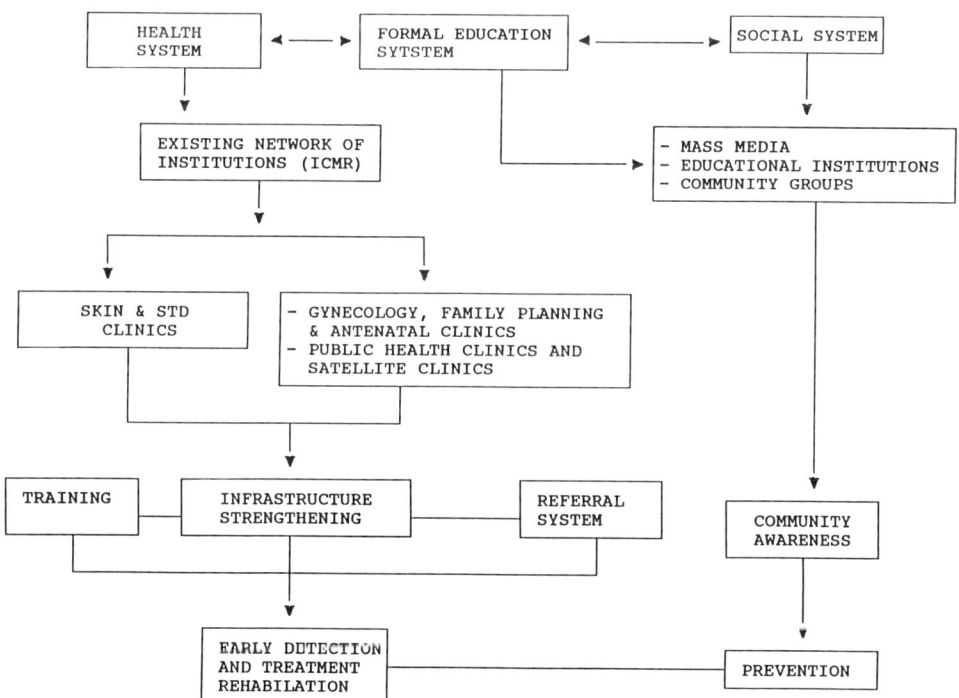

Figure 3. Integrated RTI Prevention and Control:
Mechanisms for Implementation

join researchers to define and achieve mutual objectives. On the one hand, the health sector must reorient existing services—for example, by closer integration between the national MCH program and the national cancer control program for cervical cancer control. On the other hand, the nonhealth sectors are needed to help generate community awareness and demand use of these facilities. A "pull approach" by the health sector and a "push approach" by related sectors would help substantially to prevent and control RTIs.

REFERENCES

1. Bali PA. Study of clinico-epidemiological investigations of vaginal discharge in rural women, 1991. Unpublished data.
2. Bang RA, Bang AT, Baitule M, Choudhary Y, Sarmukaddam S, Tale O. High prevalence of gynaecological diseases in rural Indian women. Lancet 1989; 1:85–6.
3. Bhalla P. A clinical, microbiological and cytological study of nonspecific vaginitis. Progress report of ongoing ICMR research project, 1990. Unpublished data.
4. Bhalla P, Rewari N, Chadha P. Gardnerella vaginalis in CuT 200 users. Indian J Med Res 1989; 89:80–6.
5. Bhargava NC. Sexually transmitted diseases in India. Presented at STD Media Orientation Workshop, Jaipur, India, 1988.
6. Bhaskaran CS. Prevalence of genital chlamydial infection in symptomatic and asymptomatic women. Progress report of ongoing ICMR research project, 1990. Unpublished data.
7. Bhatt R, Gogate A, Deodhar L. Mycoplasma infection in genital tract with special reference to immunofluorescence. J Postgrad Med 1989; 35:40–2.
8. Bhujwala RA. Role of Chlamydia trachomatis in pelvic inflammatory disease: detection of antigen and antibody by enzyme immunoassay. Progress report of ongoing ICMR research project, 1990. Unpublished data.
9. Bhujwala RA, Department of Microbiology, All India Institute of Medical Sciences, New Delhi. Personal communications, 1990.
10. Bhujwala RA, Bhargava NC, Biswas T, Narain S, Pandhi RK. Antimicrobial sensitivity of N. gonorrhoeae to spectinomycin and rosoxacin. Indian J Med Res 1987; 86:702–6.
11. Bhujwala RA, Buckshee K, Shriniwas. Gardnerella vaginitis and associated aerobic bacterials in nonspecific vaginitis. Indian J Med Res 1985; 81:251–6.
12. Bhujwala RA, Mishra B, Bhargava NC et al. Nongonococcal urethritis in men and its response to therapy. Indian J Med Res 1984; 79:728.
13. Bhujwala RA, Pandhi RK, Bhargava NC et al. N. gonorrhoeae, its sensitivity to pencillin and tetracycline over a decade. Indian J Med Microbiol 1983; 1:43–8.
14. Health Information India. Central Bureau of Health Intelligence, Director General of Health Services, Ministry of Health and Family Welfare, Government of India, New Delhi, 1988.
15. Chakraborty S, Munni M. Serological survey for syphilis amongst antenatal cases in selected hospitals of Delhi. Indian J Public Health 1989; 33:33.
16. Chowdhury A. A bacteriological study of Gardnerella vaginitis isolated from patients, 1985. Unpublished data.
17. Das BC, Sehgal A, Murthy MS et al. Human papilloma virus and cervical cancer in Indian women. Lancet 1989; 2:1271.

18. Deodhar LP. Study of Ureaplasma urealyticum from male genital tract infections, and detection of specific antibodies to U. urealyticum serotypes by ELISA. Progress report of ongoing ICMR research project, 1990. Unpublished data.

19. Department of Women and Child Development, Ministry of Human Resource Development. National perspective plan for women, New Delhi, 1988.

20. Dhall K, Sarkar A, Sokhey C, Dhall GI, Ganguly NK. Incidence of gonococcal infection and its clinicopathological correlation in patients attending gynaecological outpatient department. J Obstet Gynecol India 1990; 40:410–3.

21. Family Welfare Programme in India. Ministry of Health and Family Welfare Year Book, New Dehli: Government of India, 1987–88.

22. Ghosh S. A strategy for basic minimal health care. Bull Nutr Found India 1990; 11:1.

23. Gopalkrishnan K, Hinduja IM, Anand Kumar TC. Semen characteristics of asymptomatic males affected by Trichomonas vaginalis. J Invitro Fertil Embryol Trans 1990; 7:165–7.

24. Gupta MM, Sharma BK, Singh V, Luthra UK. Immunocytological demonstration of HSV-II antigen on exofoliated cells from precancerous and cancerous lesions of the uterine cervix. Diagn Cytopathol 1988; 4:48–9.

25. Indian Council of Medical Research. HIV infection—ongoing studies and future research plans. ICMR Bull 1988; 18:109–19.

26. Indian Council of Medical Research. Illegal abortion in rural India. Report of a collaborative study, New Delhi, 1989.

27. Indian Council of Medical Research. Evaluation of quality of family welfare services at PHC level. Report of a collaborative study, New Delhi, 1992 (in press).

28. Institute of Cytology and Preventive Oncology, Indian Council of Medical Research. Uterine cervical dysplasia study. Part II. Progress report, New Delhi, 1990.

29. Institute of Cytology and Preventive Oncology, Indian Council of Medical Research. Community control of cervical cancer. A feasibility study. Progress report, 1990. Unpublished data.

30. Jacob M, Rao PS, Sridharan G, John TJ. Epidemiology and clinical profile of genital herpes. Indian J Med Res 1989; 89:4–11.

31. Luthra UK, Bhatnagar P, Das DK et al. Condylomatous lesion (HPV infection) of uterine cervix. Ann Biol Clin 1989; 47:283–6.

32. Luthra UK, Roy ML, Sehgal A. Clinical downstaging of uterine cervix by paramedical personnel. Lancet 1988; 1:1401.

33. Luthra UK, Mitra AB, Prabhakar AK, Bhatnagar P, Agarwal SS. Copper containing intrauterine devices and cervical carcinogenesis—48 months follow up. Indian J Med Res 1980; 72:659–64.

34. Luthra UK, Sehgal A. Control of cervical cancer. Proceedings of 15th International Cancer Congress, Hamburg, August 16–22, 1990. J Cancer Res Clinic Oncol, 1990; 116.

35. Mishra MK, Sinha TK. Cytologic screening for the detection of cancer in the uterine cervix. A survey in Patna (India). Cancer Lett 1990; 52:21.

36. Mishra JS, Engineer AD, Tandon P. Cytopathological changes in human cervix and endometrium following prolonged retention of copper-bearing intrauterine contraceptive devices. Diagn Cytopathol 1989; 5:237–42.

37. Mishra JS, Tandon P, Engineer AD. Results of cytological monitoring of cervical smears in gynaecology outpatients and contraceptive users, 1990. Unpublished data.
38. Murthy MS, Sehgal A, Satyanarayana L et al. Risk factors related to biological behaviour of precancerous lesions of the uterine cervix. Br J Cancer 1990; 61:732–6.
39. National Cancer Registry Programme, Indian Council of Medical Research. Annual report, New Delhi, 1987.
40. Pandit DV. Gardnerella vaginalis in the etiology of bacterial vaginosis or nonspecific vaginosis. Progress report of ongoing ICMR research project. Unpublished data.
41. Pandit DV, Barve SM, Deodhar LP. Biotypes of Gardnerella vaginalis isolated from non-specific vaginitis patients in Bombay. Indian J Med Res 1989; 89:435–8.
42. Sehgal VM, Jain MK. Pattern of epidemics of donovanosis in the "nonendemic" region. Int J Dermatol 1989; 27:396–9.
43. Sehgal VM, Koranne RV, Srivastava SB, Gupta MM, Luthra UK. Clinicopathology and immunohistochemistry of genital warts. Int J Dermatol 1988; 27:690–4.
44. Sharma M, Nayak N, Malhotra S, Kumar B, Hemal A. Chlamydiazyme test for rapid detection of Chlamydia trachomatis. Indian J Med Res 1989; 89:4–11.
45. Sharma N, Kumar B, Agarwal KC, Sharma SK, Surinder Kaur. Penicillinase producing strains of N. gonorrhoeae from Chandigarh. Indian J Med Res 1984; 80:512–5.
46. Thirumoorthy T. The epidemiology of sexually transmitted diseases in Southeast Asia and the Western Pacific. Semin Dermatol 1990; 90:102–4.
47. Urmil RC, Dutta PK, Basappa K, Ganguly SS. A study of morbidity patterns among prostitutes attending a municipal clinic in Pune. J Indian Med Assoc 1989; 87:29–31.

REPRODUCTIVE TRACT INFECTIONS IN MOZAMBIQUE: A CASE STUDY OF INTEGRATED SERVICES

Rui Bastos dos Santos, M.D.
Professor Auxiliair de la Fac. Med.
Directeur du Programme National de Butte Contre les Mst.
Au Ministere de la Sante
Directeur du Service de Dermatologia de L'Hopital Central de Maputo
P.O. Box 1164, Hospital Central de Maputo
Maputo, Mozambique

Elena Maria Pereira Folgosa, M.D.
Professor Auxiliair de la Fac. de Med.
Microbiologue du Laboratoire de Reference pour les Mst.
P.O. Box 257, Faculdade de Medicina
Maputo, Mozambique

Lieve Fransen, M.D., Ph.D.
AIDS Task Force, European Economic Community
67A Rue Josef II
Brussels 1040, Belgium

INTRODUCTION

Sexually transmitted diseases (STDs) were not acknowledged or properly dealt with in Mozambique, as in the majority of developing countries, until the AIDS problem, recognized in the mid-1980s, highlighted the importance of controlling STDs in the context of primary health care.

The social and economic situation in Mozambique is extremely bad, mainly because of the long-lasting war, which has displaced more than one third of the total population of approximately 10 million inhabitants. Some 1.5 million people have sought refuge in neighboring countries. Of the remaining population, 60 percent live under the poorest and most violent conditions one can imagine. War and displaced populations are causing the breakup of families and social structures; fueling promiscuity and commercial sex; and increasing the risk of STD and human immunodeficiency virus (HIV) infection, which are spreading widely and rapidly. In addition, the precarious state of the general health services, caused by the same difficulties, precludes early detection, diagnosis, and treatment of STDs,

Reproductive Tract Infections, Edited by A. Germain *et al.*
Plenum Press, New York, 1992

thus further increasing the possibilities for spread, as well as for severe and costly complications and sequelae, mainly among women and children.

Few data are available about STDs in the pre-AIDS era because very little attention was given to the problem. Table 1 summarizes the available data on syphilis among pregnant women and reveals a range of seroprevalence of 5–18 percent.[1,2] It is also noteworthy that in 1984, in the central hospital of Maputo, 8 percent of the 153 perinatal deaths were due to syphilis (not shown).[3] In 1987, 3 percent of 190 STD patients in Maputo were found to be HIV-positive; this prevalence was four times that among blood donors and five times that among the general population.

To control the spread of HIV in Mozambique, a national program for AIDS control was initiated in 1987 with the support of the World Health Organization/Global Program on AIDS (WHO/GPA). Support from the European Economic Community (EEC) was requested to develop a national STD control program as part of the AIDS control program, and to assist its implementation, financially and technically. From the beginning, STD control has been a major strategy to control the spread of AIDS, as well as to reduce the impact of STDs in Mozambique. The STD and AIDS control program, although organized as a discrete entity, totally integrates its activities into the national health service infrastructure, which includes both preventive and curative services and is the predominant source of health care.

Health services in Mozambique are organized in four levels. Primary health care centers (centros de saude and postos de saude) are the main pillars of the system, and most people go to these facilities for the majority of their health problems. Education, prevention, and counseling programs are also provided through these centers. Access to a functional primary health care system has been drastically reduced by the destruction of nearly half of the health centers in the country. The second level in the structure consists of the rural and general hospitals, the third level consists of five provincial hospitals; and the fourth includes three central hospitals (in Nampula, Beira, and Maputo).[2] Additionally, many Mozambicans seek health services from traditional healers. In Maputo Province alone, where the population is approximately one million, there are also 3,500 traditional healers. However, data about visits of patients to traditional healers for STD problems are not known.

Table 1. Syphilis Seroprevalence among Pregnant Women

Year	Test	N	Result (% positive)
1982–83[1]	Venereal Disease Research Laboratory (VDRL)	—	5–15
	Treponema Pallidum Haemagglintination (TPHA); Flourescent Treponema Antibody Absorbative (FTA.abs)	—	2–10
1986[2]	Rapid Plasma Reagin (RPR)	227	18

Methodology

In July 1988, the national STD and AIDS control program began an 18-month pilot phase in Maputo City and Province. STD and AIDS control activities were integrated into the structure of primary health care (see Figure 1), and syndromic diagnosis was used. The pilot project addressed the following nine components of control activities.

1. Planning and management structure. At the level of the Ministry of Health and with the support of WHO/GPA, a special unit was created for the management of the AIDS control program. Within this unit, a sub-unit was created to plan, manage, and direct the STD control program dealing with reproductive tract infections (RTIs), and an STD and AIDS program manager was appointed to oversee this division while continuing to fulfill his duty as a clinical expert on STDs at the central hospital in Maputo.

2. Expert unit. An expert unit was created, composed of experts from the reference and research laboratories, the reference clinic, the central hospital of Maputo, and the educational unit of the National Directorate for Health. Experts in clinical management, training, laboratory techniques, and educational and epidemiological methodology collaborate within this unit while they continue to fulfill their other duties. The expert unit, jointly with the STD control program manager, elaborated a national control plan, and an operational plan for the first phase was finalized with support of the EEC's AIDS Task Force. Syndromic patient management was designed on the basis of WHO guidelines, the few epidemiological data available in the country, and a minimum of laboratory support. On the basis of the few epidemiological data available, 14 management strategies for patients and their partners were designed by the expert unit (see appendices for the four main algorithms), a manual with those strategies was printed, and the list of essential drugs available in Mozambique was adapted to include 12 drugs for STD management. The essential drugs available for treatment were benzathine penicillin tablets, Cotrimoxazole tablets, doxycycline tablets, erythromycin tablets, erythromycin (pediatric) syrup, Gentian violet solution, Kanamycin injections, Metronidazole tablets, Nystatin vaginal ovules, tetracycline tablets, tetracycline ointments, and spectinomycin injections (at referral level or under special conditions).

3. Training. Training was undertaken for clinicians; nurses; laboratory technicians; and persons in charge of education in primary health care centers, laboratories, and the reference clinic of Maputo. The health centers involved in the program were equipped, and the personnel were trained to perform Gram stains, rapid plasma reagins (RPRs), and wet mount; to manage a separate pharmacy with STD drugs and condoms; and to give health education and informative leaflets to patients. A logical sequence of developing strategies and algorithms, producing a manual, making the necessary supplies available, and training all personnel to use the strategies and supplies was followed to assure that trained personnel were able to practice as soon as possible after the training. Monthly supervision was organized at the different levels to assure the appropriate and exact use of the strategies, to analyze problems encountered, and to give feedback about surveillance data analyzed.

4. Procurement of supplies. A national procurement and distribution agency (Medimoc) was made responsible for organizing restricted calls for tender, and for purchasing and distributing drugs and diagnostics.

5. Organization of clinical services and cost recovery. At the central hospital in Maputo, one clinical referral center was strengthened to take care of referred patients, and to monitor, train, and supervise the technical activities in the health centers. In the centers

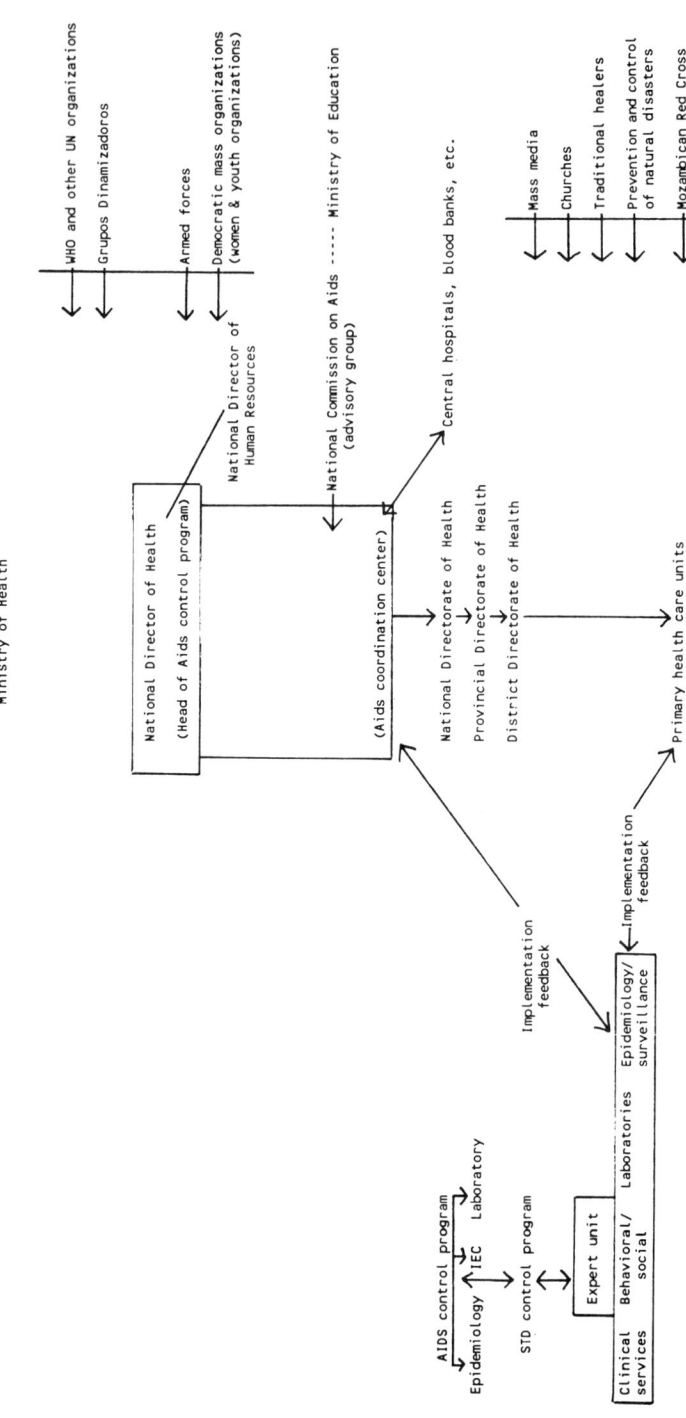

Figure 1. Organization of National STD/AIDS Control Program, Mozambique

where perinatal consultations are performed, RPRs were made available to test pregnant women systematically. During the first phase of implementation, consultations for management of STDs and AIDS were organized daily in 20 primary health care centers in the city and in Marracuene, Maputo Province. Patients received treatment on the basis of syndromic algorithms and, when possible, paid a minimal fee covering the real cost (not including tax and distribution) of the drugs. At this moment, the funds are going into the general fund for drugs of the Ministry of Health, but the plan is for them to be used to restock the drugs used in the STD and AIDS program consultations. The majority of the patients are able to pay for treatment.

6. *Counseling and partner notification.* Before the medical consultation, patients now receive information, counseling, free condoms, and an educational booklet about STDs and HIV. Patients are also asked to refer their sexual contacts to a clinic, using a special anonymous leaflet for this purpose. Educational and preventive messages are repeated briefly during consultation. Patients who do not improve after treatment, although their contacts have been treated, or who experience complications, are referred to the central hospital. There, etiological diagnoses can be made with the support of the reference laboratory, and additional drugs, such as spectinomycin, are available.

7. *Mandatory prevention and case finding.* All newborns delivered in centers or hospitals are to receive one dose of tetracycline ointment after their eyes are cleared. All pregnant women presenting at prenatal consultations are to have blood drawn for RPR testing and receive treatment for syphilis if positive.

8. *Surveillance activities.* The STD consultations are being used for epidemiological surveillance and monitoring of RTI syndromes, HIV, and their complications. Using a special form, all centers submit monthly reports on patients seen to the city authorities, who report to the program authorities. The program authorities discuss the data and give feedback to the city authorities and the centers. A few of the STD consultations are also used as sentinel posts for the surveillance of HIV. Studies of the relative frequency of various etiologies for specific syndromes are being performed to adapt the syndromic strategies in use to local reality, but analysis of these data is not yet available.

9. *Monitoring and evaluation.* Specific targets were set up during the planning process based on discussion with health workers in the services. Targets for the first year and a half were to fully equip 20 health centers, the reference clinic and the laboratory, and to train all personnel involved in implementation and supervision. Additional targets included the use of the algorithm for all patients and screening of all pregnant women for syphilis. Referral of patients is being monitored, with an anticipated decrease by half. Monthly reports about the achievement are made using standardized forms. Indicators for effectiveness will be analyzed on the basis of the targets achieved, and efficiency will be analyzed on the basis of the effectiveness and the real costs of interventions.

Regular supervision visits are made to monitor the quality, regularity, and acceptance of the education and information sessions given. The number of partners presenting with a contact slip is recorded to gauge the effectiveness of partner notification efforts. Some of the recorded indicators are to be used for the process evaluation that is planned after the program has been in operation for 18 months. The HIV seroprevalence in the sentinel surveillance, the syphilis seroprevalence among pregnant women, and the incidence of complications presenting in gynecology and ophthalmology clinics are to be used for monitoring.

RESULTS

Patients Managed

Over a period of one year (July 1988–July 1989), the program reported that 38,867 patients and contacts consulted for RTIs in the 20 health centers. This total represents approximately 6 percent of the sexually active population of the area served. In this first year, these visits accounted for 10–15 percent of all visits to the primary health centers in the province. Because records were totally inaccurate before the program was installed, this number cannot be compared with previous data. Of the patients seen, 46 percent were men, and 54 percent were women. In the second year of activity (August 1989–August 1990), of the persons were seen, 48 percent were men, and 52 percent were women.

In the first year of activity, 33 percent of the men seen presented with urethral discharge. Only 46 percent of the men with urethral discharge were assessed by Gram stain. Of these, 75 percent had intracellular Gram-negative diplococci. Of the women seen, 40 percent presented with vaginal discharge; 6 percent presented with abdominal pain and were managed with the pelvic inflammatory disease (PID) syndromic approach. Overall, 10 percent of patients presented with genital ulcerations, and the prevalence for men was twice as high as for women; 7 percent of the patients had another STD or another diagnosis altogether. No significant difference was found between rural and urban areas in this sample.

Both the number of referrals and the proportion of referrals with gonococcal infection declined dramatically in the first year of activity. Of the 38,867 patients seen, fewer than 5 percent were referred to the clinic at the central hospital for further investigation and treatment. Before the inauguration of the STD control program, 8 percent were referred over a similar period of time, and 42 percent of these referrals had gonococcal urethritis. Of the patients referred after the program was installed, only 23 percent had gonococcal urethritis. This decline demonstrates the important and rapid effect of using appropriate algorithms and strategies at the first level.

The impact of the program was not measurable during the first year of activity in terms of declining cases of congenital syphilis. In that year, 0.9% of neonates in the central hospital of Maputo were found to have congenital syphilis at birth; in the second year of activity, the number was also 0.9% of neonates.[3] The approximate number of births per year in the province is 50,000, but the number of pregnant women consulting at prenatal care clinics was not recorded the first year, and the RPR test, in spite of being planned for, was not systematically used because of lack of logistic support.

Eye infections caused by STDs remained very common, probably because most infants are born at home and therefore do not receive eye prophylaxis at birth. It also is striking how many adults had gonococcal eye infections, probably caused by self-contamination. From January through September 1989, 89 adults, 35 children older than one month, and 136 children younger than one month were seen in the ophthalmology department with purulent conjunctivitis. Of these adults and children, 84 percent had *Neisseria gonorrhoea* isolated from the eyes (confirmed with sugar tests). Some 26 adults and two children lost sight in one or both eyes as a result. On average, 15 percent of the patients consulting in all centers were the sexual partners of STD patients and had partner notification slips.

Recurrent Costs of the Program

The principal components of the recurrent costs to implement this program at the peripheral level (management of patients, excluding program management, research, or training) during the first phase are described in Tables 2–6.

Table 2 demonstrates that the cost of consumables used in the management strategies was 69,132.5 ECUs, or US$82,959. The main cost item was screening of all pregnant women for syphilis.

In general, the drugs and diagnostics purchased by Medimoc cost the regular price in Europe or less. The time between the start of the restricted call for tender and the delivery took approximately one year. Table 3 demonstrates that the total cost for drugs to manage the patients presenting during one year was 71,613.5 European Count Units (the ECU is the European Economic Community's money unit), or US$ 85,936. The main cost item was spectinomycin, which was, for the period discussed, the second-line treatment for urethral discharge, vaginal discharge, and PID.

Table 2. Costs of Diagnostics for Management of Patients and Partners

Syndrome	Diagnostic	Patients and partners	Cost per unit (ECU)	Total cost (ECU)	US$ (ECU x 1.2)
Urethral discharge	Gram stain	13,479	0.2	2,696	3,235
	RPR*	15,600	0.7	10,920	13,104
Vaginal discharge	Wet mount	15,600	0.1	1,560	1,872
	RPR*	10,920	0.7	7,644	9,173
Vaginal discharge and PID	Wet mount	2,340	0.1	234	281
	Neisseria gonorrhoeae culture	4,680	1.4	6,552	7,862
	Gram stain	585	0.2	117	140
	RPR*	585	0.7	409.5	491
Ophthalmia neonatorum	Gram stain	20,000	0.2	4,000	4,800
Syphilis screening during pregnancy	RPR*	50,000	0.7	35,000	42,000
Total				69,132.5	82,959

* Quantitative.

Table 3. Cost of Drugs for Treatment of RTIs per 1 Million Population*

Syndrome	Drug	Formula unit	Dose per disease period	Patients and partners	Cost per treatment unit (ECU)	Total cost (ECU)	US$ ECUx1.2
Urethral discharge	Kanamycin	2 g IM	1 dose	13,835	0.35	4,848	5,818
	Spectinomycin	2 g IM	1 dose	2,372	2.7	6,404	7,685
	Doxycycline	100 mg tablets	1 pd/14 days	4,157	0.4	1,662.8	1,994
	Erythromycin	500 mg tablets	4 pd/7 days	267	2.24	598	718
	Benzathine pen.	2.4 MU.IM	1 dose	1,560	0.5	780	936
Vaginal discharge	Metronidazole	250 mg tablets	8 tablets in 1 dose	1,560	0.06	93.6	112
	Metronidazole	2 g	2 days	3,120	0.12	374.4	449
	Gentian violet	?	3 days	1,560	0.6	93.6	112
	Nystatin	Vaginal ovules	3 days	560	0.02	11.2	13
	Kanamycin	2 g IM	1 dose	9,264	0.35	3,242	3,980
	Spectinomycin	2 g IM	1 dose	3,276	2.7	8,845	10,614
	Benzathine pen.	2.4 MU.IM	1 dose	1,419	0.5	709.5	851
	Erythromycin	500 mg tablets	4 pd/7 days	3,276	2.24	7,338.5	8,806
Venereal disease and PID	Spectinomycin	2 g IM	2 doses	2,340	5.4	12,636	15,163
	Erythromycin	500 mg	4 pd/7 days	2,340	2.24	5,241	6,289
	Kanamycin	2 g IM	1 dose	293	0.35	102	122
	Doxycycline	100 mg	2 pd/7 days	293	0.4	117	140
	Benzathine pen.	2.4 MU.IM	1 dose	59	0.5	29.5	35
Genital ulcer disease	Benzathine pen.	2.4 MU.IM	1 dose	4,169	0.5	2,084.5	2,501
	Tetracycline	100 mg	3 pd/10 days	219	0.9	193.9	233
	Cotrimoxazole	80/400	4 pd/2 days	4,169	1.2	5,002	6,002
	Erythromycin	500 mg	4 pd/7 days	219	2.24	491	589
Bubo Inguinale	Doxycycline	100 mg	1 pd/14 days	1,594	0.4	638	766
	Erythromycin	500 mg	4 pd/28 days	131	2.24	303	364
Ophthalmia Neonatorum	Tetracycline	Ointment	2 tubes 14 days	10,000	0.5	5,000	6,000
	Kanamycin	/ kg IM	1 dose	2,500	0.35	875	1,050
	Erythromycin	Syrup	14 days	1,250	0.56	1,400	1,680
RTI	Benzathine pen.	2.4 MU.IM	1 dose	5,000	0.5	2,500	3,000
Total						71,613.5	86,023.2

* Costs for transport, taxes, and distribution not included.
Note: pd = per day.

Table 4. Diagnostics for Surveillance and Algorithm Development

	Test	Number	Cost per unit	Total cost (ECU)
Male: urethral discharge	Gram stain	500	0.2	100
	HIV	500	2.3	1,150
	RPR	500	0.7	350
	TPHA	50	1.1	55
	Gonorrhea	500	1.4	700
	Chlamydia trachomatis ELISA	500	5.0	2,500
			Subtotal	4,855
Female: vaginal discharge	Gonorrhea	500	1.4	700
	Chlamydia trachomatis ELISA	500	5.0	2,500
	Wet mount	500	0.1	50
	RPR	500	0.7	350
	TPHA	50	1.1	55
	HIV	500	2.3	1,150
	Papanicolaou smear	500	0.35	175
			Subtotal	4,980
Female: pregnant women	Same as above		Subtotal	4,980
Genital ulcer disease: ulcers	RPR	500	0.7	350
	TPHA	50	1.1	55
	HIV	500	2.3	1,150
	Chancroid	500	2.0	1,000
			Subtotal	2,555
Total				17,370

Table 5. Personnel Time Required for Management of RTI Syndromes

Syndrome	Number of visits		Total time (hours)*	
Urethral discharge	Men: Women:	25,959 7,988	Men: Women:	4,327 1,997
Vaginal discharge	Women: Men:	53,040 3,276	Women: Men:	13,260 546
Venereal disease and PID	Women: Men:	9,360 1,170	Women: Men:	2,340 195
Genital ulcer disease	Men: Women:	7,020 1,756	Men: Women:	1,170 439
BUBO	Men: Women:	3,000 500	Men: Women:	500 125
ONN	Baby:	20,000	Baby:	5,000
Total				29,899

* Visit of men: total mean duration of 10 minutes; visit of women: total mean duration of 15 minutes.

Table 4 shows the costs of the diagnostic tests used to perform minimal RTI/HIV surveillance and to perform simple prevalence studies to adapt the management strategies. A total of 17,370 ECUs, or US$20,844, is needed per year.

Table 5 summarizes the minimum time necessary to manage patients. An estimate of all the personnel time used to manage a patient visit during a disease episode suggests that 214 person-months (20 paramedical workers, full-time per year) were required to manage patients for a population of one million inhabitants.

Table 6 presents a synthesis of the major recurrent costs. The total cost was 355,466 ECUs, or US$426,558, for a total of 38,867 patients seen at the STD consultation in the primary health care setting and 50,000 pregnant women to be tested for syphilis during a period of one year. The cost was approximately 9 ECUs, or US$10.80, per patient managed (not shown).

DISCUSSION

This paper describes a carefully executed model of an integrated STD/AIDS control program and of integrated RTI services and activities in a functioning primary health care structure in a developing country. The experience highlights that, if carefully designed, a joint STD/AIDS control program is feasible and can be beneficial. A condition for integration of interventions and activities into the existing primary health care structure is a functioning primary health care structure including referral, supervision, and feedback.

Table 6. Recurrent Costs for Minimal Requirements at Primary Health Care Centers

Essential supplies (patients and partners)	Total cost (ECU)	US$ (ECU x 1.2)
Administrative and secretarial	20,000	24,000
Diagnostics	86,352.5	103,622
Therapeutic	74,113.5	88,936
Condom/education	65,000	78,000
Needles/syringes	20,000	24,000
Laboratory, slides, tubes	20,000	24,000
Transport, taxes, distribution (supplies)	32,000	38,400
Subtotal	317,466	380,958
Services		
Telephone	7,000	8,400
Fuel	13,000	15,600
Subtotal	20,000	24,000
Maintenance		
Transport	5,000	6,000
Buildings	13,000	15,600
Subtotal	18,000	21,600
Grand Total	355,466	426,558

The planning process of the program was shown to be very important and involved all interested parties in ministries, laboratories, and health services. Targets, indicators, and acceptable reporting systems and records were discussed and agreed upon, and feedback was organized. The whole process was managed by a highly motivated manager and a fully committed team and expert unit who have been able to motivate and sustain interest among all participants. Quality control was important not only for laboratory services but also for clinical and educational management of patients and partners.

In one year, the number of patients visiting the reference clinic decreased drastically, allowing for more specialized care for the more difficult cases. The pathology seen at the reference center became more appropriate for it because selection at the first level was more effective. Improving STD management at the first level of the primary health care system enables the reference center to manage patients screened prior to referral and thus spend less at the second and third levels, where resources are more precious and expensive. The organization of short and appropriate training of health service workers at a time when the program was ready to be implemented was also important to enable the trained personnel to immediately practice the skills learned.

This experience also demonstrates the importance and feasibility of adapting essential drug lists to include drugs for RTI management. In the first stage, drugs were kept in special pharmacies to enable program activities to adequately start. It is clear that long-term solutions have to be sought to assure regular provision of all essential drugs, including drugs for RTI. However, it is important to highlight the fact that this program respected national guidelines and decisions about drug procurement and did not create competition and confusion by setting up parallel procurement channels outside the nationally acceptable procedures and priorities. It will therefore be easier to sustain at a later stage by the existing procedures in the country. Cost recovery for RTI drugs was attempted, and it was demonstrated that, in the urban area at least, most of the patients and their contacts were able and willing to pay a minimal fee for the drugs. Although the program plans to use the recovered funds to buy RTI drugs in the future, this is a difficult measure to implement because of Ministry of Planning regulations. The study also demonstrates that procurement and distribution of essential drugs and diagnostics can sometimes be achieved more rapidly and cheaply by national services within a country than by European or multilateral agencies.

Some weaknesses, however, were identified during the first phase of implementation. For example, while vertical programming allows rapid implementation, it may be more expensive and less sustainable than an integrated initiative. In addition, syndromic management strategies do not enable medical personnel to make etiological diagnoses and thus do not permit them to distinguish between STDs and other causes of RTIs. Although using syndromes and algorithms is not as exact as using etiological diagnostic methods, it is cheaper, more feasible, and much less labor-intensive. This enables overburdened health services in developing countries to deal with STDs at the primary health care level. Using syndromic assessment to manage women's complaints makes it possible to reach more of the at-risk female population.

However, syndromic strategies are not well adapted and do not work as well for female populations with RTIs as for male populations. Using the syndromic approach also makes it difficult to know if the woman's male partners have to be notified or epidemiologically treated. It was therefore decided after the first stage to perform some etiological studies to tailor the strategies to the spectrum of RTIs found in Mozambique. Further clinical and operations research is needed to improve algorithms for women and to address the issue of partner notification. Better and more appropriate screening devices for women with RTIs are urgently needed to improve the algorithms used, because when syndromes and algorithms are used, it is important to develop strategies that can be adapted regularly to the regional pathology and prevalence of diseases. Therefore, regular and appropriate epidemiological and etiological studies are needed, and the results must be used to adapt the algorithms.

It is important to notice that with this approach, women are consulting as frequently as men, whereas if special STD clinics are the major focal points for STD management, men are usually the main clients. Although symptomatic men are supposed to notify their female partners, they usually do not. Data in developing countries demonstrate that a maximum of only 15 percent of men bring their female partners for consultation. Very often, the man leaves out the regular partner, for fear of straining the relationship.

Education and behavior modification activities targeted at the patients were not always adequate, and the impact was difficult to monitor or evaluate. The first-year experience demonstrates the need to design and evaluate effective strategies to take care of this important aspect of the program. The data reported during this phase demonstrate that RTIs and STDs are an important problem in the city and cause a serious burden to the health system. These findings also show the possible threat of an explosive spread of HIV infection in the population. Program experience thus far suggests that the proportion of the sexually active population consulting for RTIs during one year (6 percent) is high compared with rates from a similar program in Senegal, where only 1 percent of the total consultations were for STD.[4]

Preventive interventions, such as eye prophylaxis with tetracycline ointment for newborns and syphilis screening for pregnant women at prenatal consultations, have not been optimally implemented and remain to be improved. Despite allocations of substantial resources to prevention efforts, serious complications such as infant blindness and neonatal syphilis are still very common. This is partly because the strategies were not fully implemented in the first year, partly because such operational aspects as coverage still need to be resolved, and partly because it is too early in the process to see a real impact on complications of STDs such as these. More research on development of focused screening strategies for pregnant women would be useful to decrease cost.

The frequent presentation with PID-like symptoms probably also demonstrates that management of the diseases among women is not yet adequate. At the same time, because clinical diagnosis was used in the syndromic approach, overdiagnosis is probable and further research is also urgently needed here.

Future trends regarding the recurrent costs of the program will have to be monitored. Only drugs and diagnostics are accounted for here, although program management, planning, training, equipment, and other recurrent costs also have to be financed. Even when taking such costs into account, we estimate 9 ECUs, or US$10.80, per patient with an STD is needed. This estimate may seem high for a country like Mozambique, but considering the benefits of limiting serious and costly complications, it is actually low. This project also demonstrates that in the city, patients are often able to pay part of the costs, such as the real costs (without tax, distribution, and so forth) of the drugs. The balance, however, still must be financed by others, such as the government and donors.

The project is now being extended to the provinces and some districts, following the same scheme as in the first phase, with improvement of the clinical and educational

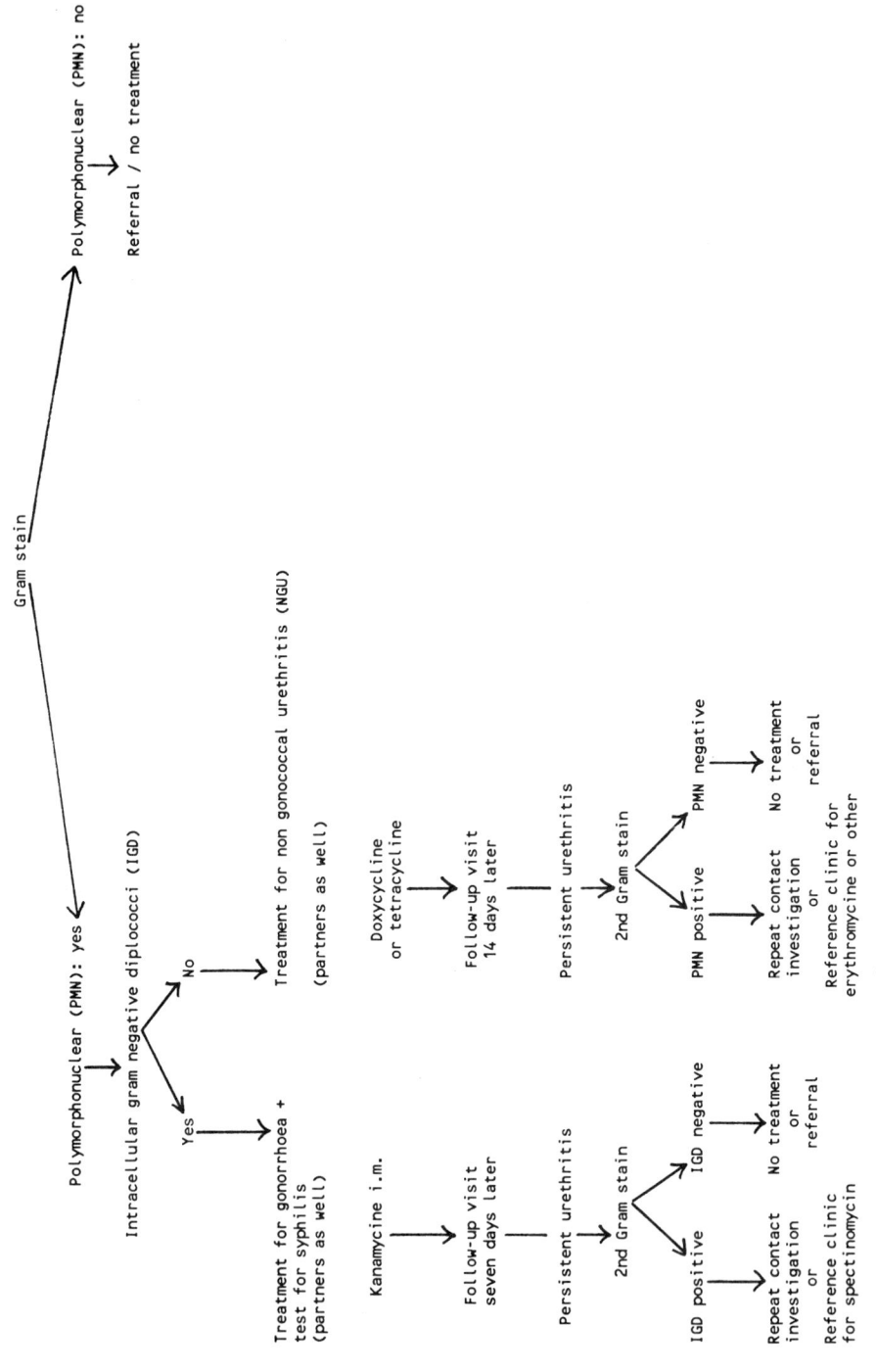

Appendix 1. Case Management for Urethritis (Dysuria or Discharge)

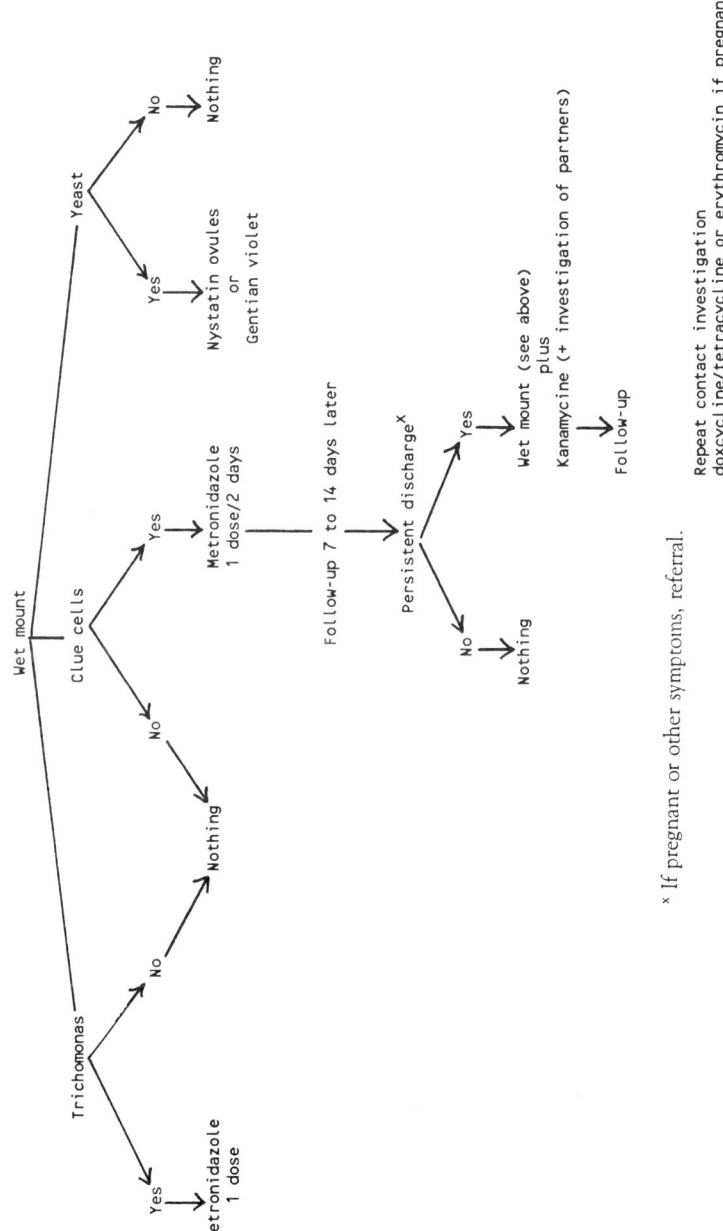

Appendix 2. Case Management for Vaginal Discharge

x If pregnant or other symptoms, referral.

Appendix 3. Case Management for PID or Lower Abdominal Pain

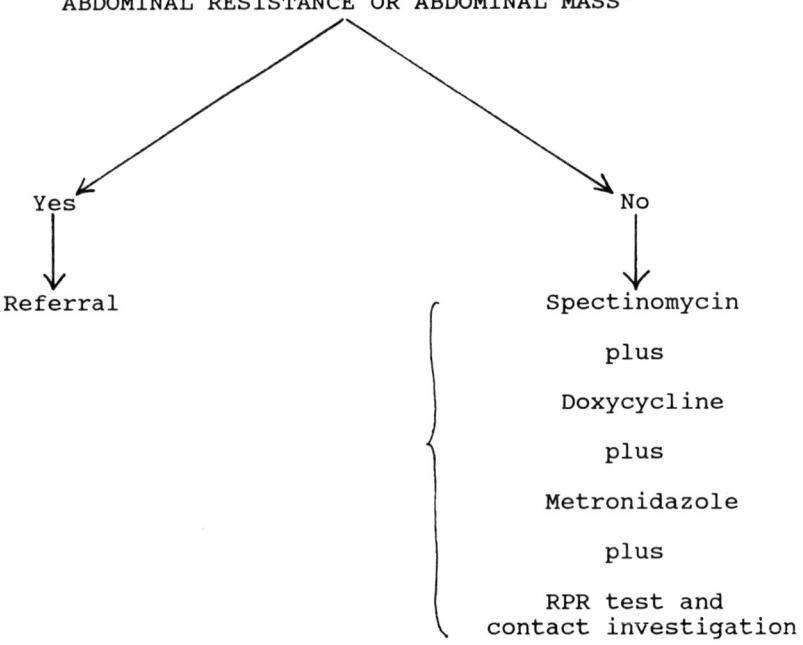

ABDOMINAL RESISTANCE OR ABDOMINAL MASS[x]

Yes   No

Referral   Spectinomycin

                                                      plus

                                                  Doxycycline

                                                      plus

                                                 Metronidazole

                                                      plus

                                               RPR test and
                                            contact investigation

[x] If pregnant or post-abortion, immediate referral.

Appendix 4. Case Management for Genital Ulcer Disease

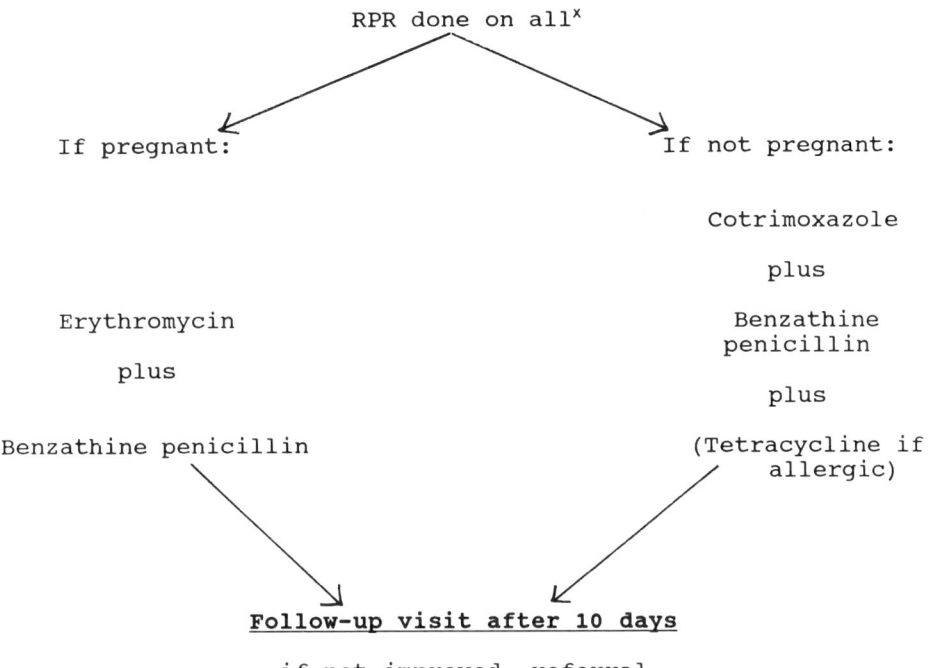

```
                    RPR done on all^x


   If pregnant:                        If not pregnant:

                                          Cotrimoxazole

                                              plus

   Erythromycin                           Benzathine
                                          penicillin
        plus
                                              plus

Benzathine penicillin                  (Tetracycline if
                                          allergic)


           Follow-up visit after 10 days

              if not improved, referral
```

^x For follow-up and epidemiological treatment of contacts.

Appendix 5. Case Management for BUBO

```
                  Doxycycline

                       or

          Erythromycin if pregnant


       Follow-up visit after 10 days


          If not improved, referral
```

strategies on the basis of further research and monitoring. More attention is also being given to special risk groups, such as migrant laborers, commercial sex workers, military personnel, and displaced people.

REFERENCES

1. Bastos dos Santos R, Palha de Sousa C, Barreto J et al. Prevalence of HIV-1 and
      HIV-2 infection in STD patients, Maputo 1987. Sixth International
      Conference on AIDS, Abstract No. 5556, Stockholm, June 12–16, 1988.
2. Razak A, Ministry of Health. Evaluation of the health system in Mozambique,
      Maputo, 1990.
3. Ministry of Health. Central hospital of Maputo, annual report, 1990.
4. Van der Veen F, AIDS Task Force expert. Personal communication, October 1990.

APPENDICIES

APPENDIX 1
RECOMMENDATIONS FOR ACTION

The following recommendations are excerpted from the Bellagio conference report
Reproductive Tract Infections in Women in the Third World:
National and International Policy Implications. *The full report is available from*
the International Women's Health Coalition, 24 East 21 Street, New York, NY 10010.

Conference participants concluded that actions are urgently required, at the national and international levels simultaneously, to put reproductive tract infections (RTIs) on existing health agendas. It is essential that each country take initiative to define its own needs, priorities, and strategies. Given competition for limited or shrinking resources, the prevailing ignorance about and neglect of RTIs, and the lack of informed and effective political constituencies to promote work on RTIs, international actions are needed to provide both expertise and political impetus to make RTIs visible and to foster action by existing health programs. The basic objectives are to prevent infection and, where it has already occurred, to treat both the infected person and those at risk of exposure in order to prevent the personally devastating and socially costly consequences of infection. Additional data will be useful to identify and implement more effective actions to prevent and control RTIs and to mobilize the political will needed to support those actions. Meanwhile, the research needed to act is minimal and is best undertaken by initiating actions that are carefully monitored and evaluated for responsiveness to women's concerns, for efficacy, and for costs.

Conference participants strongly recommended close interaction at all levels among policymakers, women's health advocates, service providers, and researchers from both biomedical and social disciplines. They made suggestions for immediate action at the national and international levels. Tables 1 and 2 outline the measures that are most feasible and are more cost-effective than other health activities currently receiving priority.

GENERAL RECOMMENDATIONS FOR NATIONAL
AND INTERNATIONAL ACTION

1. Support women to mobilize as a key constituency to advocate policy development and to participate in the design, implementation, and evaluation of programs. The group recommended that the International Women's Health Coalition foster initial efforts in this direction.

Table 1. Priority Actions to Prevent and Control RTIs

Social Action and Education

- Give higher priority to public health and other social services in national budgets, and work to adjust gender power relations and attitudes toward women. Two goals are particularly important here:

  1. Enabling women to control when and with whom they have sexual relations, and to protect themselves against infection by practicing safer sex, especially negotiating condom use; and

  2. Encouraging men to adopt sexual behaviors that are respectful of their own health and of women's health, dignity, and bodily integrity.

- Reduce gender discrimination so that girls and women have the same access as boys and men to education and health services and to employment. When women gain such opportunities, they will not have to resort to selling sex or trading sex for favors.

- Provide sex education and counseling, including analysis of gender roles, to children, young people, and the general public through a variety of channels.

Modifications in Ongoing Health,
Family Planning, and STD/HIV Programs

- Minimize procedure-related infections by providing training, supervision, regular supplies, and rewards for service quality.

- Provide safe abortion and delivery services.

- Promote condom use through all health and family planning services, as well as through the mass media and other channels.

- Designate and fund a specific person or mechanism to direct a national STD program, including coordination with other health and education sectors, and special efforts to provide diagnosis, treatment, and counseling for groups at particularly high risk of acquiring and transmitting STDs.

- Provide syndromic diagnosis and screening for RTIs and other gynecologic problems in all public health services, especially family planning and MCH services. Expand the diagnostic and treatment capacities of these health services, especially for gonorrhea, syphilis, and genital ulcer disease, and develop protocols for management of common STD syndromes.

- Strengthen partner notification and treatment by all programs that undertake diagnosis, including STD/HIV, family planning, and MCH services.

Technology Development and Research

- Improve and develop new female-controlled methods to protect against infection.

- Develop simpler, inexpensive diagnostic tests and treatment regimens especially for chlamydia and gonorrhea.

- Evaluate the efficiency and cost-Effectiveness of prophylactic antibiotics for IUD insertion and termination of pregnancy.

- Develop means to monitor the prevalence of RTIs and their antibiotic resistance patterns, the incidence of consequences, patterns of sexual and health-care-seeking behaviors, and the costs of RTIs.

- Evaluate experimental programs to prevent and control RTIs.

2. Renew governmental and international agency commitment to create broader social conditions in which women can manage their sexual health, and men and women can adopt the responsible and respectful sexual relationships necessary for emotional and physical sexual health. An important means is to use existing mechanisms, such as "women in development" offices, to assess the implications of social and economic development strategies and projects for women's health, as well as for women's status.

3. Support existing health (child survival, safe motherhood, MCH, HIV/AIDS, STD) and family planning programs to integrate a concern for RTIs into their routine work, including the following objectives:

    ■ Develop and implement standards, training, and supervision to minimize procedure-related infections; educate and supervise staff to provide information on sex and on condoms to all individuals regardless of age or marital status, to prevent sexually transmitted and endogenous infections.

    ■ Adopt and carefully implement uniform guidelines and training for staff to diagnose, counsel, and treat infection; to promote condom use; and to provide partner notification and services when diagnosis of infection is firm.

    ■ With regard to sexually transmitted infections, simple, inexpensive diagnostics exist for syphilis, HIV, and common vaginal infections. The validity of syndromic assessment needs to be evaluated, but is probably reasonable for genital ulcer disease and urethritis in men; simple, inexpensive treatment regimens are known for syphilis, chancroid, gonorrhea, chlamydia infection, and vaginal infections. Syphilis, gonorrhea, bacterial vaginosis, trichomonas, and, in many parts of the world, chancroid require only a single dose of treatment. Single-dose therapies for chlamydia are now under development. Demonstration projects should be developed at the national level, with international assistance as necessary, to determine the human resources needed, logistics requirements, costs, and outcomes.

4. Compare the effectiveness, acceptability, quality, costs, and cost-effectiveness of community-based, integrated primary care efforts with those of vertical programs to prevent and control RTIs; assess the benefits of incorporating RTI prevention and control into health, AIDS, and family planning programs.

5. Assess the viability of providing RTI information and services through the private and informal sectors; design and evaluate cost-sharing approaches to services.

6. Develop and test simple, low-cost diagnostics for gonorrhea and chlamydia.

7. Develop bacterial STD treatment regimens that are financially and technically appropriate for Southern countries; survey antimicrobial resistance patterns in various populations; and develop RTI treatments that are effective despite HIV infection and are safe during pregnancy.

8.   Develop and test female-controlled methods to protect against STDs.

9.   Invest in human resources for policies, programs, and services, especially at the national level. Emphasize recruitment and training of health providers, particularly women, in sexual health, gender equity, and RTI prevention; include not only clinical skills, but also counseling and partner notification.

10.   Invest in biomedical and social research capacity in Southern countries. Train professionals in methodology, proposal writing, all stages of research implementation, data analysis, and report writing. Strengthen basic institutional capacity, including laboratory facilities; technical skills; and improved financial, professional, and academic remuneration for research. Identify research priorities attuned to program and policy needs, as well as to the views of consumers. Fund research in Southern countries.

NATIONAL POLICY RECOMMENDATIONS

1.   Convene national commissions and other such bodies, including women's health advocates, to address various aspects of the situation:

- To generate public support for action to prevent and control RTIs (among other women's health issues).

- To define local goals and priorities.

- To mobilize necessary financial resources locally and internationally.

- To review policies that foster infection and their consequences, including policies that restrict access of certain groups (especially children, adolescents, and the unmarried) to necessary information and services, and policies that restrict safe abortion services.

2.   Develop one or more specific mechanisms for national program development and coordination that would work with and through women's health advocates, existing health and family planning programs, and health professionals to accomplish the following:

- Develop suitable training and treatment guidelines, and recommend appropriate constellations of services for the various service programs.

- Facilitate drug supply and distribution, including adding drugs necessary for RTI control to essential drug lists.

- Facilitate condom and spermicide supply and distribution.

- Define and oversee achievement of standards for the quality of health and family planning services.

- Foster development of necessary laboratory facilities.

- Outline a priority research agenda, including basic biomedical studies, research on sexual behavior and socioeconomic factors, and operations research to assess costs and other factors.

- Design a feasible means of data collection for monitoring the prevalence of RTIs, patterns of sexual behavior, and program activities and costs.

- Disseminate information (from program evaluations, research, and basic monitoring systems) to the general public, health providers, decision makers, and women's organizations.

3. Undertake studies to assess the prevalence of RTIs; to evaluate the incidence and medical, social, and economic costs of their consequences for women, for health services, and for health objectives; and to assess the capacity of existing health services to prevent and control RTIs.

INTERNATIONAL SUPPORT FOR NATIONAL ACTION

1. Develop an international advocacy group on RTIs with broad participation by women's health advocates, especially from Southern countries.

2. Provide technical advice to countries on policies, programs, and research through existing programs, such as the World Health Organization's programs on women's health, human reproduction, AIDS, and STDs; increase the participation of women's health advocates; and strengthen RTI knowledge, skills, and financial resources within these programs.

3. Provide financial and other material resources for national program and research development.

4. Model the likely costs and impacts of feasible actions, and their cost-effectiveness relative to that of other health priorities or actions to improve women's health and public health.

5. Map current national and international funding for RTI-related activities.

BEHAVIORAL AND OPERATIONS RESEARCH NEEDED
(Research recommendations also appear under other headings.)

1. Assess gender power relations, including the economic, social, cultural, and political roots of power imbalances between women and men, along with women's strategies to achieve self-esteem.

2.   Explore human sexuality, including cultural and social factors that influence choice, number, and characteristics of partners; differences in sexual behavior between men and women; and the meanings of sexuality and sexual behavior in social life and for individuals.

3.   Assess women's perceptions of and experiences with RTIs, including the social meanings of infection, treatment sought, knowledge of causes, and consequences.

4.   Determine the cultural, social, and personal conditions that affect motivation to use (or not use) condoms and other barrier methods among subgroups of the population.

5.   Assess obstacles to women's use of health services; develop and evaluate specific actions to remove these obstacles. Give special attention to women who are less educated or otherwise disadvantaged, to adolescents, and to older women. Consider, for example, timing and location of services; personal treatment; quality of medical services; and partner, family, or community pressure.

6.   Assess the obstacles to men's use of STD services, their participation in partner notification, and their attitudes toward condom use not only with commercial sex workers, but also with other partners.

7.   Develop, test, and evaluate means to ensure that providers implement RTI screening and services as mandated, minimize procedure-related infection, and provide appropriate and sympathetic risk-reduction counseling.

8.   Design, test, and evaluate humane, efficient, and cost-effective approaches to counseling of infected women and men, to partner notification, and to treatment.

9.   Evaluate Pap smear screening programs in Southern countries for effectiveness and cost.

PROGRAM-SPECIFIC RECOMMENDATIONS

Building on these generally applicable recommendations, participants identified activities that existing service programs are specifically qualified to undertake.

Family Planning

Because the most effective contraceptives provide little if any protection against infection, and some increase the risk of infection, service providers need to help each client choose a contraceptive regimen with the appropriate balance between contraceptive efficacy and protection against infection. Possible choices—depending on the client's circumstances and preferences, and the availability of safe abortion services—include use of a highly effective contraceptive together with condoms and use of barrier methods and spermicides with recourse to safe abortion. Programs can take a number of steps:

1. Prevent iatrogenic infection. More careful implementation of standards of care for IUD and Norplant® insertion and for sterilization, appropriate screening of clients for contraindications, and elimination of unnecessary procedures (e.g., misuse of cesarean section as a means to obtain of sterilization in Brazil) will help achieve this goal.

2. Provide safe early abortion services. Such services will reduce a major cause of maternal morbidity and mortality and allow freer choice of barrier methods of contraception, which protect against infection.

3. Assess the utility of antibiotic prophylaxis in surgical abortion and of medical abortifacients in reducing the risk of infection from induced abortion.

4. Evaluate the effectiveness and cost-effectiveness of antibiotic prophylaxis for IUD insertion.

5. Develop and test means to promote condom use that are effective both for disease prevention and for contraception; assess empirically the specific groups able to use condoms effectively.

6. Evaluate in various subgroups the use-effectiveness (for disease prevention and contraception) and the cost-effectiveness of simultaneous use of two contraceptive methods.

7. Evaluate the impact of specific contraceptives (e.g., hormonal methods, IUDs, spermicides) on RTIs, including the impact on HIV transmission and the safety of current contraceptives where RTIs are endemic.

8. Develop effective female-controlled contraceptives that also protect against infection.

MCH, Child Survival, and Safe Motherhood

Available technologies and cost assessments indicate clearly that MCH programs should screen and treat pregnant women for syphilis, and routinely provide prophylaxis to newborns to prevent ophthalmia neonatorum (which can lead to blindness). The cost-effectiveness of screening and treating pregnant women for other sexually transmitted infections is less clear, largely because demonstration programs have not been mounted, and because the diagnostic and treatment techniques are either more expensive or more difficult. Cost-benefit analyses have tended to assess the outcomes for the child only (sometimes the woman only), whereas treatment of the pregnant woman would benefit both the woman and the child and raise estimates of cost-effectiveness. These programs should undertake several activities:

1. Reduce trauma and infection in the reproductive tract. Programs can accomplish this by continuing and expanding safe delivery services at all levels of the health system; by training and equipping traditional birth attendants; and by reducing unnecessary invasive procedures.

Table 2. Summary of Program Specific Actions

Type of Action	Family planning	MCH	STD/HIV control	Primary health care*	Public education
HEALTH SERVICES Ophthalmia neonatorum: provide prophylaxis for eye infections		X		X	
Syphilis: screening programs	X	X	X	X	
Genital ulcer disease and cervical, vaginal, and urethral discharge: syndromic diagnosis and therapy	X	X	X	X	
Cervical cancer: Pap smears or visual inspection of cervix for premalignant lesions (following World Health Organization guidelines)	X	X	X	X	
Birth prevention: Safe surgical contraception (IUDs, implants, sterilization, and safe abortion)	X	X		X	
Puerperal infection: Prenatal care, safe delivery, and postnatal care		X		X	
EDUCATIONAL INTERVENTIONS Individual/group counseling to increase condom use and partner notification, and improved health care utilization for RTIs	X	X	X	X	
Information, education, and communication to foster sexual health, more egalitarian gender roles and responsible sexual relationships, and condom use	X	X	X	X	X

*Participants suggested that primary health care services could effectively provide integrated reproductive health care that includes family planning, MCH, and STD/HIV control. They discussed two possible models: combined family planning/MCH/STD service at the primary health care level (a reproductive health clinic) with one or more specialized staff; and special clinics at the urban level that do both family planning and RTI work (including STD/HIV programs).

2.   Provide safe abortion services or referral.

3.   Screen and treat all pregnant women (and their partners) for syphilis. This will require simple laboratory facilities on-site, operations research to ensure quality, and evaluation of partner notification strategies.

4.   Develop carefully documented demonstration projects to screen and treat pregnant women for other genital ulcer diseases, gonorrhea, chlamydial infections, and trichomoniasis.

5.   At all levels of health delivery, including through traditional birth attendants, administer prophylaxis to newborns to prevent ophthalmia neonatorum.

6.   Assess the feasibility and efficacy of training auxiliary health workers and traditional birth attendants to recognize symptoms of RTIs in women and children and to refer for care.

7.   Assess the impact of specific RTIs and their treatments on the health of pregnant women, as well as on fetal wastage, prematurity, and intrauterine growth retardation.

AIDS and STD Prevention and Control

A clear consensus emerged that AIDS and STD control programs should be integrated at all levels, given that STDs and HIV infection have synergistic relationships that the mode of transmission is the same for each, and that they share behavioral factors. In general, these programs have served primarily "high-risk groups"—commercial sex workers and their clients in the case of HIV programs; men with sexually transmitted infections, and to a lesser extent commercial sex workers, in the case of vertical STD programs. It is essential to reach these groups to limit the spread of infection into the general population. STD programs have, however, generally failed to identify and assist the female partners of men who receive diagnoses and treatment. These women are at very high risk of infection. In general, much more needs to be done to encourage men who are possibly infected to seek diagnosis and treatment, and to encourage those who are infected to notify their partners and support them to seek diagnosis and care. Partner notification is an especially effective way to identify women with STDs who are asymptomatic. STD/HIV programs can seek to achieve the following:

1.   Invest more in partner notification and services, carefully documenting the efficacy of alternative strategies.

2.   Improve access to services by expanding service sites and working with other health and family planning programs, and by conducting community education and outreach, especially for men of all ages.

3.   Develop attractive, accessible, comprehensive services for priority groups, such as commercial sex workers, their clients, and adolescents, and evaluate the impact on RTI control in the general population.

4.   Provide syndromic management of genital ulcer disease and urethritis in men in all health services.

5.   Develop and evaluate RTI treatment regimens that are effective in HIV-infected individuals.

Public Education

Mass media campaigns are a common public health tool, but their efficacy in changing sexual and gender role behavior has yet to be demonstrated. In most countries, information and education programs for children and youths, in and out of school, are controversial. Conference participants emphasized the importance of carefully documenting and evaluating efforts to accomplish several goals:

1.   Support women's organizations to inform their constituencies and mobilize them to advocate policy and program development for RTI prevention, and to manage their own sexuality and health, which includes seeking appropriate health care.

2.   Identify influential men's groups and work with them on issues of sexual behavior and relationships, gender roles and power relations, and RTI prevention.

3.   Design and provide education to children and youth on human sexuality, gender equity, and prevention of RTIs.

4.   Utilize mass media and traditional communication channels to educate the public on safer sexual behavior, promote condom use, encourage health-care seeking, and generate respectful and responsible sexual and gender relations.

5.   Evaluate the efficacy and cost-effectiveness of each of the above actions.

APPENDIX 2.
LIST OF AUTHORS AND PARTICIPANTS
AT THE BELLAGIO CONFERENCE

Dr. Adeyemi O. Adekunle
Senior Lecturer in Obstetrics
  and Gynecology
Department of Obstetrics and Gynecology
College of Medicine
University of Ibadan
University College Hospital
Ibadan, Nigeria

Dr. Sevgi O. Aral
Division of Sexually Transmitted
  Diseases/STD Prevention
Centers for Disease Control
Freeway Park (Mailstop E44)
Atlanta, GA 30333

Dr. Carmen Barroso
Director
Population Program
The John D. and Catherine T.
  MacArthur Foundation
140 South Dearborn Street
Chicago, IL 60603

Dr. Rui Bastos dos Santos
Professeur Auxiliare de la Fac. Med.
Directeur du Programme National de
  Lutte Contre les MST
  Au Ministère de la Sante
Directeur du Service de Dermatologie de
  L'Hôspital Central de Maputo
P.O. Box 1164
Hôspital Central de Maputo
Mozambique

Dr. Stuart M. Berman
Special Assistant for Perinatal
  and Adolescent Studies
Division of STD/HIV Prevention
Centers for Disease Control
Freeway Park (Mailstop E44)
Atlanta, GA 30333

Dr. N. C. Bhargava
Regional STD Centre
Safdarjung Hospital
New Delhi 110 029, India

Professor Robert C. Brunham
Chairman
Department of Medical Microbiology
University of Manitoba
Basic Medical Sciences Building
Room 543
730 Willias Avenue
Winnipeg, Manitoba
Canada R3E DW3

Dr. Willard Cates, Jr.
Director
Division of STD/HIV Prevention
Centers for Disease Control
Freeway Park (Mailstop E44)
Atlanta, GA 30333

373

Dr. Josef Decosas
AIDS Specialist
Canadian International
  Development Agency
200 Promenade du Portage
Hull, Quebec
Canada K1A OG4

Ms. Carmen Díaz-Olivo
Executive Assistant to
  the Vice President
International Women's
  Health Coalition
24 East 21 Street
New York, NY 10010

Dr. Joanne Embree
Assistant Professor
Departments of Pediatric Child Health
  and Medical Microbiology
University of Manitoba
Basic Medical Sciences Building
Room 530
730 Winnipeg, Manitoba
Canada R3E OW3

Dr. Mahmoud Fathalla
Director
Special Programme of
  Research on Human Reproduction
World Health Organization
1211 Geneva 27, Switzerland

Dr. Aníbal Faúndes
Senior Associate Representative
The Population Council and
  University of Campinas
Caixa Postal 6181
13081 Campinas
São Paulo, Brazil

Dr. Elena Maria Pereira Folgosa
Professeur Auxiliaire de la Fac. de Med.
Microbiologique Laboratoire de
Reference pour les MST
P.O. Box 257
Faculdade de Medicina
Maputo, Mozambique

Dr. Lieve Fransen
AIDS Task Force
European Economic Community
67A, Rue Joseph II
Brussells 1040, Belgium

Ms. Adrienne Germain
Vice President
International Women's
  Health Coalition
24 East 21 Street
New York, NY 10010

Ms. Ann Hamilton
Director
Population and Human
  Resources Department
The World Bank
1818 H Street NW, Room 6055
Washington, DC 20016

Dr. Ellen Hardy
Assistant Professor
Department of Obstetrics and Gynecology
School of Medical Sciences
University of Campinas
Caixa Postal 1170
13100 Campinas
São Paulo, Brazil

Dr. King K. Holmes
Director
Center for AIDS and STDs
University of Washington
1001 Broadway, Suite 215
Seattle, WA 98122

Dr. Mukesh Kapila
Senior Health and Population Advisor
Overseas Development Administration
Elan House, Stag Place
London SW18 6DH, England

Professor Oladapo A. Ladipo
Professor of Obstetrics and Gynecology
Department of Obstetrics and Gynecology
College of Medicine
University of Ibadan
University College Hospital
Ibadan, Nigeria

Dr. Marie Laga
Epidemiologist
Department of Microbiology
Institute of Tropical Medicine
Nationalestraat 155
2000 Antwerp, Belgium

Dr. Katherine Laguardia
Research Scientist
The Rockefeller Foundation
1133 Avenue of the Americas
New York, NY 10036

Dr. Usha K. Luthra
Additional Director General
Indian Council of Medical Research
Director
Institute of Cytology and
  Preventive Oncology
P.O. Box 4508, Ansari Nagar
New Delhi 110 029, India

Dr. A. B. Ndugga Maggwa
Research Fellow/Lecturer
Department of Obstetrics and Gynecology
College of Health Sciences
University of Nairobi
P.O. Box 20835
Nairobi, Kenya

Dr. André Meheus
Program Manager
Sexually Transmitted Diseases Programme
World Health Organization
1211 Geneva 27, Switzerland

Dr. Suman Mehta
Indian Council of Medical Research
Ansari Nagar
New Delhi 110 029, India

Mr. N. S. Murthy
Institute of Cytology and
  Preventive Oncology
Maulana Azad Medical College
New Delhi 110 002, India

Dr. Elizabeth Ngugi
Lecturer
Department of Community Health
College of Health Sciences
University of Nairobi
P.O. Box 19676
Nairobi, Kenya

Dr. Nancy Pielemeier
Deputy Director
Office of Health Bureau for
  Science and Technology
U.S. Agency for International
  Development
Washington, DC 20232

Professor Peter Piot
Head
Department of Microbiology and
  World Health Organization
  Collaborating Center on AIDS,
Institute of Tropical Medicine
Nationalestraat 155
2000 Antwerp, Belgium

Dr. Prema Ramachandran
Indian Council of Medical Research
Ansari Nagar
New Delhi 110 029, India

Dr. Allan Ronald
Professor and Head
Department of Internal Medicine
Health Science Centre, Room GC430
University of Manitoba
700 Willias Avenue
Winnipeg, Manitoba
Canada R3E 0Z3

Dr. Jane Rowley
Department of Pure and
  Applied Biology
Imperial College
University of London
Prince Consort Road
London SW7 2BB

Dr. Badri Saxena
Senior Deputy Director General
Indian Council of Medical Research
Ansari Nagar
New Delhi 110 029, India

Dr. Joann M. Schulte
Medical Epidemiologist
Division of STD/HIV Prevention, CPS
Centers for Disease Control
Atlanta, GA   30333

Mr. Kenneth F. Schulz
Associate Director
International Activities
Division of STD/HIV Prevention
Centers for Disease Control
Freeway Park (Mailstop E44)
Atlanta, GA   30333

Dr. Sheldon Segal
Director
Population Sciences Division
The Rockefeller Foundation
1133 Avenue of the Americas
New York, NY   10036

Dr. A. Sehgal
Institute of Cytology and
  Preventive Oncology
Maulana Azad Medical College
New Delhi 110 002, India

Dr. Katherine M. Stone
Clinical Research Investigator
Division of STD/HIV Prevention
Centers for Disease Control
1600 Clifton Road (Mailstop EO2)
Atlanta, GA   30333

Dr. Ana Cristina Tanaka
Professor
Faculty of Public Health
University of São Paulo
Av. Dr. Arnaldo, 715
01255 São Paulo, Brazil

Dr. Judith N. Wasserheit
Chief
Sexually Transmitted Disease Branch
Microbiology and Infectious
  Diseases Program
National Institute of Allergy
  and Infectious Diseases
National Institutes of Health
Westwood Building, Room 749
Bethesda, MD   20892

INDEX